Endogenous Mediators of Gastrointestinal Disease

Editor

John L. Wallace, Ph.D.

Associate Professor
Department of Medical Physiology
University of Calgary
Calgary, Alberta, Canada

CRC Press, Inc.
Boca Raton, Florida

Library of Congress Cataloging-in-Publication Data

Endogenous mediators of gastrointestinal disease/ editor, Wallace, John L.
p. cm.
Includes bibliographies and index.
ISBN 0-8493-4574-X
1. Peptic ulcer—Etiology. 2. Gastric mucosa—Pathophysiology. 3. Digestive organs—Secretions. I. Wallace, John L. [DNLM: 1. Gastric Mucosa—metabolism. 2. Gastrointestinal Diseases—immunology. WI 100 E555]
RC821.E53 1989 616.3'3071 89-9851

Direct all inquires to CRC Press, Inc., 2000 Corporate Blvd., N.W., Boca Raton, Florida, 33431.

International Standard Book Number 0-8493-4574-X

Library of Congress Card Number 89-9851
Printed in the United States

PREFACE

Whether the gastrointestinal mucosa ulcerates can be viewed as a balance between aggressive factors present in the lumen and the mucosal defense system. Several of these aggressive factors, such as acid, bile, and pepsin, are endogenous substances. Similarly, several endogenous substances exert control over mucosal blood flow and secretion and thus are important mediators of mucosal defense. The synthesis and release of these factors may therefore be very important in the pathogenesis of mucosal injury. In this volume, experts in this field (basic scientists and clinicians) have contributed chapters on some of the most important of these endogenous mediators, including histamine, prostaglandins, leukotrienes, and platelet-activating factor. The potential contribution to gastrointestinal disease has been assessed, as has the role of these mediators in gastrointestinal side effects of drugs (i.e., nonsteroidal anti-inflammatory drugs). These mediators have also been discussed in the context of the mechanism of action of drugs used clinically for the treatment of maladies of the digestive system.

THE EDITOR

John L. Wallace, Ph.D., is Associate Professor, Department of Medical Physiology, University of Calgary, Calgary, Alberta, Canada. He received his M.Sc. from Queen's University, Kingston, and his Ph.D. from the University of Toronto in 1983.

Prior to his appointment at the University of Calgary, he served as Assistant Professor in the Department of Physiology at Queen's University. In 1986, Dr. Wallace was a Visiting Lecturer at the Medical School of Ribeirao Preto in São Paolo, Brazil, and a postdoctoral fellow at the Institut Pasteur, Paris, and the Wellcome Research Foundation, Beckenham, England.

Dr. Wallace has received a number of awards for his work in the field of gastroenterology, including the MRC of Canada Scholarship, the Queen's National Scholarship, an Alberta Heritage Foundation Medical scholarship, Young Investigator Award from the World Congress of Gastroenterology, the Ontario Graduate Scholarship, Health Sciences Research Award from the University of Toronto, and a research fellowship from The Mount Sinai Institute, and has authored or coauthored over 75 articles in professional journals and books.

CONTRIBUTORS

Adrian Allen, D.Phil.
Professor of Physiological Biochemistry
Department of Physiological Sciences
University of Newcastle-Upon-Tyne
Newcastle-Upon-Tyne, England

Paul L. Beck, Ph.D.
Research Associate
Department of Biology
Queen's University
Kingston, ON, Canada

Max M. Cohen, M.D.
Surgeon-in-Chief
The Graduate Hospital
Philadelphia, Pennsylvania

Paul H. Guth, M.D.
Faculty of Medicine
University of Calgary
Calgary, AB, Canada

David A. Hutton, B.Sc.
Department of Physiological Sciences
University of Newcastle-Upon-Tyne
Newcastle-Upon-Tyne, England

Stanislaw J. Konturek
Director
Institute of Physiology
Academy of Medicine
Krakow, Poland

Eric R. Lacy, Ph.D.
Associate Professor
Department of Anatomy and Cell Biology
Medical University of South Carolina
Charleston, South Carolina

Andrea J. Leonard, B.Sc.
Department of Physiology
University of Newcastle-Upon-Tyne
Newcastle-Upon-Tyne, England

Thomas A. Miller, M.D.
Professor
Department of Surgery
University of Texas Medical School
Houston, Texas

Gerald P. Morris, Ph.D.
Professor
Department of Biology
Queen's University
Kingston, ON, Canada

K. D. Palitzsch, M.D.
Visiting Research Fellow
Chemical Pathology Research Division
Harvard Medical School
Boston, Massachusetts

Jeffrey P. Pearson, Ph.D.
Department of Physiological Sciences
University of Newcastle-Upon-Tyne
Newscastle-Upon-Tyne, England

Brigitta M. Peskar, M.D.
Head
Department of Experimental Clinical Medicine
Ruhr-University of Bochum
Bochum, West Germany

L. A. Sellers, Ph.D.
Laboratory of Protein Structure
Medical Research Council
National Institute for Medical Research
London, England

Sandor Szabo, M.D., Ph.D.
Head
Chemical Pathology Laboratory
Brigham and Women's Hospital
Boston, Massachusetts

Brant E. Victor, M.D.
Research Fellow
Department of Surgery
University of Texas Medical School
Houston, Texas

John L. Wallace, Ph.D.
Associate Professor
Department of Medical Physiology
University of Calgary
Calgary, AB, Canada

Brendan J. R. Whittle, Ph.D.
Head
Department of Pharmacology
Wellcome Research Laboratories
Kent, England

Naoji Yasue, M.D.
1st Department of Internal Medicine
Nagoya City University School
of Medicine
Nagoya, Japan

TABLE OF CONTENTS

Chapter 1

EFFECTS OF BILE ON THE GASTRIC MUCOSA

Gerald P. Morris, Eric R. Lacy, and Max M. Cohen

TABLE OF CONTENTS

I. INTRODUCTION

There is ample evidence that exposure of the gastric mucosa to constituents commonly found in the duodenal contents, such as bile salts and lysolecithin, can cause acute damage in both humans and animals. Such damage is manifested by focal hemorrhage, erythema, and the characteristic signs of a broken gastric mucosal barrier (net sodium and potassium efflux, loss of luminal hydrogen ion, and a decrease in transmucosal potential difference). It is not clear, however, whether prolonged exposure of the gastric mucosa to refluxed intestinal contents at concentrations which are actually found in the stomach can cause peptic ulcer.

The roles of acid alone, or in combination with refluxed duodenal contents, in causing gastrointestinal damage are also open to question. There is no doubt that either inhibition of acid secretion by H_2 receptor antagonists or neutralization of secreted acid by regular intake of antacids will accelerate the healing of existing peptic ulcer. There is, however, a high rate of relapse following such therapy and it is apparent that although these treatments allow the mucosal healing response to restore the integrity of the luminal epithelium, they are not removing the underlying causes of the chronic ulceration.[1] The effects of treatments which elevate intragastric pH on the possible damaging effects of refluxed intestinal contents are particularly complex, since the potentially damaging agents have markedly different pH-dependent effects.

II. COMPOSITION OF BILE

Bile acids represent the active constituent of bile. The bile acids form mixed micelles with fatty acids and monoglycerides, thus facilitating the diffusion of these molecules through the unstirred layer to the surfaces of the intestinal epithelial cells. Bile acids are also essential for adequate absorption of fat-soluble vitamins and permit the elimination of cholesterol.[2] Bile also contains lecithin (phosphatidylcholine) which is converted by pancreatic phospholipase A_2 to lysolecithin.

The primary bile acids, cholic and deoxycholic, are synthesized from cholesterol in the liver and conjugated with glycine or taurine prior to release into the intestine. Some of the conjugated bile acids are deconjugated by bacterial enzymes. Although most deconjugation occurs in the colon, some occurs in the ileum. The production of secondary and deconjugated bile acids may be of particular importance in the small bowel in the presence of bacterial overgrowth, with resulting entry of increased quantities into the enterohepatic circulation.[3]

The composition of the intestinal contents which may be refluxed into the stomach varies widely depending on age, diet, feeding, and the presence of disease. The taurine-conjugated bile acid taurocholic acid or the corresponding bile salt have been most widely used in experimental studies. Taurocholate is, however, only one of six bile acids which predominate in human bile. The experiments of Duane et al.[4-6] are unique in that they have employed a mixture of conjugated bile acids (with and without added fatty acids, lysolecithin, and cholesterol) which, they state, simulates those present in human bile. Their mixture contains 14% taurocholic, 14% taurochenodeoxycholic, 5.3% taurodeoxycholic, 28% glycocholic, 28% glycochenodeoxycholic, and 10.7% glycodeoxycholic acid.

When studying the acute effects of bile acids, fatty acids, and lysolecithin on the gastric mucosa, it is also important to appreciate the range of concentrations which might be found in clinically relevant situations. For general purposes, an upper limit for total intragastric bile acid concentrations of perhaps 5 to 10 m*M* can be considered as realistic, although individuals with bile acid concentrations of more than 30 m*M* have been described.[4] Intragastric concentrations of lysolecithin greater than 2.0 m*M* are rare.

The damaging effects of bile acids at a given pH are concentration dependent; however, bile acids also differ in their capacity to produce mucosal damage. For instance, the dihydroxy secondary bile acid taurodeoxycholate is more damaging in the stomach[7-10] and in the intestine[11] than the trihydroxy primary bile acid, taurocholate. It is by no means certain that a cause-effect relationship exists, but deoxycholate and its taurine conjugates were found to form a significantly higher fraction of the bile acid complement in patients with chronic atrophic gastritis than in those with either normal mucosae or chronic superficial gastritis.[12]

Differences in luminal pH will also affect the extent to which bile acids and their salts can damage the gastric mucosa, and may alter the mechanisms by which damage is produced. The effects of whole bile on the gastric mucosal barrier of dogs were greatest at pH 2 and least at pH 8;[13] however, the salts of conjugated bile acids (taurodeoxycholate and taurocholate) damaged the canine gastric mucosal barrier at both pH 2.0 and 7.0, whereas the unconjugated salts of cholate and deoxycholate had no effect at pH 2.0, but did produce damage at pH 7.0.[7] These results reflected the relative solubilities of the bile salts. Taurine-conjugated bile salts with pKa of 1.9 were soluble at acid pH, while the unconjugated bile salts with pKa of 5 were precipitated and inactive. Taurocholate remains soluble below its pKa, and at a 10 m*M* concentration, both ionized (pH 7.0) and protonated (pH 1.1) forms produced endoscopically visible erosions and damage to the mucosal barrier of humans.[14] While ionized bile salts may disrupt the gastric mucosal barrier by dissolution of mucosal lipids, protonated taurocholate may produce damage subsequent to binding to membrane components or entry into mucosal cells.[5,15]

The ability of bile to damage the gastric mucosa is also dependent on the concentration of nondamaging lipids such as lecithin. Addition of excess lecithin or cholesterol to solutions containing 2 m*M* lysolecithin diminished or prevented the ability of lysolecithin to damage the gastric mucosal barrier at both acid and neutral pH.[16] Cholesterol and lysolecithin formed an insoluble complex, whereas the formation of soluble mixed micelles of lecithin and lysolecithin probably reduced dissolution of mucosal lecithin. Similarly, Martin et al.[17] found that the equimolar lecithin significantly reduced the effects of taurodeoxycholate on net cation fluxes, potential difference (PD), formation of hemorrhagic erosions, and visible mucus efflux in chambered rat gastric mucosae. This was also considered to be a result of mixed micelle formation, which reduced the ability of the bile acid to interact with epithelial phospholipids.

III. EFFECTS OF CHRONIC EXPOSURE TO BILE

Alkaline reflux gastritis is defined as a distinct postgastrectomy syndrome, characterized by abdominal pain, bilious vomiting, weight loss, and severe inflammation of the gastric mucosa.[18,19] This syndrome supposedly occurs in patients in whom prior gastric surgery permits free duodenogastric reflux. The pH of the gastric juice is high (usually above pH 5.0 and often near neutral) and gastric aspirates contain elevated levels of bile acids and lysolecithin.[4] Despite the finding of high bile acid concentrations in the intestines of symptomatic patients and the reproduction of symptoms by intragastric infusion of autologous intestinal contents, Meshkinpour et al.[20] found that there was little response of symptomatic patients to artificial bile acid solution. They concluded that there is no simple relationship between refluxed bile acids and alkaline reflux gastritis. Other constituents of the refluxed intestinal contents such as lysolecithin, fatty acids, and lecithin may be necessary for the production of symptoms.

Medical treatment of alkaline reflux gastritis is relatively unsuccessful and surgery is necessary, though not always effective, in severe cases.[21,22] Recent controlled trials have demonstrated that while Roux-en-Y diversion can eliminate enterogastric reflux and produce significant improvement of symptoms, recurrent pain, nausea, and vomiting remain in many of the patients.[23,24] In a recent review, Ritchie[3] stated that it is still uncertain whether, in fact, "a specific symptom complex exists as a consequence of excessive enterogastric reflux".

There is some evidence from studies on both humans and animals that prolonged or repeated exposure of the gastric mucosa to refluxed duodenal contents, especially bile, is involved in the etiology of gastric ulcer (GU). Pyloric sphincter dysfunction, possibly related to failure of closure in response to cholecystokinin,[25,26] and increased reflux of bile into the stomach, have been described in gastric ulceration in humans.[27,28] During duodenogastric reflux, the luminal pH of GU patients was also significantly higher (pH >5.0) than in normal subjects or duodenal ulcer (DU) patients.[26] An association between duodenogastric reflux and DU has also been described. Thomas[29] found increased duodenogastric reflux in 11 of 15 patients with DU and 12 of 14 patients with GU. Scintigraphic assessment allowed detection of the area of the stomach affected by reflux. This was usually limited to the antrum and distal stomach in patients with DU, but in GU patients, duodenal contents refluxed up the lesser curvature. Histological assessment of biopsies revealed gastritis in the body of the stomach only in patients with GU and it was claimed that the degree of gastritis correlated with the degree of reflux. Niemela et al.[30] also used a scintigraphic technique to quantify postprandial duodenogastric bile reflux in 107 nonoperated patients with dyspepsia. They found a significant association between increasing bile reflux and severity of superficial inflammatory cell infiltration and foveolar hyperplasia in both the antrum and the body.

Experiments on dogs, using surgical preparations involving chronic diversion of duodenal contents into the gastric mucosa, have shown that these procedures produce increased cell proliferation, histologic gastritis,[31-33] elevated serum gastrin levels, and enhanced maximal acid secretory capacity.[34] Witt et al.[19] inserted a denervated tube of gastric corpus into the duodenum of dogs and found after 4 months mucus cell hyperplasia, gland distortion, and parietal cell atrophy, but only a mild inflammatory response. The extent of gastritis and parietal cell atrophy was increased in animals with antrectomy and Billroth I gastroduoenostomy, lending support to earlier work suggesting that the gastric antrum exerts a protective effect on gastric mucosa which is chronically exposed to duodenal contents.[35] The remarkable feature of these experiments is that ulceration was never observed, despite the prolonged (more than 2 years, in some experiments) exposure of the gastric mucosa to duodenal contents. As Meyer[36] has pointed out, however, these models would not reproduce the qualitative changes in bile composition, such as increases in the proportion of unconjugated bile salts and secondary bile acids, which have been implicated in the etiology of GU by some studies.

In contrast to studies on dogs, surgical implantation of both the lower and upper bile duct into the stomach of rats (such that pancreatic juice and bile or bile alone entered the stomach) produced chronic-type gastric ulcers over a period of up to 5 months.[37] Kaminishi et al.[38] have recently described the production of chronic-type antral ulcers in rats by a surgical preparation involving anastomosis of the upper jejunum to the forestomach, and subsequent transsection of the duodenum distal to the entry of the bile duct and pancreatic duct. Chronic-type antral ulcers were present at 3 weeks after the initiation of reflux by duodenal transsection and continued to grow in size and depth over a period of 30 weeks. The appearance of these ulcers was accompanied by increases in intragastric pH, elevated serum gastrin levels, and increases in total intragastric bile salt concentration (to levels of 12 to 21 m*M*).

IV. GASTRIC MUCOSAL BLOOD FLOW AND SUSCEPTIBILITY OF MUCOSAE TO DAMAGE BY REFLUXED DUODENAL CONTENTS

It is well established that reductions in mucosal blood flow will increase the susceptibility of the gastric mucosa to topical bile.[39-41] Several studies have demonstrated that both hypovolemia and high, but physiological, levels of luminal acid are tolerated by gastric mucosae. If, however, bile salts are added to the luminal surface, the result is production of a series of changes which range from physiological signs of a "broken gastric mucosal barrier" accompanied by histological evidence of superficial epithelial damage,[41] to the rapid production of extensive hemorrhagic erosions.[42-44]

Bowen and LeDoux,[42] using ultramicroelectrodes placed in epithelial cells, found that exposure of the surface epithelium to 1 to 5 m*M* sodium taurocholate (or to 10% ethanol) produced first a reduction in transmucosal PD, and later (10 to 20 min), a decline in pO_2. This was interpreted as reflecting initial alterations in cell membranes, with subsequent alterations of the subepithelial microcirculation. Total blood flow to the stomach did not change during their experiments. Bowen and Fairchild[45] have coined the term "functional arteriovenous shunting" to describe the situation in which epithelial disruption of the type produced by bile salts is followed by focal microcirculatory disruption and local hypoxia. Such localized microvascular disruption can take place in the presence of greatly increased gastric mucosal blood flow. In fact, when gastric mucosae from normotensive animals are exposed to high concentrations of bile salts, extensive erosions form, but are accompanied by up to a fourfold increase in gastric mucosal blood flow.[41,46] This protective hyperemic response is prevented by hemorrhagic shock, vasopressin-induced hypovolemia, or parenterally administered nonsteroidal antiinflammatory drugs (NSAID).[40,41,43,44,47] The essential feature of these observations is that the production of damage by luminal bile salts does not require a reduction in gastric mucosal blood flow. The failure of the mucosa to respond by hyperemia is sufficient to render the mucosa vulnerable.

V. EFFECTS OF BILE SALTS ON GASTRIC MUCOSAL ENERGY METABOLISM

The gastric mucosa has very low levels of glycogen and is thus much more susceptible than many tissues and organs to reduced blood flow. Menguy et al.[48-50] demonstrated that a reduction in blood volume to the gastric mucosa of approximately 30% caused, within 15 min, a 75% reduction in adenosine triphosphate (ATP) concentrations and an almost complete reduction in glycogen reserves. The antrum was found to be less susceptible than the corpus or fundus.[50] It is significant that in studies on isolated mitochondria, taurocholate at concentrations as low as 250 μ*M* acted as an uncoupler of oxidative phosphorylation, while concentrations from 1 to 8 m*M* inhibited gastric mucosal ATPase.[51] Ohe et al.[52] have confirmed the ability of taurocholate to reduce mucosal energy charge in Ussing chamber preparations of guinea pig gastric mucosae, and have shown that a 50% reduction in PD is correlated with a significant decrease in energy charge. Serosal acidification only occurred subsequent to the decline in PD and decrease in energy charge.

The gastric mucosa can also be rendered susceptible to the damaging effects of topically applied bile salts by dietary insufficiency. Oram-Smith and Rosato[53] showed that rats fed orally or parenterally for 7 d did not differ in the susceptibilities of their gastric mucosae to damage caused by exposure to acidified 6.5 m*M* sodium taurocholate; however, rats fed a "semistarvation" diet developed extensive gastric erosions and had significantly greater loss of luminal hydrogen ion ("back-diffusion").

VI. CAN REFLUXED INTESTINAL CONTENTS DAMAGE THE GASTRIC MUCOSA?

Many experimental studies which have as their objective the study of potentially "cytoprotective" agents use concentrations of bile acids and luminal acid (100 m*M* taurocholate in 0.2 *M* HCl, for instance)[54-56] which are far above those encountered by the gastric mucosa under physiological conditions. These studies are valuable in demonstrating the ability of the mucosa to resist assault under extremely damaging conditions, and they have revealed much useful information about the nature of the mucosal defenses. They do not, however, tell us to what extent similar damage may be expected to occur in the gastric mucosa of humans.

A. LEVELS OF BILE ACIDS AND BILE SALTS IN THE STOMACH

Although duodenogastric reflux must be considered a normal event,[57,58] the concentrations of various constituents of the refluxed intestinal juice can reach very high levels in patients with upper gastrointestinal disease and are, indeed, capable of producing acute mucosal injury. Rhodes et al.[27] found bile salts at mean concentrations up to 5.3 m*M* in GU patients after feeding, compared with 0.13 m*M* in controls. Patients symptomatic for reflux gastritis syndrome had a mean intestinal bile acid concentration of 2.7 m*M*, more than twice that of the asymptomatic group.[20] Duane et al.[4] determined total and soluble concentrations of bile acid, lysolecithin, fatty acid, and lecithin in gastric aspirates from subjects with Billroth II anastomosis and from normal controls. They found a marked difference between bile acid and lysolecithin concentrations in gastric aspirates taken postprandially and in the fasting state from the Billroth II subjects. During fasting, the median soluble bile acid concentration was 2.49 m*M*, and that of lysolecithin was 0.26 m*M*. These fell postprandially to median values of 0.76 m*M* and 0.02 m*M*, respectively. Similar mean concentrations of bile acid (5.0 m*M*) and lysolecithin (0.37 m*M*) have been described in the gastric juice of GU patients after cholecystokinin-induced reflux.[26]

Moore et al.[59] studied patients with type I GU who were in clinical and endoscopic remission. These patients had a higher gastritis index than healthy controls or DU patients, but the groups did not differ significantly in fasting gastric pH or bile acid concentrations; however, two of the seven GU patients did have relatively high total bile acid concentrations (0.56 and 1.02 m*M*). This study raises the possibility that persistent gastritis and antral hypomotility predispose to ulceration with gastritis presumably resulting from some cause unrelated to duodenogastric reflux. It can also be argued that stress-induced changes in hormonal or central nervous control over motility,[60] which could produce an increase in the concentration of intragastric bile or lysolecithin in an already inflamed stomach, may be an initiating event in relapse.

B. LEVELS OF LYSOLECITHIN AND PHOSPHOLIPASE A_2 IN THE STOMACH

Johnson and McDermott[61] found that GU patients had mean peak concentrations of lysolecithin of about 0.9 m*M* and mean concentrations in all samples of about 0.4 m*M*. DU patients had much lower levels, which were in most cases well below the critical micellar concentration (CMC) of 0.2 m*M*.[62] Similarly, Sarosiek et al.[63] found that basal gastric secretions from GU patients contained mean lysolecithin concentrations of 0.93 m*M*. This was significantly higher than levels found in DU patients, and in the GU group, patients with antral ulcer had higher gastric concentrations of lysolecithin than those with ulcers in the middle portion of the lesser curvature. Following pentagastrin stimulation; however, the mean lysolecithin concentration in the GU patients showed a twofold decrease. This study also showed a significant correlation between concentrations of lysolecithin and glyceroglucolipids in the gastric juice of GU patients,[63] leading to speculation that lysolecithin may be involved in solubilization of presumably protective gastric mucus. In a separate study on purified pig gastric mucus, Slomiany et al.[64] found that lysolecithin at concentrations of 0.1 to 1.0 m*M* reduced the viscosity of mucus by 33 to 52%.

Phospholipase A_2 is also found in higher concentrations in cholecystokinin-induced refluxed gastric juice of GU patients than in normals.[26] Pancreatic phospholipase A_2 actively converts biliary lecithin into lysolecithin only at pH approaching neutrality, but the enzyme is not irreversibly inactivated by acid pH. Boyle et al.[26] point out that the contribution of phospholipase A_2 to gastric injury would be expected to become increasingly important as chronic gastritis progresses and acid secretion decreases. In their study, the mean pH of gastric juice from GU patients during duodenogastric reflux (pH 5.3) was significantly higher than that of normal subjects (pH 3.7) and of DU patients (pH 2.7).

C. ACUTE EFFECTS OF PHYSIOLOGICALLY RELEVANT LEVELS OF BILE ACIDS AND LYSOLECITHIN

The most convincing demonstrations that the above levels of refluxed duodenal contents are capable of producing gastric damage have come from animal studies, although studies on humans have also demonstrated the ability of clinically relevant levels of bile salts to damage the gastric mucosal barrier.[65-68]

Duane et al.[4] used a canine Heidenhain pouch model to determine that minimal injurious levels of bile acids and lysolecithin were about 2.5 and 0.2 to 0.4 m*M*. respectively. At these concentrations, there was significant efflux of Na^+ into the lumen and loss of hydrogen ion. Long chain fatty acids (palmitic, stearic, oleic, and linoleic) did not potentiate the effects of a minimally damaging mixture of bile acid and lysolecithin or cause appreciable disruption of the mucosal barrier up to a concentration of 7 m*M*. Using these criteria, about half of the Billroth II subjects studied by Duane et al.[4] had potentially toxic fasting concentrations of bile acids and lecithin. It should be noted that in this study, the pH of gastric aspirates from Billroth II patients was always greater than 3.0 and usually more than 5.0. Thus, even though lowering the pH has been shown in some studies to exacerbate the damaging effects of bile on the gastric mucosa,[13,69] damage is most likely to occur only at higher pH in this population. As was mentioned above, it is at higher pH that the damage due to lysolecithin is likely to be most significant.

Fromm and co-workers[70,71] studied the effects of 1 and 5 m*M* taurocholate at pH 7.4 on isolated cells from the rabbit gastric mucosa. A 10-min exposure to 1 m*M* taurocholate destroyed about 50% of the surface cells, but did not significantly alter survival of glandular cells. At a concentration of 5 m*M*, taurocholate destroyed all of the surface cell population and about 50% of the glandular cells. The glandular cell population contained 63% parietal cells, but it was not determined whether this population was more or less resistant than chief cells or mucous neck cells.

Exposure of the guinea pig stomach to 2 m*M* lysolecithin in neutral solution for 2 h has been shown to produce extensive hemorrhagic erosions.[72] Lysolecithin caused loss of surface epithelial cells, edema and vascular damage including the formation of platelet thrombi and neutrophil margination, and extravasation. The ability of low concentrations of lysolecithin (0.04 m*M*) to potentiate ADP-induced platelet aggregation has been previously described,[73] and Maksem et al.[72] suggest that this effect on vascular integrity, coupled with the cytolytic effect of high luminal concentations, may be an initiating factor in lysolecithin-induced damage.

D. DO REFLUXED INTESTINAL CONTENTS HAVE A ROLE IN DRUG- AND STRESS-INDUCED ACUTE ULCER FORMATION?

Experiments on rats have shown that bile duct ligation reduces the extent of acute erosions produced by aspirin,[74] restraint stress,[75] and lateral hypothalamic lesions,[76] however, all of these agents and procedures have been shown to be capable of producing gastric erosions by effects on gastric secretion, motility, or blood flow. The demonstration by Guth et al.[77] that bile duct ligation markedly inhibits gastric acid secretion in the rat, suggests that this is the primary consequence of this procedure, and a role for duodenal contents cannot be claimed in these models. In addition, Meeroff et al.[78] found no significant differences in the incidence of gastric lesions resulting from cold-restraint stress in rats with or without bile duct ligation.

There is some evidence from animal studies that prior exposure to 20% ethanol can increase the susceptibility of the gastric mucosa to damage by lysolecithin. This finding is of particular interest because of other studies which show that 20% ethanol is capable of producing "adaptive cytoprotection".[79] Neiderhiser and Maksem[80] found that neither 20% ethanol nor 1 m*M* lysolecithin produced macroscopic damage to the guinea pig stomach (although each did produce signs of a "broken barrier"); however, when exposure to 20% ethanol was followed 1 h later by orogastric lysolecithin, there was a significant increase in the extent of hemorrhagic erosions. They suggested that this synergistic effect could be due to ethanol-induced increases in permeability which could allow lysolecithin micelles access to the lamina propria. In contrast to the effects of ethanol, pretreatment of guinea pigs with aspirin did not augment the damage produced by 2 m*M* lysolecithin.[72]

Lysolecithin has also been implicated in the development of stress ulcers subsequent to hemorrhagic shock. Kivilaakso et al.[81] described a significant increase in intragastric lysolecithin in piglets following hemorrhagic shock and prevention of gastric ulceration in animals in which duodenogastric reflux was prevented by duodenal exclusion and Roux-en-Y gastrojejunostomy. Orogastric replacement of lysolecithin resulted in the development of gastric lesions in shocked animals.

VII. EFFECTS OF BILE ON MUCOSAL DEFENSES AND REPAIR

A. THE "MUCUS-BICARBONATE BARRIER" AND THE UNSTIRRED WATER LAYER

It is widely believed that the stomach and duodenum are protected by a "mucus-bicarbonate barrier". As proposed by Heatley,[82] this barrier requires a continuous coat of gastroduodenal mucus and secretion of alkali from the mucosa into this layer. In its most generally accepted form, the hypothesis predicts that mucus, which is released from luminal epithelial cells, forms a continuous "mixing barrier" within which luminal acid is neutralized by secreted or released bicarbonate.[83,84] Evidence for the continuous nature of the mucus coat is based primarily on *in vitro* measurements of mucus continuity and thickness from thick sections of unfixed mucosa.[85,86] The measured mean thickness of the mucus coat varies from about 50 to 150 μm, depending on the species[85] (Figure 1). There is still considerable uncertainty about the extent and continuity of the mucus coat,[87,88] and it is possible that the apparently continuous adherent coat is an artefact resulting from the optical technique used to visualize it.[89] There is general agreement that the coat, whether continuous or discontinuous, is very thin over much of the stomach (5 μm or less),[85,87] and would not, even as part of a mucus-bicarbonate barrier, provide significant protection against mucosal damaging agents such as bile and lysolecithin. It is, however, considered to provide a primary defense for the luminal epithelial cells against acid and pepsin (see Chapter 3). The cells of the gastric glands, which are not covered by mucus and which are exposed to the highest concentrations of acid and pepsin, are assumed to be protected by some unknown membrane-mediated process.[83]

The most convincing case for the clinical relevance of the bicarbonate component of the mucus-bicarbonate barrier can be made for the proximal small intestine. The proximal duodenum, in particular, secretes large quantities of bicarbonate,[90,91] and patients with duodenal ulcer disease have both decreased basal bicarbonate output and decreased output following luminal acidification relative to normal subjects.[91] Known ulcerogenic agents such as NSAID also decrease both bicarbonate secretion and prostaglandin synthesis.[92]

1. Do Bile Salts Inhibit Mucosal Secretion of Bicarbonate and Thus Impair the Mucus-Bicarbonate Barrier?

There are conflicting data regarding the direct effects of bile acids on the ability of the gastric mucosa to secrete or release bicarbonate. Ross et al.[93] described an "opacification" of gastric mucus following exposure to acidified 10 m*M* taurocholate but did not detect a drop in the surface pH unless the mucus was physically removed. *In vitro* studies have demonstrated that low concentrations of taurocholate at neutral pH converted net alkalinization to transient acidification in both isolated rabbit and amphibian gastric mucosae;[94,95] however, the net acid secretion resulted from exposure to a concentration (1 m*M*) which did not affect mucosal resistance or PD, and subsequent exposure to taurocholate did not produce acidification. In addition, the ability of relatively high concentrations of taurocholate (9 to 20 m*M*) to inhibit carbonic anhydrase *in vitro* and *in vivo* has led to the suggestion that this may contribute to its ulcerogenic action.[96]

In vivo studies suggest, however, that the response of the gastric mucosa to "irritating" doses of bile salts is to secrete alkaline fluid, which may account for the adaptive cytoprotection conferred by exposure of gastric mucosae to 20 m*M* taurocholate.[97] This outpouring of alkaline

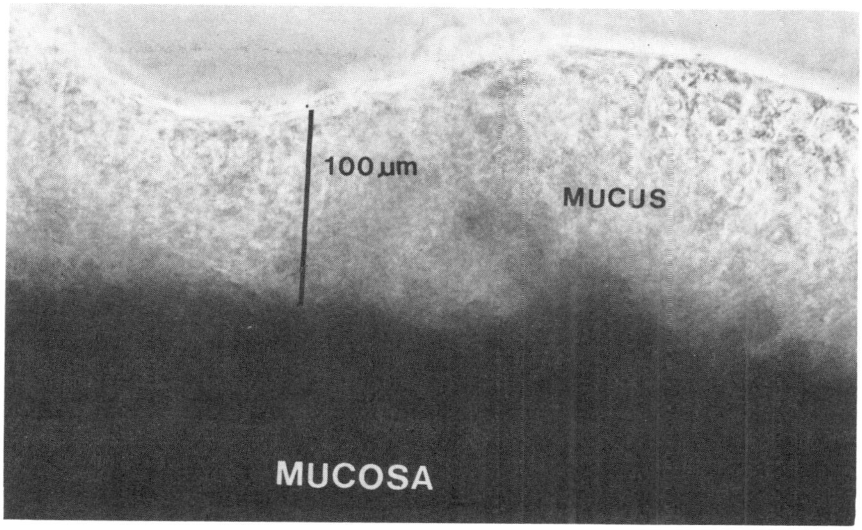

FIGURE 1. Extracellular mucus coat of rat gastric mucosa as viewed by the technique of Kerss et al.[85] A 1.5-mm thick section of rat gastric mucosa was mounted transversely on a microscope slide and viewed by phase contrast microscopy.

secretion is not only a property of bile salts. At high doses, 16,16-dimethyl PGE_2 produces a similar release and also produces a comparable drop in the transmucosal potential difference.[98] The ability of taurocholate to provide adaptive cytoprotection and to produce alkaline secretion is inhibited by parenteral indomethacin at doses (5 mg/kg in rats) which also prevent the hyperemic response.[47]

2. Effects of Bile on the Unstirred Water Layer

It is possible that the extracellular mucus coat forms a part of the unstirred water layer which exists at the surface of the gastric mucosa.[99] The unstirred water layer has been calculated to be about 880 µm thick over the rat gastric mucosa.[6] This closely matches the thickness of the pH gradient which has been measured over the surfaces of gastric and duodenal mucosae from several species, including humans.[100-104] The extent of the unstirred water layer at any point in time would be a consequence of the rate of flux of the sodium-rich alkaline fluid from the underlying mucosa,[105] the thickness of the adherent coat of gelatinous or fibrous mucus, the possible contribution of partly degraded (but still viscous) mucus from the adherent layer,[99] and shear forces exerted by gastrointestinal motility.

Duane et al.[6] have demonstrated that mixing of an intragastric solution of bile salts by continual withdrawl and injection with a syringe can reduce the thickness of the unstirred water layer from more than 800 to about 450 µm. Mixing the bile salt solution increased net fluxes of cations and increased the efflux of phospholipid and cholesterol, changes which were interpreted as indicating increased mucosal damage. We have carried out studies, using a rat gastric chamber preparation, on the effects of stirring the luminal solution on the susceptibility of the mucosa to acute damage by acidified sodium taurocholate.[106] When the bile salt is added to mucosae which have had the luminal solution stirred during the previous 10 min period, there is a highly significant increase in damage. Conversely, the protection afforded when the bile salt is added to a mucosa exposed to a previously unstirred solution is abolished by prior parenteral injection of indomethacin at a dose (5 mg/kg) which inhibits gastric cyclooxygenase activity by about 85%.

The role of mucus in contributing to the unstirred water layer is, however, not clearly proven.

Thomson and Dietschy[104] argue that for the intestine at least, most studies indicate that intestinal mucus and the glycocalyx do not significantly impair the absorption of solutes or contribute to the effective resistance of the unstirred water layer.

B. EFFECTS OF BILE AND ACID ON REPAIR BY RESTITUTION

The gastric mucosa responds to topical exposure to various damaging agents, including bile acids, by exfoliation of luminal epithelial cells, release of intracellular mucus stores from surviving cells, and plasma shedding.[88,107-109] The result is a rapidly formed, local coat of shed cells and mucus, which is further stabilized by a network of fibrin strands.[87,110] In the absence of extensive microvascular congestion, the integrity of the epithelium is soon restored by epithelial migration (restitution) over the exposed basal lamina.[107,111,112] In the presence of an intact vascular supply, the efflux of bicarbonate-rich fluid (occurring during the period of bile-induced hyperemia) will coincide with the period of epithelial restitution,[113] and can neutralize influxing luminal acid within the "mixing barrier" provided by the adherent mucus cap.

1. Microvascular Architecture of the Gastric Mucosa

The microvascular architecture of the gastric mucosae of rats and of humans is fundamentally similar.[114-116] Mucosal arterioles arise from submucosal vessels, penetrate the muscularis mucosae, and branch laterally to form terminal arterioles which, in turn, undergo up to three levels of branching before giving rise to an ascending capillary network (Figure 2). Capillaries do not connect laterally with the collecting venules and below the luminal epithelium, the capillaries form a continuous, interconnected network which surrounds the foveolar openings (Figure 3). Capillaries drain into collecting venules which may extend through the mucosa without branching until they approach the luminal surface, or which may form two or more major branches which converge to form a single collecting venule (Figure 4). The location of the capillary-collecting venule loop at a point immediately beneath the luminal epithelial cells makes this a particularly vulnerable site since blockade at this point will produce localized stasis throughout the depth of the mucosa.[110] The collecting venules drain into a complex, interconnecting collecting venule plexus which lies within the muscularis mucosae[117] (Figure 5). This plexus then drains into the submucosal venular plexus.

Thus, the mucosal microarchitecture is basically that of a hairpin, with interconnections between capillaries and collecting venules being limited to the region immediately beneath the luminal epithelium. The complex network of interstitial and surface capillary interconnections allows perfusion of regions immediately adjacent to localized microvascular damage and the extensive terminal branching of the mucosal collecting venules also allows the mucosa to tolerate numerous isolated sites of microvascular occlusion; however, when occlusion extends below the upper $^1/_3$ of the mucosa, or is widespread, the entire affected region is rendered ischemic.[115]

2. Acute Effects of Bile Acids on Gastric Mucosal Morphology

Very few studies have examined the ultrastructure of the gastric mucosa in the period immediately after the topical application of constituents of bile, at the time when physiological studies show rapid damage to the gastric mucosal barrier. Eastwood[69] examined the effects of taurocholate and glycochenodeoxycholate on the mouse gastric mucosa and described the appearance, within 2 min of irreversible damage to surface epithelial cells, marked by clumping of nuclear chromatin and loss of cytoplasmic density. Damage of this type could be attributed to the effects of the 100 m*M* HCl used in some experiments, rather than being unique to a particular barrier breaker.[107] Sawyer et al.[118] described cytoplasmic vacuolation and condensation, nuclear pyknosis, and occasional loss of intracellular mucus 15 min after exposure of human gastric mucosae to chenodeoxycholate. Carter et al.[119] described extensive exfoliation of

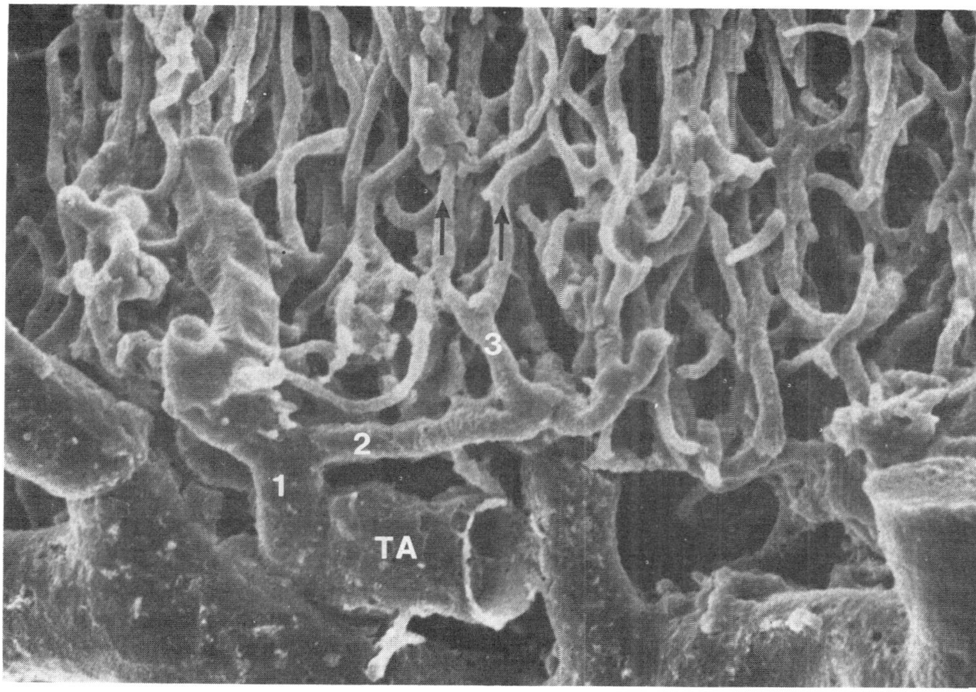

FIGURE 2. Scanning electron micrograph of corrosion cast preparation of rat gastric mucosa. Terminal arterioles (TA) at the base of the mucosa form primary (1), secondary (2), and tertiary (3) branches which give rise to the ascending capillaries (arrows). (Magnification × 500.)

canine surface epithelial cells following exposure of the mucosae to taurocholate in 100 m*M* HCl. The extent of damage was not quantified, but was reported to be concentration-dependent.

We have examined the effects of seven different barrier breakers, including sodium taurocholate (10 and 50 m*M* in 50 m*M* HCl), on various physiological indicators of gastric mucosal barrier integrity in the rat.[120] Our results indicated that taurocholate, isobutyric acid, and 3 *M* glucose differed from the other barrier breakers tested (40% ethanol, thermal injury, aspirin and aspirin/ethanol) in that the group of agents which included bile salt produced much less extensive hemorrhagic erosions than did the ethanol/salicylate/thermal injury group, when the changes in PD and net K^+ efflux were equivalent. This was interpreted as reflecting the relatively greater ability of the latter group of agents to produce vascular stasis in addition to destruction of surface epithelial cells.

Exposure of the rat gastric mucosa to 10 or 50 m*M* taurocholate in 50 m*M* HCl causes a rapid, dose-dependent drop in PD (Figure 6). Microscopical examination of tissue from 7 mucosae fixed 5 min after exposure of the mucosae to 10 m*M* taurocholate revealed that 11.8 ± 3.4% of the fundic surface epithelium was destroyed at this time. The earliest stages of damage involved swelling of the apical mucus cap and dissolution of mucus granules (Figures 7 and 8). This was followed by apical rupture and release of mucus into the lumen (Figure 9) and subsequently, exfoliation of the destroyed cells. Less extensive ultrastructural studies were carried out on the effects of 50 m*M* taurocholate, but tissue examined at 1 min after topical application of the bile salt showed the same extensive epithelial destruction. In this model system, damage is extremely rapid, and it is probable that the rapid decline in PD is paralleled by destruction of epithelial cells. After mucosae had been exposed to taurocholate for 10 min, and after a subsequent 1 h period

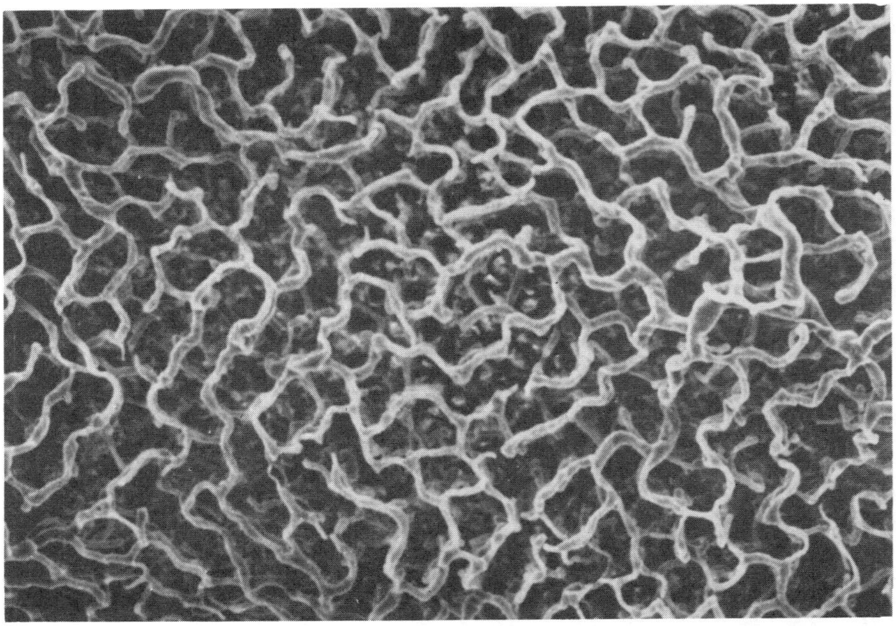

FIGURE 3. Scanning electron micrograph of corrosion cast of luminal microvasculature of rat fundic mucosa showing honeycomb-like pattern of interconnected capillary network which surrounds gastric glands. (Micrograph courtesy of T.T. Hynna. Magnification × 140.)

in which the gastric chamber contained 50 m*M* HCl, hemorrhagic erosions covered approximately 5% of the glandular mucosae.

3. Effects of Bile and Acid on Restitution

There is no information on the effects of continued exposure to bile constituents on the process of epithelial restitution. In our studies, we found that the depression in transmucosal PD produced by taurocholate persisted for the period in which taurocholate was in the chamber (10, 20, or 30 min). Subsequent to the removal of taurocholate/HCl and replacement with HCl, the PD rose to control levels. This may reflect effects on the restitution process or continued cell death during exposure to taurocholate. The more prolonged exposures to the bile acid did not; however, result in significant increases in the areas of hemorrhagic erosions at the end of the experiments.

Rutten and Ito[121] have shown, using an *in vitro* preparation, that at pH 1 both morphological and physiological indicators of restitution are impaired. We have emphasized the permissive rather than causal role of acid in the development of acute damage.[110] In the absence of an intact microvascular supply and resulting efflux of bicarbonate-rich fluid, or in the presence of high concentrations of luminal acid, the influxing acid can destroy otherwise viable cells,[107] promote hemorrhage,[122] accelerate loss of the mucus cap by destroying the stabilizing fibrin network,[107] and break down the basal lamina which provides a necessary substrate for restitution.[123]

We have also examined the process of restitution in the human gastric mucosa following exposure to 10 m*M* taurocholate in 100 m*M* HCl. Mucosal biopsies were obtained from the antral mucosae of volunteers using standard pinch biopsy forceps during endoscopy 45 min after intragastric infusion of the acid/taurocholate. The mucosae showed sites where the luminal epithelium had been destroyed and where epithelial continuity had not yet been restored, as well as sites where restitution had covered previously denuded interfoveolar epithelium (Figures 10 to 12). The transmucosal PD was not recorded in our study, but the apparent extensive recovery

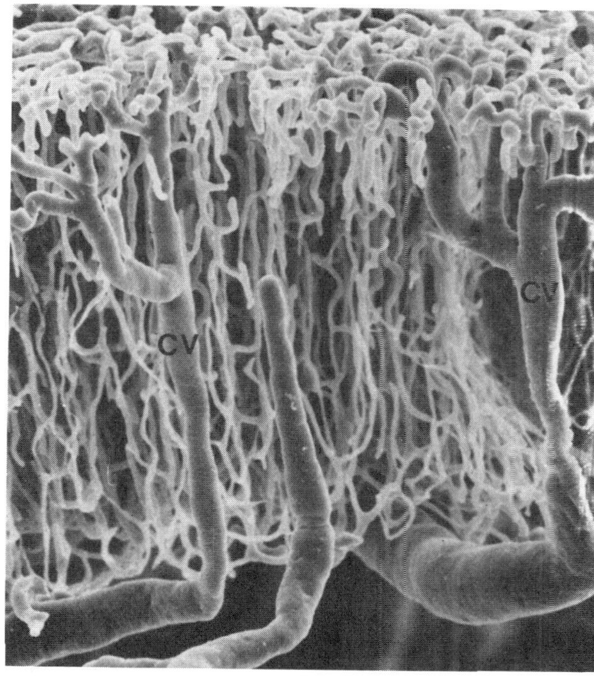

FIGURE 4. Scanning electron micrograph of corrosion cast of rat fundic mucosa. This lateral view shows different levels of branching in the collecting venules (CV). Interconnections between capillaries and branches of collecting venules are limited to the region immediately beneath the mucosal surface. (Magnification × 270.)

in epithelial integrity at a time 45 min after infusion of the taurocholate/acid solution correlates well with numerous studies on animals in which restitution is paralleled by a recovery in PD and the study of Geall et al.[66] in which recovery in PD was underway 30 min after exposure of the gastric mucosae of volunteers to whole bile.

C. EFFECTS OF BILE ON MUCUS

Lysolecithin and bile salts have been shown to decrease mucus viscosity[64,124] and to reduce the ability of mucus to retard hydrogen ion diffusion;[125] however, Bell et al.[126] detected no significant effects on the mechanical properties of gastric or duodenal mucus following incubation with pig gallbladder bile for 18 h over a range of pH 2 to 8. Addition of exogenous phospholipids to mucus glycoprotein may enhance the diffusion barrier properties of gastric mucus,[127] and it has been suggested that this may account for the protection conferred by added lecithin; however, the protection afforded by lecithin against the damaging effects of lysolecithin in the study of Martin et al.[17] was accompanied by an obvious decrease in the quantity of mucus released.

It is, in fact, unlikely that effects on the physical properties of mucus have any role in the development of acute damage induced by the constituents of bile. We have found that extensive damage to the luminal epithelium, as assessed by both decreases in PD and ultrastructural examination, occurs within a few seconds to 5 min. The remarkable change in appearance of the gastric mucus from a clear, gelatinous layer to an opaque, thick layer following exposure to taurocholate results not from effects of bile on the extracellular mucus coat, but rather is a consequence of extensive and rapid cell death and exfoliation.[89]

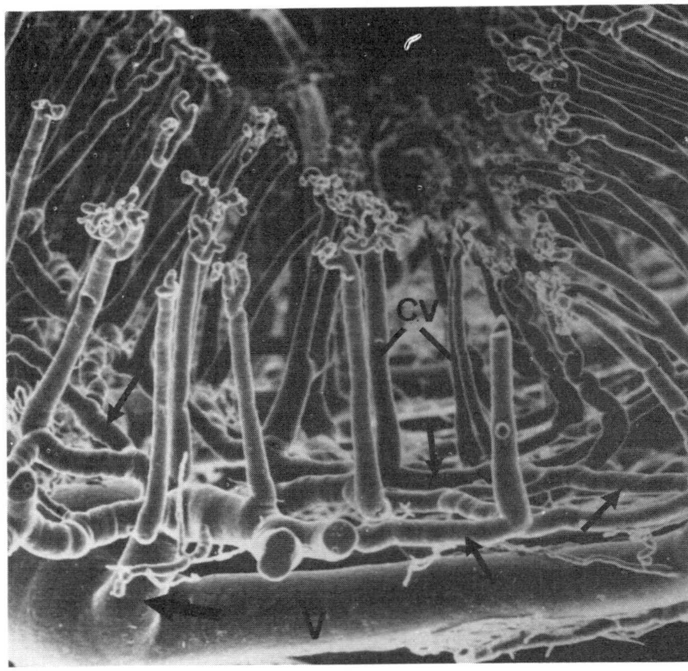

FIGURE 5. Scanning electron micrograph of corrosion cast of "valley" region (between mucosal folds) of rat fundic mucosa. This is a partial retrograde cast, in which liquid plastic was perfused through the superior mesenteric vein and perfusion was stopped before the capillary bed was filled. Collecting venules (CV) drain into an interconnected venous plexus (small arrows) located within the muscularis mucosae. The large arrow indicates a draining vein which penetrates the muscularis mucosae and joins a submucosal vein (V). (Micrograph courtesy of T.T. Hynna. Magnification × 80.)

VIII. THE EFFECTS OF CIGARETTE SMOKING ON BILE REFLUX

A high incidence of both gastric and duodenal ulcers is found in chronic cigarette smokers.[128-130] Cigarette smokers show increased bile salt reflux and gastric bile salt concentrations, which may partly explain the apparent proulcerogenic effect of smoking.[131] The bile salt concentrations measured in the study of Muller-Lissner and Fraass[131] were well below those shown by others to cause acute damage,[4] although the concentrations of other possibly damaging constituents of refluxed duodenal contents, such as lysolecithin, were not measured. In addition, the chronically increased duodenogastric reflux found in smokers will occur in a context of decreased gastric mucosal prostaglandin synthesis,[132,133] with consequent reduced mucosal defenses.

IX. *CAMPYLOBACTER* AND DUODENOGASTRIC REFLUX

Considerable attention has been directed recently to the association of *Campylobacter*-like organisms (*C. pylori*) with gastritis and peptic ulcer.[134,135] *C. pylori* has been shown to be associated with histologically active gastritis,[136] elevated fasting gastric pH,[137] and peptic ulceration.[138,139] There is not, however, any apparent association between *C. pylori* and duodenogastric reflux. In their study of 107 nonulcer dyspepsia patients, Karttunen et al.[140]

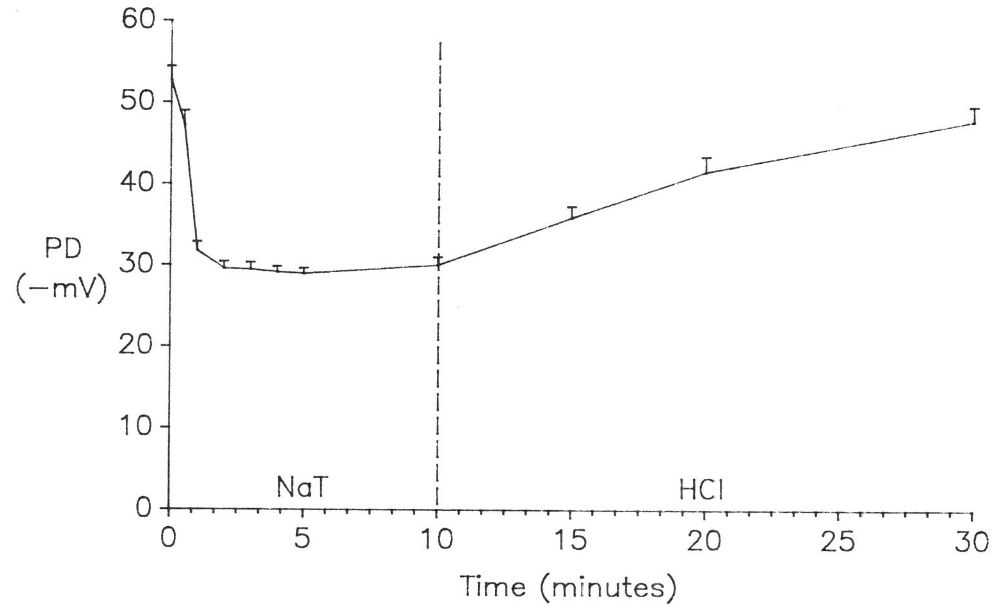

FIGURE 6. Transmucosal potential difference (PD) plotted at 0 time (before application of taurocholate), 30 s, 1 to 5 min, and 10, 15, 20, and 30 min after instillation of 10 mM taurocholate in 50 mM HCl. The acid/taurocholate remained in the chamber for 10 min and was replaced (11 to 30 min) with 50 mM HCl in 0.2 M mannitol. Values plotted are the mean ± SEM for 14 animals (time 0 to 5 min), and for 7 animals (15 to 30 min). Samples of fundic mucosae from 7 animals (4 tissue samples from each animal) were fixed for light and electron microscopy after exposure to acid/taurocholate for 5 min. Note the extremely rapid decline in PD, with baseline values of -29 to -30 mV being obtained within 1 to 2 min after exposure to taurocholate. The PD remained at this level while the taurocholate was in the chamber, but returned to control levels over the succeeding 20 min.

found *Campylobacter*-like organisms to be significantly associated with superficial gastritis in the body and atrophic gastritis in the antrum, but not with intragastric bile acid or lecithin concentration, degree of duodenogastric reflux, or intragastric pH.

X. PROTECTION AGAINST BILE-INDUCED GASTRIC DAMAGE

The obvious candidate for therapy, which has as its intent the lessening of bile-induced damage to the gastric mucosa, is alkaline reflux gastritis. As was mentioned above, both surgical and medical treatments have proven less than satisfactory (see Ritchie[3] for an excellent recent review). In particular, the use of agents such as cholestyramine and antacids which bind bile acids have been ineffective in both humans[141,142] and in studies on acute damage in animals.[143]

The recent focus on cytoprotection has given rise to numerous studies in humans and in animals in which the abilities of a range of cytoprotective agents to prevent acute damage by bile have been studied. With one exception in which whole bile of unstated origin was used as a necrotizing agent,[144] all of these studies examined the effects of sodium taurocholate. Protection against acute damage was[145] and was not[146] conferred by 100 mg/kg cimetidine in rats, was[147] and was not[145] conferred by 125 and 200 mg sucralfate, respectively, in rats, was[148] and was not[67,68,149] conferred by prostaglandins in humans, and was[150] and was not[151] conferred by combined H_1 and H_2 blockers in dogs. Antacids,[56,152,153] mild irritants,[154] and inhibitors of thromboxane synthesis[54,55] are consistently effective at protecting the mucosa against the rapidly developing hemorrhagic erosions which follow the topical application of high concentrations of acidified taurocholate.

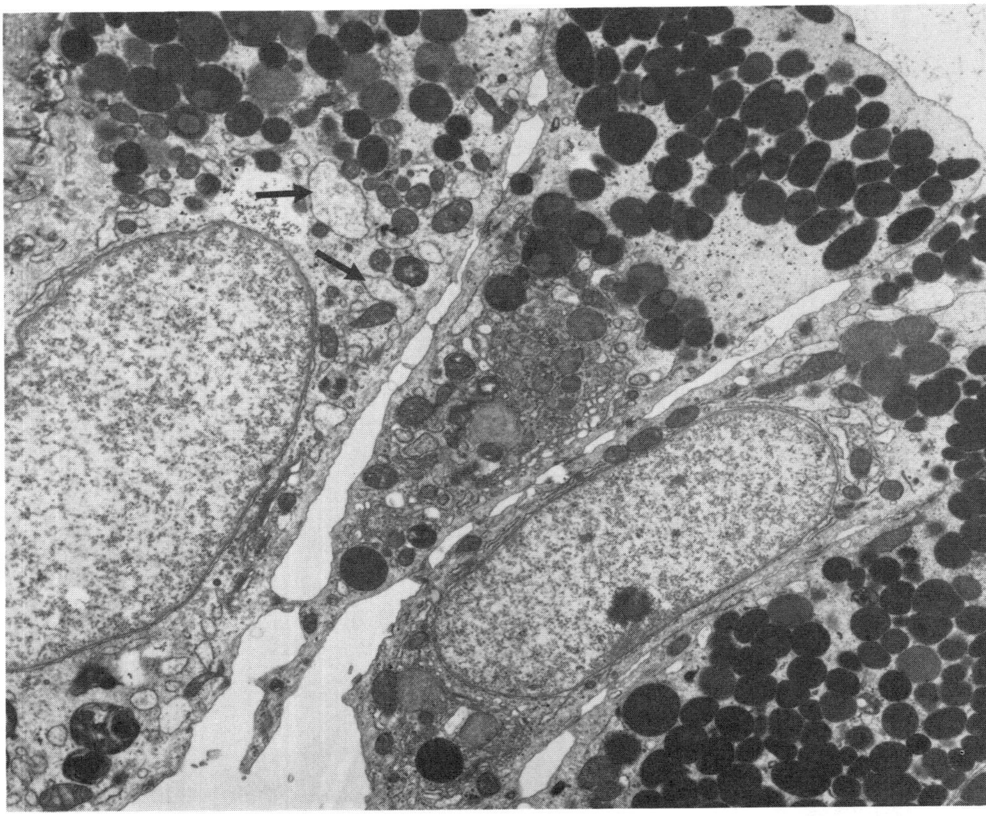

FIGURE 7. Transmission electron micrograph of surface epithelial cells from rat gastric mucosa after exposure to 10 m*M* taurocholate in 50 m*M* HCl for 5 min. Note swelling of apical cytoplasm and localized swelling of endoplasmic reticulum (arrows). Nuclei are swollen relative to control tissue and to unaffected cells. (Magnification × 6200.)

It is, however, questionable to what extent the above studies have clinical relevance. Prostaglandins have been shown to be effective in the treatment of peptic ulcer when administered at antisecretory doses.[155-157] Whether they will ultimately prove to be "a major therapeutic advance for the treatment of acid peptic disease"[158] or remain "a promise unfulfilled"[159] has yet to be determined.

There are some indications based on studies of isolated cell membranes and cultured cells which suggest that prostaglandins may have a specific protective role against bile acids at the cellular level. Exposure of isolated plasma membranes from rat gastric mucosal cells to a very high concentration of taurocholate (100 m*M*) enhanced the fluidity of the membranes as determined by electron spin resonance spectroscopy.[160] The observed changes were completely prevented by preincubation with PGE_2. Terano et al.[161] demonstrated significant protection by 16,16-dimethyl PGE_2 and $PGF_{2\alpha}$, in cultures of rat gastric mucosal cells, against 10 m*M* taurocholate. These studies provide a basis for speculating that changes in levels of endogenous prostaglandin synthesis may, in fact, be of importance in maintaining gastric mucosal integrity. At present, the situation remains one in which the constituents of bile have proven cytolytic activities, but it is not yet possible to state with certainty that this has significance in terms of the development of chronic gastric disease or that the protective effects shown in the *in vitro* studies are relevant to cytoprotection (more accurately, organoprotection) as shown *in vivo*.

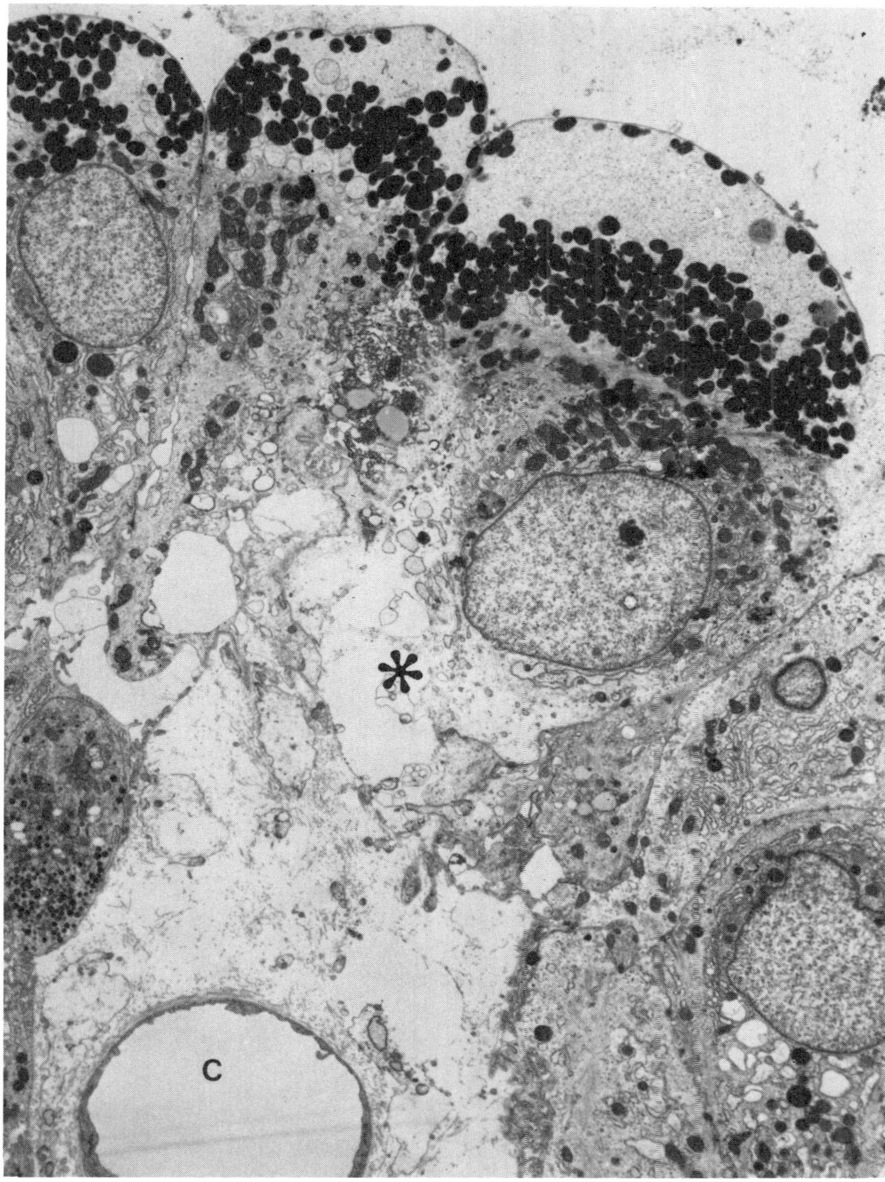

FIGURE 8. Interfoveolar surface epithelial cells from rat gastric mucosa 5 min after exposure to acid/taurocholate. Note apical swelling and dissolution of mucus granules. Asterisk indicates a site of basal cytoplasmic swelling and rupture of the plasma membrane C, subepithelial capillary. (Magnification × 2400.)

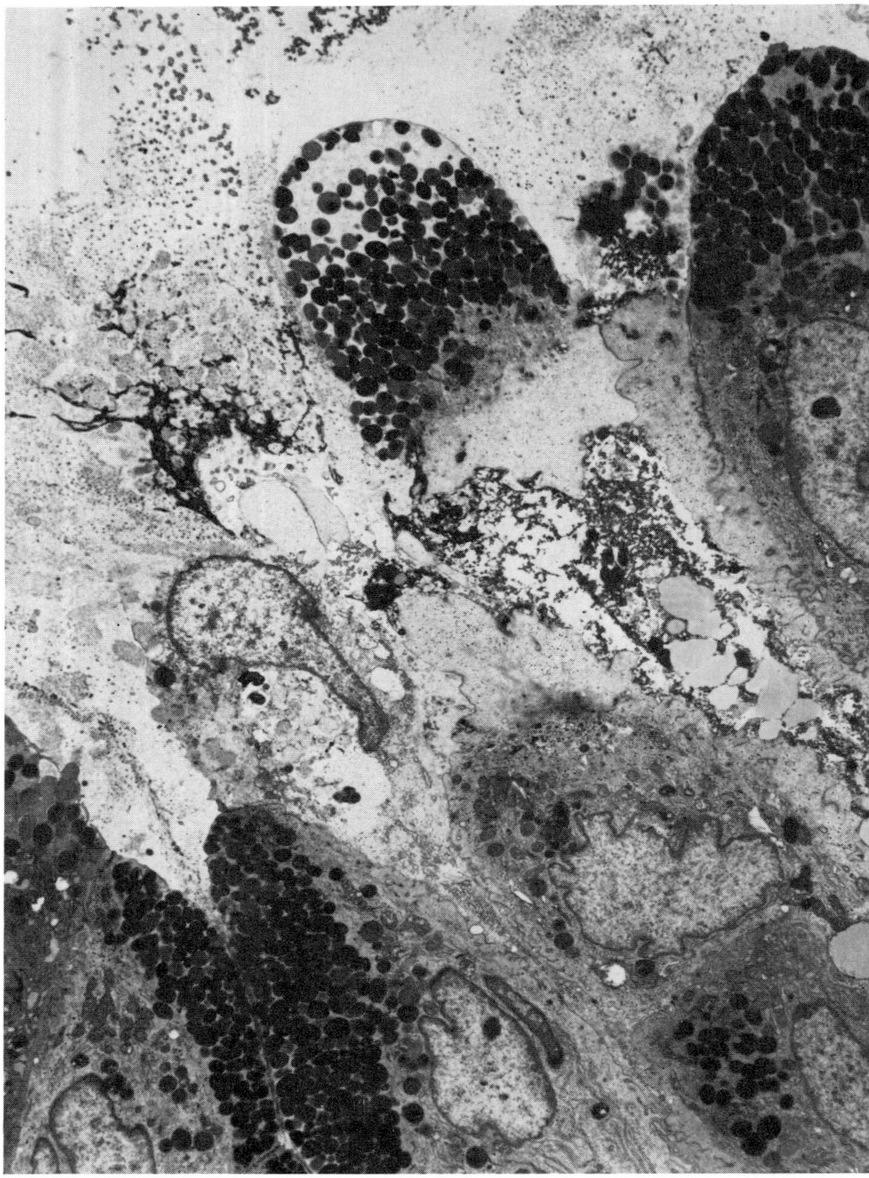

FIGURE 9. Apical rupture and release of mucus from epithelial cells of rat gastric mucosa after a 5-min exposure to acid/taurocholate. Epithelial cells lining upper gastric pit (lower portion of micrograph) appear unaffected. (Magnification × 2400.)

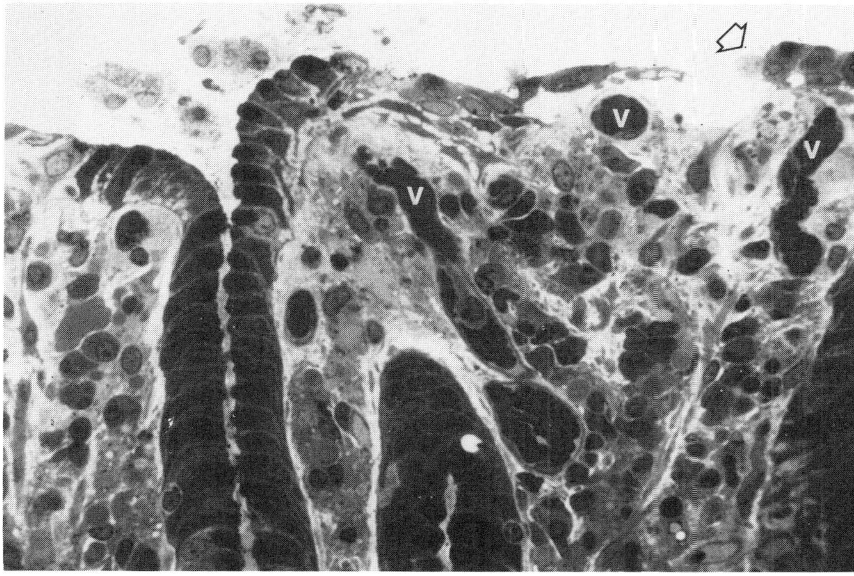

A

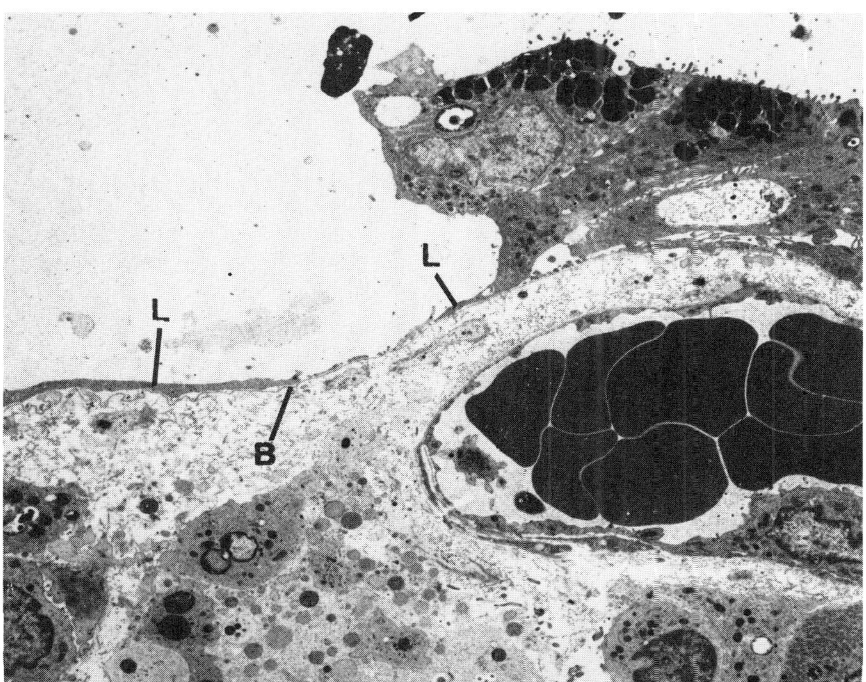

B

FIGURE 10. Light micrograph of toluidine blue-stained section (A) and corresponding transmission electron micrograph (B) from biopsy of human antral mucosa. Tissue was removed and fixed for microscopical study 45 min after exposure of the stomach to 10 m*M* taurocholate in 100 m*M* HCl. Arrow on light micrograph indicates site which is shown in detail on electron micrograph. Restitution had not been completed at the indicated site (A). Note the congested blood vessels (**V**) beneath the damaged site. Surface epithelial cells adjacent to the exposed basal lamina (**B**) are extending lamellipodia (**L**) which have already covered much of the exposed surface. (Magnifications: A, × 510; B, × 2800.)

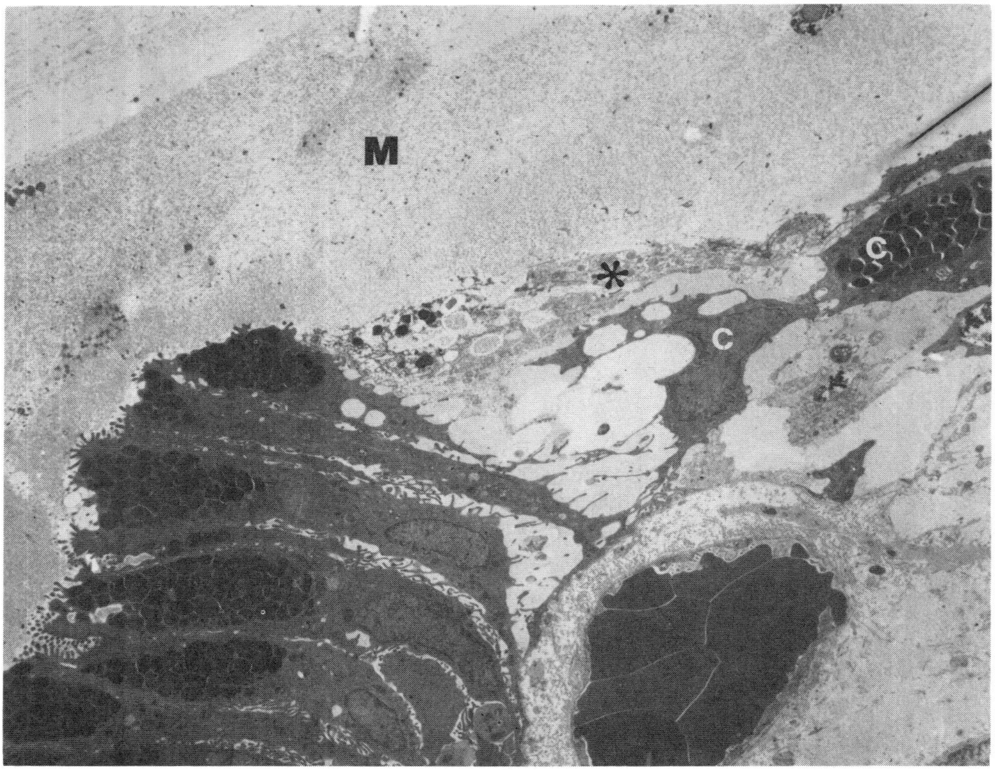

FIGURE 11. Transmission electron micrograph of interfoveolar region of human antral mucosa exposed to taurocholate and processed as described in caption to Figure 10. At this site, the cells are covered with an adherent cap of released mucus (M). Epithelial continuity has been restored by stretched epithelial cells (C). Note congested capillary beneath site of restitution and remnants of destroyed epithelial cell (indicated by asterisk). (Magnification X 2600.)

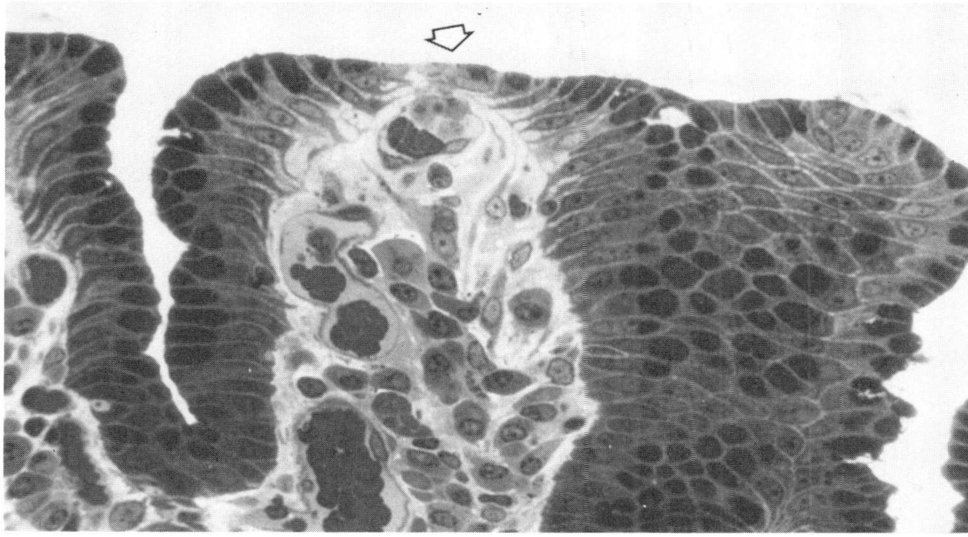

A

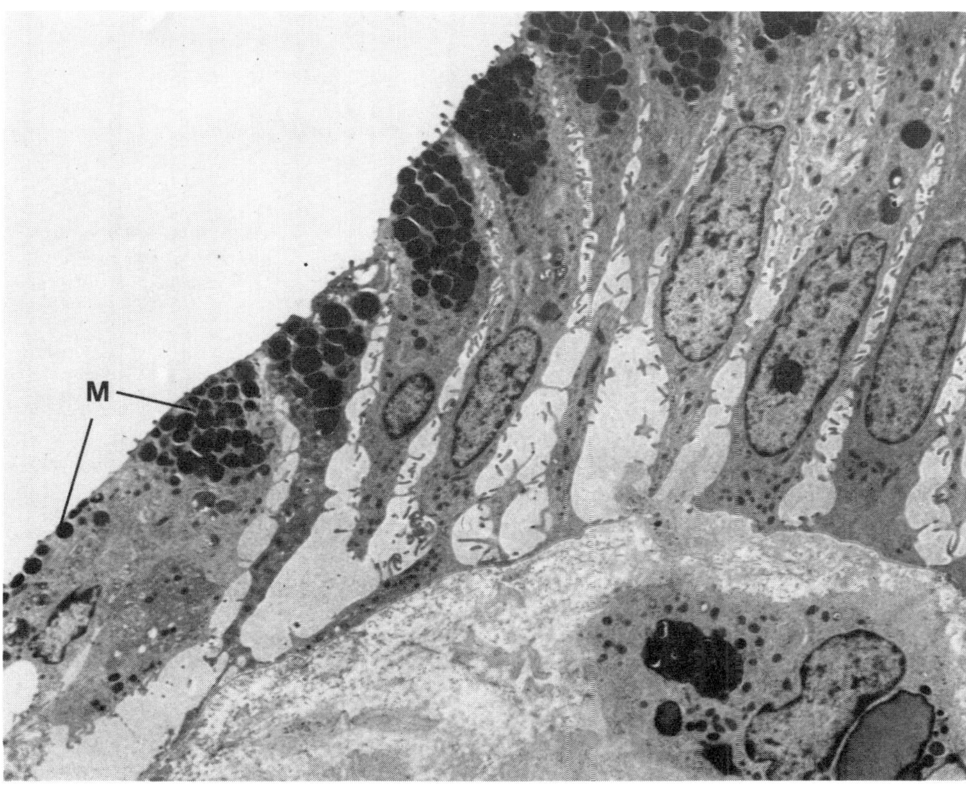

B

FIGURE 12. Light micrograph of toluidine blue-stained section (A) and transmission electron micrograph of region indicated by arrow (B), from human antral mucosa exposed to taurocholate and processed as described in caption to Figure 10. Restitution is complete at this site, although the epithelial cells over the interfoveolar site are still stretched relative to the normal columnar configuration. Note the loss of much of the apical intracellular mucus cap (M) in cells which have covered the previously denuded basal lamina. (Magnifications: A, X 520; B, X 3100.)

REFERENCES

1. **Wormsley, K. G.,** Duodenal ulcer: does pathophysiology equal aetiology?, *Gut,* 24, 775, 1983.
2. **Hoffman, A. F.,** The enterohepatic circulation of bile acids, in *Gastrointestinal Disease: Pathophysiology, Diagnosis, Management,* Sleisenger, M. H. and Fordtran, J. S., Eds., W. B. Saunders, Philadelphia, 1978, 92.
3. **Ritchie, W. P.,** Other causes of GI mucosal injury: upper intestinal content, *Clin. Invest. Med.,* 10, 264, 1987.
4. **Duane, W. C., Wiegand, D. M., and Gelberstadt, M. L.,** Intragastric duodenal lipids in the absence of a pyloric sphincter: quantitation, physical state, and injurious potential in the fasting and postprandial states, *Gastroenterology,* 78, 1480, 1980.
5. **Duane, W. C. and Wiegand, D. M.,** Mechanism by which bile salt disrupts the gastric mucosal barrier in the dog, *J. Clin. Invest.,* 66, 1044, 1980.
6. **Duane, W. C., Levitt, M. D., Staley, N. A., McHale, A. P., Wiegand, S. M., and Fetzer, C. A.,** Role of the unstirred layer in protecting the murine gastric mucosa from bile salt, *Gastroenterology,* 91, 913, 1986.
7. **Harmon, J. W., Doong, T., and Gadacz, T. R.,** Bile acids are not equally damaging to the gastric mucosa, *Surgery,* 84, 79, 1978.
8. **Harmon, J. W., Lewis, C.D., and Gadacz, T. R.,** Bile salt composition and concentration as determinants of canine gastric mucosal injury, *Surgery,* 89, 348, 1981.
9. **Ritchie, W. P. and Felger, T. S.,** Differing ulcerogenic potential of dihydroxy and trihydroxy bile acids in canine gastric mucosa, *Surgery,* 89, 342, 1981.
10. **Felger, T. S. and Ritchie, W. P.,** Ulcerogenic potential of 1° vs 2° bile acids in gastric mucosa, *Surg. Forum,* 33, 324, 1982.
11. **Gullikson, G. W., Cline, W. S., Lorenzsonn, V., Benz, L., Olsen, W. A., and Bass, P.,** Effects of anionic surfactants on hamster small intestinal membrane structure and function: relationship to surface activity, *Gastroenterology,* 73, 501, 1977.
12. **Masci, E., Testoni, P. A., Fanti, L., Guslandi, M., Zuin, M., and Tittobello, A.,** Duodenogastric reflux: correlations among bile acid pattern, mucus secretion, and mucosal damage, *Scand. J. Gastroenterol.,* 22, 308, 1987.
13. **Black, R. B., Hole, D., and Rhodes, M. D.,** Bile damage to the gastric mucosal barrier: the influence of pH and bile acid concentration, *Gastroenterology,* 61, 178, 1971.
14. **Stern, A. I., Hogan, D. L., and Isenberg, J. I.,** Effect of sodium taurocholate on the human gastric mucosa at acid and neutral pH's, *Gastroenterology,* 87, 1272, 1984.
15. **Duane, W. C., Wiegand, D. M., and Sievert, C. E.,** Bile acid and bile salt disrupt gastric mucosal barrier in the dog by different mechanisms, *Am. J. Physiol.,* 242, 95, 1982.
16. **Duane, W. C., McHale, A. P., and Sievert, C. E.,** Lysolecithin-lipid interactions in disruption of the canine gastric mucosal barrier, *Am. J. Physiol.,* 250, G275, 1986.
17. **Martin, G. P., Newbery, R. S., Turner, N. C., and Marriott, C.,** Gastric mucosal injury by bile acids: the influence of phospholipids, *Gastroenterol. Clin. Biol.,* 9, 80, 1985.
18. **Himal, H. S.,** Alkaline gastritis and alkaline esophagitis: a review, *Can. J. Surg.,* 20, 403, 1977.
19. **Witt, T. R., Roseman, D. L., and Banner, B. F.,** The role of the gastric antrum in the pathogenesis of reflux gastritis, *J. Surg. Res.,* 26, 220, 1979.
20. **Meshkinpour, H., Marks, J. W., Schoenfield, L. J., Bonnoris, G. C., and Carter, S.,** Reflux gastritis syndrome: mechanism of symptoms, *Gastroenterology,* 79, 1283, 1980.
21. **Boren, C. H. and Way, L. W.,** Alkaline reflux gastritis: a reevaluation, *Am. J. Surg.,* 140, 40, 1980.
22. **Bondurant, F. J., Maull, K. I., Nelson, H. S., and Silver, S. H.,** Bile reflux gastritis, *South. Med. J.,* 80, 161, 1987.
23. **Malagelada, J. R., Phillips, S. F., Shorter, R. G., Higgins, J. A., Magrina, C., van Heerden, J. A., and Adson, M. A.,** Postoperative reflux gastritis: pathophysiology and long term outcome after Roux-en-Y diversion, *Ann. Intern. Med.,* 103, 178, 1985.
24. **Ritchie, W. P.,** Alkaline reflux gastritis: late results of a controlled trial of diagnosis and treatment, *Ann. Surg.,* 203, 537, 1986.
25. **Fisher, R. S. and Cohen, S.,** Pyloric-sphincter dysfunction in patients with gastric ulcer, *N. Engl. J. Med.,* 288, 273, 1973.
26. **Boyle, J. M., Neiderhiser, D. H., and Dworken, H. J.,** Duodenogastric reflux in patients with gastric ulcer disease, *J. Lab. Clin. Med.,* 103, 14, 1984.
27. **Rhodes, J., Barnardo, D. E., Phillips, S. F., Rovelstad, R. A., and Hofmann, A. F.,** Increased reflux of bile into the stomach in patients with gastric ulcer, *Gastroenterology,* 57, 241, 1969.
28. **Rhodes, J. and Calcraft, B.,** Aetiology of gastric ulcer with special reference to the roles of reflux and mucosal damage, *Clin. Gastroenterol.,* 2, 227, 1973.
29. **Thomas, W. E. G.,** The possible role of duodenogastric reflux in the pathogenesis of both gastric and duodenal ulcers, *Scand. J. Gastroenterol.,* 19(Suppl. 92), 151, 1984.

30. **Niemela, S., Karttunen, T., Heikkila, J., and Lehtola, J.,** Characteristics of reflux gastritis, *Scand. J. Gastroenterol.*, 22, 349, 1987.
31. **Lawson, H. H.,** Effect of duodenal contents on the gastric mucosa under experimental conditions, *Lancet*, 1, 469, 1964.
32. **Menguy, R. and Max, M. H.,** Influence of bile on the canine gastric-antral mucosa, *Am. J. Surg.*, 119, 177, 1970.
33. **Robbins, P. L., Broadie, T. A., Sosin, H., and Delaney, J. P.,** Reflux gastritis. The consequences of intestinal juice in the stomach, *Am. J. Surg.*, 131, 23, 1976.
34. **Thomas, W. E. G.,** Functional changes in acid secretion produced by duodenogastric reflux, *Gut*, 21, 413, 1980.
35. **Lawson, H. H.,** The role of the pyloric antrum and Hofmeister valve in the development of the chronic gastric mucosal reaction, *Br. J. Surg.*, 63, 592, 1976.
36. **Meyer, J. H.,** Reflections on reflux gastritis, *Gastroenterology*, 77, 1143, 1979.
37. **Kirk, R. M.,** Experimental gastric ulcers in the rat: the separate and combined effects of vagotomy and bile-duct implantation into the stomach, *Br. J. Surg.*, 57, 521,1970.
38. **Kaminishi, M., Sadatsuki, H., Johijima, Y., Oohara, T., and Kondo, Y.,** A new model for production of chronic gastric ulcer by duodenogastric reflux in rats, *Gastroenterology*, 92, 1913, 1987.
39. **Moody, F. G., McGreevy, J. M., Zalewsky, C. A., Cheung, L. Y., and Simons, M.,** The cytoprotective effect of mucosal blood flow in experimental erosive gastritis, *Acta Physiol. Scand.*, Spec. Suppl., 35, 1978.
40. **Gaskill, H. V., Sirinek, K. R., and Levine, B. A.,** Prostacyclin-mediated gastric cytoprotection is dependent on mucosal blood flow, *Surgery*, 92, 220, 1982.
41. **Ritchie, W. P.,** Acute gastric mucosal damage induced by bile salts, acid, and ischemia, *Gastroenterology*, 68, 699, 1975.
42. **Bowen, J. C. and LeDoux, J. C.,** Effect of taurocholate and ethanol on metabolism and oxygenation of gastric mucosa, *J. Surg. Res.*, 26, 326, 1979.
43. **DenBesten, L. and Hamza, K. N.,** Effect of bile salts on ionic permeability of canine gastric mucosa during experimental shock, *Gastroenterology*, 62, 417, 1972.
44. **Whittle, B. J. R.,** Mechanisms underlying gastric mucosal damage induced by indomethacin and bile-salts, and the actions of prostaglandins, *Br. J. Pharmacol.*, 60, 455, 1977.
45. **Bowen, J. C. and Fairchild, R. B.,** Oxygen in gastric mucosal protection, in *Mechanisms of Mucosal Protection in the Upper Gastrointestinal Tract*, Allen, A., Flemstrom, G., Garner, A., Silen, W., and Turnberg, L. A., Eds., Raven Press, New York, 1984, 263.
46. **Cheung, L. Y., Moody, F. G., and Reese, R. S.,** Effect of aspirin, bile salt, and ethanol on canine gastric mucosal blood flow, *Surgery*, 77, 786, 1975.
47. **Whittle, B. J. R.,** The potentiation of taurocholate-induced rat gastric erosions following parenteral administration of cyclooxygenase inhibitors, *Br. J. Pharmacol.*, 80, 545, 1983.
48. **Menguy, R. and Masters, Y. F.,** Gastric mucosal energy metabolism and "stress ulceration", *Ann. Surg.*, 180, 538, 1974.
49. **Menguy, R., Desbaillets, L., and Masters, Y. F.,** Mechanism of stress ulcer: influence of hypovolemic shock on energy metabolism in the gastric mucosa, *Gastroenterology*, 66, 46, 1974.
50. **Menguy, R. and Masters, Y. F.,** Mechanism of stress ulcer. II. Differences between the antrum, corpus, and fundus with respect to the effects of complete ischemia on gastric mucosal energy metabolism, *Gastroenterology*, 66, 509, 1974.
51. **Menguy, R. and Masters, Y .F.,** Mechanism of stress ulcer. Influence of sodium taurocholate on gastric mucosal energy metabolism during hemorrhagic shock and on mitochondrial respiration and ATPase in gastric mucosa, *Am. J. Dig. Dis.*, 21, 1001, 1976.
52. **Ohe, K., Hayashi, K., Shirakawa, T., Yamada, K., Kawasaki, T., and Miyoshi, A.,** Aspirin- and taurocholate-induced metabolic damage in mammalian gastric mucosa *in vitro*, *Am. J. Physiol.*, 239, G457, 1980.
53. **Oram-Smith, J. C. and Rosato, E. F.,** The effects of semistarvation and parenteral nutrition on the gastric mucosa of rats, *Surgery*, 79, 306, 1976.
54. **Konturek, S. J., Brzozowski, T., Radecki, T., and Dobrzanska, M.,** Generation of endogenous prostaglandins and thromboxanes in taurocholate-induced gastric mucosal lesions, *Scand. J. Gastroenterol.*, 19(Suppl. 92), 91, 1984.
55. **Walt, R. P., Kemp, R. T., Filipowicz, B., Davies, J. G., Bhaskar, N. K., and Hawkey, C. J.,** Gastric mucosal protection with selective inhibition of thromboxane synthesis, *Gut*, 28, 541, 1987.
56. **Tanaka, H.,** Gastric cytoprotection of aceglutamide aluminium in rats, *Arzneim.-Forsch./Drug Res.*, 36(II), 1485, 1986.
57. **Muller-Lissner, S. A., Bauerfeind, P., and Blum, A. L.,** Bile in the stomach, *Gastroenterol. Clin. Biol.*, 9, 72, 1985.

58. **Muller-Lissner, S. A., Fimmel, C. J., Sonnenberg, A., Will, N., Muller-Duysing, W., Heinzel, F., Muller, R., and Blum, A. L.,** Novel approach to quantify duodenogastric reflux in healthy volunteers and in patients with type I gastric ulcer, *Gut,* 24, 510, 1983.
59. **Moore, S. C., Malagelada, J. R., Shorter, R. G., and Zinsmeister, A. R.,** Interrelationships among gastric mucosal morphology, secretion, and motility in peptic ulcer disease, *Dig. Dis. Sci.,* 31, 673, 1986.
60. **Johnson, A. G.,** Peptic ulcer and the pylorus, *Lancet,* 1, 710, 1979.
61. **Johnson, A. G. and McDermott, S. J.,** Lysolecithin: a factor in the pathogenesis of gastric ulceration?, *Gut,* 15, 710, 1974.
62. **Saunders, L.,** Molecular aggregation in aqueous dispersions of phosphatidyl- and lysophosphatidylcholines, *Biochim. Biophys. Acta,* 125, 70, 1966.
63. **Sarosiek, J., Slomiany, B. L., Slomiany, A., and Gabryelewicz, A.,** Lysolecithin and glyceroglucolipids in gastric secretion of patients with gastric and duodenal ulcer, *Scand. J. Gastroenterol.,* 18, 935, 1983.
64. **Slomiany, B. L., Sarosiek, J., Liau, Y. H., Laszewicz, W., and Slomiany, A.,** Lysolecithin affects the viscosity, permeability, and peptic susceptibility of gastric mucin, *Scand. J. Gastroenterol.,* 21, 1073, 1986.
65. **Ivey, K. J., DenBesten, L., and Clifton, J. A.,** Effect of bile salts on ionic movement across the human gastric mucosa, *Gastroenterology,* 59, 683, 1970.
66. **Geall, M. G., Phillips, S. F., and Summerskill, D. M.,** Profile of gastric potential difference in man. Effects of aspirin, alcohol, bile, and endogenous acid, *Gastroenterology,* 58, 437, 1970.
67. **Fimmel, C. J., Muller-Lissner, S. A., and Blum, A. L.,** Acute, bile salt-induced mucosal damage in man: time course and effect of misoprostol, a PGE_1-analogue, in *Mechanisms of Mucosal Protection in the Upper Gastrointestinal Tract,* Allen, A., Flemstrom, G., Garner, A., Silen, W., and Turnberg, L. A., Eds., Raven Press, New York, 1984, 341.
68. **Fimmel, C. J., Muller-Lissner, S. A., and Blum, A. L.,** Bile salt-induced, acute gastric mucosal damage in man: time course and effect of misoprostol, a PGE_1-analogue, *Scand. J. Gastroenterol.,* 19(Suppl. 92), 184, 1984.
69. **Eastwood, G. L.,** Effect of pH on bile salt injury to mouse gastric mucosa. A light- and electron-microscopic study, *Gastroenterology,* 68, 1456, 1975.
70. **Tanaka, K. and Fromm, D.,** Effects of bile acid and salicylate on isolated surface and glandular cells of rabbit stomach, *Surgery,* 93, 660, 1983.
71. **Fromm, D. and Olender, E.,** Isolated gastric mucosal surface cells: viability, effects of salicylate and bile acid, and acid disposal, in *Mechanisms of Mucosal Protection in the Upper Gastrointestinal Tract,* Allen, A., Flemstrom, G., Garner, A., Silen, W., and Turnberg, L. A., Eds., Raven Press, New York, 1984, 91.
72. **Maksem, J., Jacobson, N., and Neiderhiser, D. H.,** Lysophosphatidylcholine-induced gastric injury and ulceration in the guinea pig, *Am. J. Pathol.,* 115, 288, 1984.
73. **Bekemeier, H., Bakathir, H. A., Giessler, A. J., Hirschelmann, R., and Huhn, P.,** Effect of lysolecithin on blood vessel reactivity and of some ethers and esters on glycerophosphocholine and phosphocholine, respectively, on aggregation of rat platelets, *Agents Actions,* 11, 563, 1981.
74. **Djahanguiri, B., Abtahi, F. S., and Hemmati, M.,** Prevention of aspirin-induced gastric ulceration by bile duct or pylorus ligation in the rat, *Gastroenterology,* 65, 630, 1973.
75. **Hemmati, M., Abtahi, F., Farrokhsiar, M., and Djahanguiri, B.,** Prevention of restraint and indomethacin-induced gastric ulceration by bile duct or pylorus ligation in rats, *Digestion,* 10, 108, 1974.
76. **Grijalva, C. V., Tordoff, M. G., Geiselman, P. J., and Novin, D.,** Gastric mucosal damage induced by lateral hypothalamic lesions in rats: the potential contribution of bile, *Brain Res Bull.,* 10, 441, 1983.
77. **Guth, P. H., Paulsen, G., Lynn, D., and Aures, D.,** Mechanism of prevention of aspirin-induced gastric lesions by bile duct ligation in the rat, *Gastroenterology,* 71, 750, 1976.
78. **Meeroff, J. C., Paulsen, G., and Guth, P. H.,** The role of bile reflux in the development of cold-restraint gastric lesions, *Am. J. Dig. Dis.,* 20, 365, 1975.
79. **Robert, A., Nezamis, J. E., Lancaster, C., Davis, J. P., Field, S. O., and Hanchar, A. J.,** Mild irritants prevent gastric necrosis through "adaptive cytoprotection" mediated by prostaglandins, *Am. J. Physiol.,* 245, G113, 1983.
80. **Neiderhiser, D. H. and Maksem, J.,** Gastric mucosal damage induced by combination of ethanol and lysophosphatidylcholine, *Dig. Dis. Sci.,* 32, 628, 1987.
81. **Kivilaakso, E., Ehnholm, C., Kalima, T. V., and Lempinen, M.,** Duodenogastric reflux of lysolecithin in the pathogenesis of experimental porcine stress ulceration, *Surgery,* 79, 65, 1976.
82. **Heatley, N. G.,** Mucosubstance as a barrier to diffusion, *Gastroenterology,* 37, 313, 1959.
83. **Allen, A. and Garner, A.,** Mucus and bicarbonate secretion in the stomach and their possible role in mucosal protection, *Gut,* 21, 249, 1980.
84. **Rees, W. D. W. and Turnberg, L. A.,** Mechanisms of gastric mucosal protection: a role for the "mucus-bicarbonate" barrier, *Clin. Sci.,* 62, 343, 1982.
85. **Kerss, S., Allen, A., and Garner, A.,** A simple method for measuring thickness of the mucus gel layer adherent to rat, frog and human gastric mucosa: influence of feeding, prostaglandin, N-acetylcysteine and other agents, *Clin. Sci.,* 63, 187, 1982.

86. **McQueen, S., Allen, A., and Garner, A.,** Measurement of gastric and duodenal mucus gel thickness, in *Mechanisms of Mucosal Protection in the Upper Gastrointestinal Tract,* Allen, A., Flemstrom, G., Garner, A., Silen, W., and Turnberg, L. A., Eds., Raven Press, New York, 1984, 215.
87. **Morris, G. P., Harding, R. K., and Wallace, J. L.,** A functional model for extracellular gastric mucus in the rat, *Virchows Arch. (Cell Pathol.),* 46, 239, 1984.
88. **Morris, G. P. and Harding, P. L.,** Mechanisms of mucosal recovery from acute gastric damage: roles of extracellular mucus and cell migration, in *Mechanisms of Mucosal Protection in the Upper Gastrointestinal Tract,* Allen, A., Flemstrom, G., Garner, A., Silen, W., and Turnberg, L. A., Eds., Raven Press, New York, 1984, 209.
89. **Morris, G. P.,** The myth of the mucus barrier, *Gastroenterol. Clin. Biol.,* 9, 106, 1985.
90. **Smeaton, L. A., Hirst, B. H., Allen, A., and Garner, A.,** Gastric and duodenal HCO^{3-} transport *in vivo*: influence of prostaglandins, *Am. J. Physiol.,* 245, 751, 1983.
91. **Isenberg, J. I., Selling, J. A., Hogan, D. L., and Koss, M. A.,** Impaired proximal duodenal mucosal bicarbonate secretion in patients with duodenal ulcer, *N. Engl. J. Med.,* 316, 374, 1987.
92. **Selling, J. A., Hogan, D. L., Aly, A., Koss, M. A., and Isenberg, J. I.,** Indomethacin inhibits duodenal mucosal bicarbonate secretion and endogenous prostaglandin E_2 output in human subjects, *Ann. Intern. Med.,* 106, 368, 1987.
93. **Ross, I. N., Bahari, H. M. M., and Turnberg, L. A.,** The pH gradient across mucus adherent to rat fundic mucosa in vivo and the effect of potential damaging agents, *Gastroenterology,* 81, 713, 1981.
94. **Rees, W. D. W., Garner, A., and Turnberg, L. A.,** Studies of acid and alkaline secretion by rabbit gastric fundus *in vitro*: effect of low concentrations of sodium taurocholate, *Gastroenterology,* 83, 435, 1982.
95. **Rees, W. D. W., Garner, A., Vivian, K. H. B., and Turnberg, L. A.,** Effect of sodium taurocholate on secretion by amphibian gastric mucosa *in vitro*, *Am. J. Physiol.,* 240, 245, 1981.
96. **Kivilaakso, E.,** Inhibition of gastric mucosal carbonic anhydrase by taurocholic acid and other ulcerogenic agents, *Am. J. Surg.,* 144, 554, 1982.
97. **Takeuchi, K., Nobuhara, Y., and Okabe, S.,** Bile salts are endogenous mild irritants to rat gastric mucosa, in *Mechanisms of Mucosal Protection in the Upper Gastrointestinal Tract,* Allen, A., Flemstrom, G., Garner, A., Silen, W., and Turnberg, L. A., Eds., Raven Press, New York, 1984, 335.
98. **Swierczek, J. S. and Konturek, S. J.,** Gastric alkaline response to mucosa-damaging agents: effect of 16,16-dimethyl prostaglandin E_2, *Am. J. Physiol.,* 241, 509, 1981.
99. **Allen, A., Hutton, D., McQueen, S., and Garner, A.,** Dimensions of gastroduodenal surface pH gradients exceed those of adherent mucus gel layers, *Gastroenterology,* 85, 463, 1983.
100. **Williams, S. E. and Turnberg, L. A.,** Demonstration of a pH gradient across mucus adherent to rabbit gastric mucosa: evidence for a "mucus-bicarbonate" barrier, *Gut,* 22, 94, 1981.
101. **Bahari, H. M. M., Ross, I. N., and Turnberg, L. A.,** Demonstration of a pH gradient across the mucus layer on the surface of human gastric mucosa *in vitro*, *Gut,* 23(6), 513, 1982.
102. **Kivilaakso, E. and Flemstrom, G.,** HCO_3^- secretion and surface pH gradient in rat duodenum exposed to luminal acid, *Scand. J. Gastroenterol.,* 19(Suppl. 92), 51, 1984.
103. **Turnberg, L. A.,** pH gradients in the gastro-duodenal mucous gel, *Gastroenterol. Clin. Biol.,* 9, 13, 1985.
104. **Thomson, A. B. R. and Dietschy, J. M.,** The role of the unstirred water layer in intestinal permeation, in *Pharmacology of Intestinal Permeation II,* Csaky, T. Z., Ed., Springer- Verlag, Berlin, 1984, 165.
105. **McGreevy, J. M. and Moody, F. G.,** A mechanism for prostaglandin cytoprotection, *Br. J. Surg.,* 67, 873, 1980.
106. **Williamson, T. E. and Morris, G. P.,** Sucralfate (SU) protection against acidified taurocholate requireseither an unstirred layer or PG synthesis, *Gastroenterology,* 94, A625, 1988.
107. **Morris, G. P. and Wallace, J. L.,** The roles of ethanol and of acid in the production of gastric mucosal erosions in rats, *Virchows Arch. (Cell Pathol.),* 38, 23, 1981.
108. **Wallace, J. L., Morris, G. P., Krausse, E. J., and Greaves, S. E.,** Reduction by cytoprotective agents of ethanol-induced damage to the rat gastric mucosa: a correlated morphological and physiological study, *Can. J. Physiol. Pharmacol.,* 60, 1686, 1982.
109. **Lacy, E. R. and Ito, S.,** Ethanol-induced insult to the superficial rat gastric epithelium: a study of damage and rapid repair, in *Mechanisms of Mucosal Protection in the Upper Gastrointestinal Tract,* Allen, A., Flemstrom, G., Garner, A., Silen, W., and Turnberg, L. A., Eds., Raven Press, New York, 1984, 49.
110. **Morris, G. P.,** Prostaglandins and cellular restitution in the gastric mucosa, *Am. J. Med.,* 81(Suppl. 2A), 23, 1986.
111. **Ito, S. and Lacy, E. R.,** Morphology of rat gastric mucosal damage, defense, and restitution in the presence of luminal ethanol, *Gastroenterology,* 88, 250, 1985.
112. **Silen, W. and Ito, S.,** Mechanisms for rapid re-epithelialization of the gastric mucosal surface, *Ann. Rev. Physiol.,* 47, 217, 1985.
113. **Svanes, K., Critchlow, J., Takeuchi, K., Magee, D., Ito, S., and Silen, W.,** Factors influencing reconstitution of frog gastric mucosa: role of prostaglandins, in *Mechanisms of Mucosal Protection in the Upper Gastrointestinal Tract,* Allen, A., Flemstrom, G., Garner, A., Silen, W. and Turnberg, L. A., Eds., Raven Press, New York, 1984, 33.

114. **Gannon, B., Browning, J., and O'Brien, P.,** The microvascular architecture of the glandular mucosa of rat stomach, *J. Anat.*, 135, 667, 1982.
115. **Denis, J. G. and Morris, G. P.,** The microvascular architecture of the rat gastric mucosa, *Proc. Micros. Soc. Can.*, 10, 42, 1982.
116. **Gannon, B., Browning, J., O'Brien, P., and Rogers, P.,** Mucosal microvascular architecture of the fundus and body of human stomach, *Gastroenterology*, 86, 866, 1984.
117. **Guth, P. H.,** Microvascular structure and function in the stomach wall, *Fed. Proc.*, 43, 12, 1984.
118. **Sawyer, W. R., Ritter, E., and Faloon, W. W.,** The morphological effects of chenodeoxycholic acid on human gastric mucosa, *Am. J. Gastroenterol.*, 79, 348, 1984.
119. **Carter, K. J., Farley, P. C., and Ritchie, W. P.,** Effect of topical bile acids on gastric surface epithelial cells, *Surgery*, 96, 196, 1984.
120. **Morris, G. P., Wallace, J. L., Harding, P. L., Krausse, E. J., and Lolle, S. J.,** Correlations between changes in indicators of gastric mucosal barrier integrity at time of exposure to "barrier breakers" and extent of hemorrhagic erosions one hour later, *Dig. Dis. Sci.*, 29, 6, 1984.
121. **Rutten, M. J. and Ito, S.,** Luminal acid effects on reconstitution of damaged guinea pig gastric mucosa *in vitro*, in *Mechanisms of Mucosal Protection in the Upper Gastrointestinal Tract*, Allen, A., Flemstrom, G., Garner, A., Silen, W., and Turnberg, L.A., Eds., Raven Press, New York, 1984, 41.
122. **Green, F. W., Kaplan, M. M., Curtis, L. E., and Levine, P. H.,** Effect of acid and pepsin on blood coagulation and platelet aggregation. A possible contributor to prolonged gastroduodenal mucosal hemorrhage, *Gastroenterology*, 74, 38, 1978.
123. **Black, B. A., Morris, G. P., and Wallace, J. L.,** Effects of acid on the basal lamina of the rat stomach and duodenum, *Virchows Arch.*, 50, 109, 1985.
124. **Martin, G. P., Marriott, C., and Kellaway, I. W.,** Direct effect of bile salts and phospholipids on the physical properties of mucus, *Gut*, 19, 103, 1978.
125. **Turner, N. C., Martin, G. P., and Marriott, C.,** The influence of native porcine gastric mucus gel on hydrogen ion diffusion: the effect of potentially ulcerogenic agents, *J. Pharm. Pharmacol.*, 37, 776, 1985.
126. **Bell, A. E., Sellers, L. A., Allen, A., Cunliffe, W. J., Morris, E. R., and Ross-Murphy, S. B.,** Properties of gastric and duodenal mucus: effect of proteolysis, disulfide reduction, bile, acid, ethanol, and hypertonicity on mucus gel structure, *Gastroenterology*, 88, 269, 1985.
127. **Sarosiek, J., Slomiany, A., Takagi, A., and Slomiany, B. L.,** Hydrogen ion diffusion in dog gastric mucus glycoprotein: effect of associated lipids and covalently bound fatty acids, *Biochem. Biophys. Res. Commun.*, 118, 523, 1984.
128. **McIntosh, J. H., Byth, K., and Piper, D. W.,** Environmental factors in aetiology of chronic gastric ulcer: a case control study of exposure variables before the first symptoms, *Gut*, 26, 789, 1985.
129. **Doll, R., Jones, J. A., and Pygott, F.,** Effect of smoking on the production and maintenance of gastric and duodenal ulcers, *Lancet*, 1, 657, 1958.
130. **Ostensen, H., Gumundsen, T. E., Ostensen, M., Burhol, P. G., and Bonnevie, O.,** Smoking, alcohol, coffee, and familial factors: any associations with peptic ulcer disease? A clinically and radiologically prospective study, *Scand. J. Gastroenterol.*, 20, 1227, 1985.
131. **Muller-Lissner, S. A. and Fraass, C.,** Bile reflux is increased in cigarette smokers, *Gastroenterology*, 90, 1205, 1986.
132. **Quimby, G. F., Bonnice, C. A., Burstein, S. H., and Eastwood, G. L.,** Active smoking depresses prostaglandin synthesis in human gastric mucosa, *Ann. Intern. Med.*, 104, 616, 1986.
133. **McCready, D. R., Clark, L., and Cohen, M. M.,** Cigarette smoking reduces human gastric luminal prostaglandin E_2, *Gut*, 26, 1192, 1985.
134. **Marshall, B. J. and Warren, J. R.,** Unidentified curved bacilli in the stomach of patients with gastritis and peptic ulceration, *Lancet*, 1, 1311, 1984.
135. **Rollason, T. P., Stone, J., and Rhodes, J. M.,** Spiral organisms in endoscopic biopsies of the human stomach, *J. Clin. Pathol.*, 37, 23, 1984.
136. **Andersen, L. P., Holck, S., Povlsen, C. O., Elsborg, L., and Justesen, T.,** *Campylobacter pyloridis* in peptic ulcer disease. I. Gastric and duodenal infection caused by *C. pyloridis*: histopathologic and microbiologic findings, *Scand. J. Gastroenterol.*, 22, 219, 1987.
137. **Morris, A. and Nicholson, G.,** Ingestion of Campylobacter pyloridis causes gastritis and raised fasting gastric pH, *Am. J. Gastroenterol.*, 82, 192, 1987.
138. **Price, A. B., Levi, J., Dolby, J. M., Dunscombe, P. L., Smith, A., Clark, J., and Stephenson, M. L.,** *Campylobacter pyloridis* in peptic ulcer disease: microbiology, pathology, and scanning electron microscopy, *Gut*, 26, 1183, 1985.
139. **Lamouliatte, H., Megraud, F., De Mascarel, A., Roux, D., and Quinton, A.,** *Campylobacter pyloridis* and epigastric pain: endoscopic, histological, and bacteriological correlations, *Gastroenterol. Clin. Biol.*, 11, 212, 1987.

140. **Karttunen, T., Niemela, S., Lehtola, J., Heikkila, J., Maentausta, O., and Rasanen, O.,** Campylobacter-like organisms and gastritis: histopathology, bile reflux, and gastric fluid composition, *Scand. J. Gastroenterol.,* 22, 478, 1987.
141. **Meshkinpour, H., Elashoff, J., Stewart, H., and Sturdevant, A.L.,** Effect of cholestyramine on the symptoms of reflux gastritis. A randomized, double blind, crossover study, *Gastroenterology,* 73, 441, 1977.
142. **Wegner, J. and Heymsfield, N.,** Absorption of bile by aluminum hydroxide, *J. Clin. Pharmacol.,* 14, 163, 1974.
143. **Eastwood, G. L.,** Failure of cholestyramine to prevent bile salt injury to mouse gastric mucosa, *Gastroenterology,* 68, 1466, 1975.
144. **Mann, N .S. and Sachdev, A. J.,** Aspirin- and bile-induced acute erosive gastritis. Its prevention by metiamide therapy, *Arch. Pathol. Lab. Med.,* 101, 206, 1977.
145. **Bauer, R. F., Bianchi, R. G., Casler, J., and Goldstein, B.,** Comparative mucosal protective properties of misoprostol, cimetidine, and sucralfate, *Dig. Dis. Sci.,* 31, 81S, 1986.
146. **Utley, R. J., Salim, A. S. M., and Carter, D. C.,** Effect of cimetidine and omeprazole on aspirin- and taurocholate-induced gastric mucosal damage in the rat, *Gut,* 26, 770, 1985.
147. **Ligumsky, M., Karmeli, F., and Rachmilewitz, D.,** Sucralfate protection against gastrointestinal damage: possible role of prostanoids, *Israel J. Med. Sci.,* 22, 801, 1986.
148. **Muller, P., Simon, B., and Dammann, H. G.,** Antisecretory properties of prostaglandin analogs in man, *Dig. Dis. Sci.,* 27, 862, 1982. .
149. **Muller-Lissner, S. A., Fimmel, C. J., and Blum, A. L.,** Failure of 16,16-dimethyl-PGE_2 to protect the human stomach from taurocholate damage, *Hepatogastroenterology,* 30, 107, 1983.
150. **Rees, W. D. W., Rhodes, J., Wheeler, M. H., Meek, E. M., Williams, B., and Newcombe, R. G.,** Effect of histamine receptor antagonists on bile damage to the gastric mucosa of canine Heidenhain pouches, *Gut,* 18, 821, 1977.
151. **Davenport, H. W.,** Gastric mucosal injury by fatty and acetylsalicylic acids, *Gastroenterology,* 46, 245, 1964.
152. **Szelenyi, I., Postius, S., and Engler, H.,** Evidence for a functional cytoprotective effect produced by antacids in the rat stomach, *Eur. J. Pharmacol.,* 88, 403, 1983.
153. **Szelenyi, I.,** Functional cytoprotection by certain antacids, *Acta Physiol. Hung.,* 64, 259, 1984.
154. **Chaudhury, T. K. and Robert, A.,** Prevention by mild irritants of gastric necrosis produced in rats by sodium taurocholate, *Dig. Dis. Sci.,* 25, 830, 1980.
155. **Mazure, P. A.,** Comparative efficacy of misoprostol and cimetidine in the treatment of acute duodenal ulcer. Results of major studies, *Am. J. Med.,* 83 (Suppl. 1A), 22, 1987.
156. **Lauritsen, K. and Rask-Madsen, J.,** Prostaglandins and clinical experience in peptic ulcer disease, *Scand. J. Gastroenterol.,* 21(Suppl. 125), 174, 1986.
157. **Sontag, S. J.,** Prostaglandins and acid peptic disease, *Am. J. Gastroenterol.,* 81, 1021, 1986.
158. **Sontag, S. J.,** Prostaglandins in peptic ulcer disease. An overview of current status and future directions, *Drugs,* 32, 445, 1986.
159. **Hawkey, C. J. and Walt, R. P.,** Prostaglandins for peptic ulcer: a promise unfulfilled, *Lancet,* 2, 1084, 1986.
160. **Guldutana, S., Zimmer, G., Kurtz, W., and Leuschner, U.,** Prostaglandin E_2 directly protects isolated rat gastric surface membranes against bile salts, *Biochim. Biophys. Acta,* 902, 217, 1987.
161. **Terano, A., Ota, S., Mach, T., Hiraishi, H., Stachura, J., Tarnawski, A., and Ivey, K. J.,** Prostaglandin protects against taurocholate-induced damage to rat gastric mucosal cell culture, *Gastroenterology,* 92, 669, 1987.

Chapter 2

ROLE OF HISTAMINE AS A MEDIATOR OF GASTROINTESTINAL DAMAGE

John L. Wallace and Paul L. Beck

TABLE OF CONTENTS

I. INTRODUCTION

The name histamine is a derivation of the Greek word *histos,* meaning tissue, as a reflection of the finding that histamine is released when virtually any tissue of the body is damaged. The true chemical name for histamine is β-imidazolylethylamine. Histamine was initially synthesized as a "chemical curiosity",[1] before its biological significance was realized. Like acetylcholine, it was first found in an extract from ergot. When subsequently isolated, it was found to be a contaminant from bacterial activity. Dale and Laidlaw[2] performed the first detailed pharmacological studies on histamine. It was these studies, in part, that led to the award of the Nobel Prize in Medicine or Physiology to Sir Henry Dale in 1936. Dale was also involved in the first isolation of histamine from undamaged tissues, thus demonstrating that histamine was stored under normal circumstances [3]

Histamine is synthesized from histidine via the action of L-histidine decarboxylase. It can be catabolized by two routes: ring methylation or oxidative deamination. Histamine is ubiquitous throughout the body, mostly contained within tissue mast cells, circulating basophils, and enterochromaffin-like cells (ECL) (see below).

Among the numerous actions of histamine are its ability to contract gastrointestinal and bronchial smooth muscle, increase capillary permeability, cause systemic hypotension through capillary and venular vasodilation, and increase gastric acid secretion through direct effects on the parietal cell (discussed in detail below).

II. CELLULAR SOURCES OF HISTAMINE

Histamine is found in various cell types, with substantial variation between species. The cellular stores of histamine can be subdivided into the mobile cellular stores and the nonmobile cellular stores. The mobile cellular stores include basophils (man), platelets (rabbit), and eosinophils (dog). Nonmobile histamine stores include mast cells, ECL, some neurons of the central nervous system, and some cells involved in rapid growth or regeneration. In the following sections, the cellular stores of histamine that are more fully discussed are the mast cells, basophils, and ECL cells, since these are the histamine-containing cells of most noted importance in mediation of gastrointestinal damage.

A. MAST CELLS

Mast cells were discovered by Paul Ehrlich in 1877. Erhlich,[4] a medical student at the time, noted that mast cell granules stained metachromatically with aniline dyes and that the granules were released when the cell was exposed to aqueous solutions (Figure 1). Mast cells are found in greatest abundance in tissues exposed to the external environment, such as the gastrointestinal and respiratory tracts, the eye, and the skin. In most higher organisms, mast cells are closely associated with the vascular system.

In addition to histamine, mast cells can also release an array of other substances, including heparin, serotonin, superoxide, platelet-activating factor, leukotrienes, and prostaglandins. Degranulation can be stimulated by numerous factors, although the IgE-dependent mechanism is the most thoroughly studied. Other substances capable of stimulating degranulation of mast cells include components of the complement system, IgG_1, platelet-activating factor, adenosinetriphosphate (ATP), kinins, glucocorticoids, and VIP. Exogenous compounds such as the calcium ionophore, A23187, compound 48/80, codeine, morphine, and aspirin can also induce mast cell degranulation under appropriate circumstances.

Mast cells are found in high numbers in the gastrointestinal mucosa of most species. In the stomach of dog, for instance, there is one mast cell for every two to three parietal cells.[5]

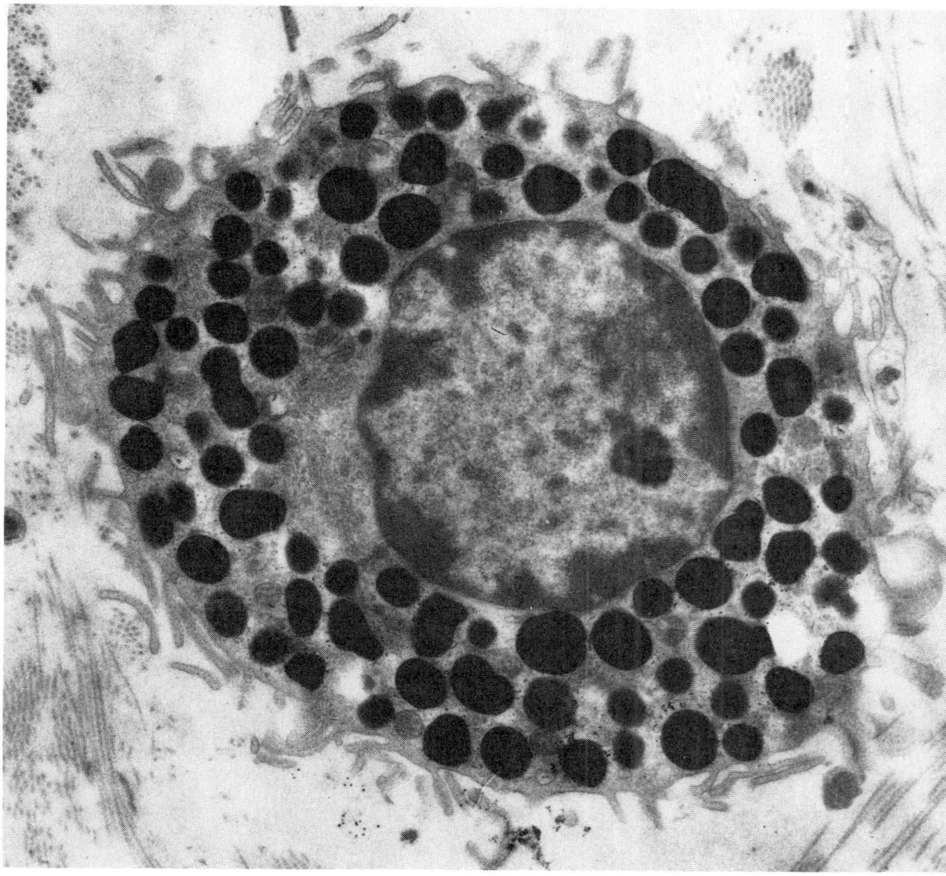

FIGURE 1. Electron micrograph of a mast cell in the rat gastric submucosa. Electron dense granules contain histamine, heparin, and other mediators.

B. BASOPHILS

Basophils represent less than 0.5% of the circulating leukocytes in man. These cells arise from the bone marrow and despite structural and functional similarities, there is no evidence that basophils and mast cells are derived from each other. Basophils do not normally leave the blood; however, they can enter tissues as part of antigen specific immunopathological processes. Basophils contain far less histamine per cell than do mast cells. They are also slower to degranulate following stimulation than are mast cells.[6]

C. ENTEROCHROMAFFIN-LIKE CELLS

In most species, there is a good correlation between the number of mast cells in a tissue, and the tissue content of histamine; however, this correlation was not found in the rat stomach.[7] Indeed, almost half of the total body content of histamine in the rat can be found in the stomach wall[8] despite a relative paucity of mast cells when compared to man, pig, or dog. Higher concentrations of histamine are found in the mucosal layer than in the submucosa or the muscularis. Rees et al.[9] found that mucosal histamine in the rat could not be depleted by the mast

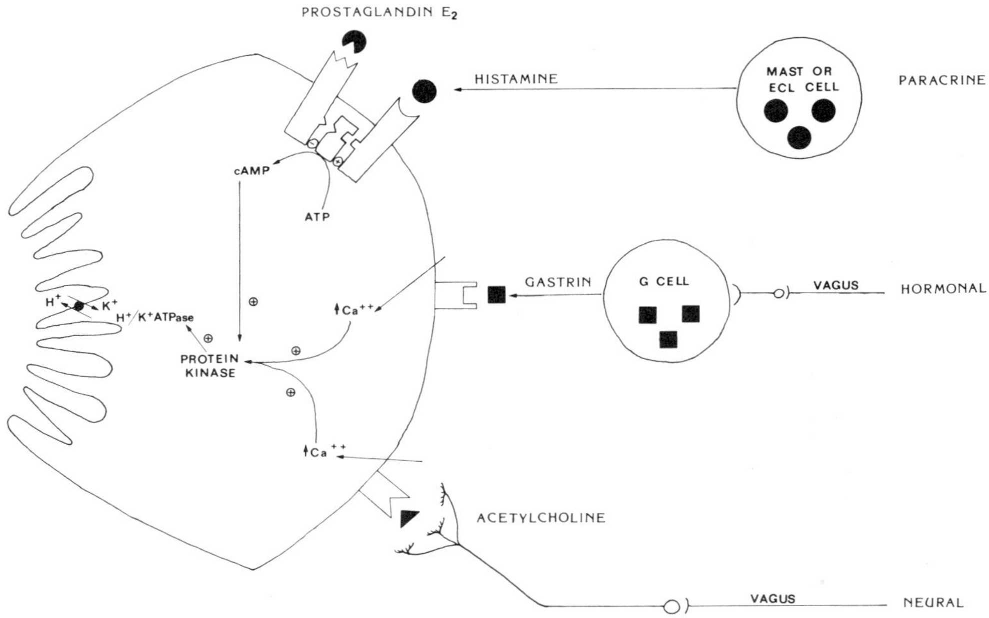

FIGURE 2. Interaction of histamine with other mediators in the regulation of parietal cell activation. (Adapted from Reference 43.)

cell degranulating agent, compound 48/80, or by antigen-antibody reactions. Soll et al.[5] demonstrated that the primary cellular store of histamine in the rat stomach was the ECL. These cells are biochemically and morphologically distinct from mast cells, and are so-named because they resemble true enterochromaffin (argentaffin) reacting cells. ECL cells are found in other species than the rat, but do not appear to be the major gastrointestinal cellular store of histmine in those species.[5]

III. ROLE OF HISTAMINE IN ANIMAL MODELS OF GASTRODUODENAL DAMAGE

Animals models of gastric and duodenal ulcer have been exploited extensively in order to examine the physiological and pathophysiological roles of histamine. Davenport[10] outlined a model for the events which take place in the early stages of gastric ulceration, and particularly emphasized the role of histamine in this process (Figure 2). The first step in his model was the breaking of the gastric mucosal "barrier" by agents such as ethanol or acetylsalicylic acid. With the barrier disrupted, luminal acid can permeate into the mucosa leading to: (1) stimulation of the intramural plexuses of the stomach and, in turn, stimulation of pepsinogen secretion, (2) stimulation of motility, (3) release of histamine from mucosal stores and stimulation of histidine decarboxylase, and (4) rupturing of mucosal capillaries, resulting in hemorrhage. Histamine levels in the interstitial fluid would reach sufficient concentrations to stimulate acid secretion, cause vasodilation, and increase capillary permeability, thereby resulting in increased loss of plasma proteins.

There are substantial data in support of Davenport's model. For instance, Johnson and Overholt[11] found that irrigating a canine gastric pouch with 100 m*M* acetic acid (a barrier breaker) resulted, within 5 min, in a marked increase in the levels of histamine in the gastric venous blood. Davenport[12] himself found that irrigation of a canine gastric pouch with 450 m*M*

HCl resulted in a large rise in venous histamine levels. In Davenport's[10] model, the stimulus which caused histamine release was back-diffusing acid; however, Tepperman and Soper[13] have shown convincingly that with ethanol-induced gastric damage, acid is not the stimulus for histamine release. They induced damage to a dog gastric mucosa by the topical application of acidified 15% ethanol and observed significant histamine release; however, when they buffered the ethanol solution to pH 7.5 and then challenged the mucosa, they still observed histamine release and damage. Interestingly, they observed reduced histamine release when the mucosa was exposed to the "cytoprotective" compound, 16,16-dimethyl prostaglandin E_2, prior to the ethanol challenge.

The concentrations of histamine released in the models described above were certainly sufficient to stimulate acid secretion and to increase vascular permeability. What is not clear from these studies is whether the histamine was released purely as a consequence of damage, or if it actually played a role in contributing to the production of damage. There is little doubt that histamine can cause gastric and duodenal damage when administered to laboratory animals. Robert et al.[14] induced duodenal ulcers in the rat by administration of a combination of histamine and carbachol at doses sufficient to stimulate acid secretion. Guinea pigs are also susceptible to histamine-induced gastric and duodenal ulceration.[15] Takeuchi et al.[16] reported that a single, intraperitoneal injection of histamine caused gastric erosions in 100% of the rats tested. This ulcerogenic action of histamine may have been only partially attributable to stimulation of gastric acid secretion, since they only observed partial protection against ulceration when they pretreated rats with high doses of the histamine H_2 antagonist, cimetidine. Hansen et al.[17] reported that intravenous infusion of histamine caused a significant augmentation of antral ulceration induced by acetylsalicylic acid in the cat.

There is substantial information on the role of histamine in stress ulcer. Release of histamine and the benefit of pharmacological manipulation of the synthesis or action of histamine has been demonstrated by several groups using the restraint model for stress ulcer in rats.[18-21] Tran and Gregg[22] performed some interesting experiments with parabiotic rats which demonstrated that an ulcerogenic factor was released into the blood during restraint stress. They found that subjecting one of a pair of parabiotic rats to restraint resulted in the development of gastric erosions in both rats. When similar experiments were performed on rats with a sham parabiotic connection, only the restrained rat developed ulcers. Gurll and Damianos[7] suggested that the blood-borne mediator causing the ulceration in the nonrestrained parabiotic rat was most likely to be histamine. Tran and Gregg[22] postulated that the likely mediator was either histamine or serotonin.

Histamine release has also been reported in hemorrhagic and septic shock,[23] both of which are associated with gastrointestinal ulceration.

A role for histamine in animal models of gastrointestinal ulceration is further supported by numerous observations of reduction of damage by histamine receptor antagonists. For instance, Rees et al.[24] found that administration of a combination of H_1 and H_2 receptor antagonists caused a significant reduction of bile salt-induced gastric damage. Several groups have reported that blockade of the H_2 receptor alone is not sufficient to reduce the gastric damage induced by bile salts.[25-27] While H_2 antagonists may be ineffective against bile salt-induced damage, they can certainly reduce damage to the stomach induced by other means. Bommelaer and Guth[28] reported that the H_2 antagonist, cimetidine, protected the rat gastric mucosa from damage induced by acetylsalicylic acid. Such protection was not augmented by concomitant administration of an H_1 receptor antagonist (mepyramine), which by itself conferred no protection. The protection induced by cimetidine in this model was still apparent when the acetylsalicylic acid was administered orally in combination with 150 m*M* HCl.[29] Cimetidine has also been shown to reduce the gastric mucosal hemorrhage which follows gastric ischemia in the rat,[30] and again, protection was still observed despite the presence in the gastric lumen of a high concentration of exogenous acid. Safaie-Shirazi et al.[31] found that another H_2 antagonist, metiamide, prevented stress-induced gastric erosions in rats even in the presence of high concentrations of luminal acid. Furthermore, Okabe et al.[32] reported that cimetidine significantly reduced the severity of aspirin-induced gastric erosions in rats or histamine-induced gastric erosions in guinea pigs without significantly reducing gastric acid secretion. These protective actions of H_2 antagonists which are clearly unrelated to inhibition of gastric acid secretion may be due to effects of these agents on the gastric vasculature (see below).

IV. ACTIONS OF HISTAMINE

A. GASTRIC ACID SECRETION

Schwarz's[33] dictum "no acid — no ulcer" was coined in 1910 and has served as the major rationale behind various forms of therapy of peptic ulcer ever since. Treatment of peptic ulcer patients with antacids, anticholinergic drugs, and by severing the vagus nerves are all aimed at reducing the amount of acid present in the lumen of the stomach. Acid contributes to the development of mucosal necrosis, interferes with hemostatic mechanisms, and prolongs repair of existing damage (these actions are discussed in detail by Morris et al. in Chapter 1). Stimulation of the intramural plexuses by acid probably contributes significantly to the pain associated with peptic ulcer,[10] thus accounting for the rapid relief of pain observed after antacid administration. The first indication that histamine plays a role in mediating gastric acid secretion was the observation of Popielski[34] that injection of histamine resulted in stimulation of acid secretion. For decades, attempts to inhibit gastric acid secretion using the classical histamine antagonists available at the time failed. It was not until 1972 that Black et al.[35] demonstrated that a second class of receptors for histamine existed in the stomach (H_2 receptors), distinct from those mediating such processes as bronchial tone, cardiac contractility, and vascular smooth muscle tone (H_1 receptors). The subsequent development of specific H_2 receptor antagonists (Figure 3) has undoubtedly been the greatest clinical advance in the treatment of peptic ulcer, and is discussed more fully later in this chapter.

While histamine is now recognized as an important mediator of gastric acid secretion, it is by no means the only such mediator. Acetylcholine and gastrin also exert potent stimulatory effects, as do caffeine, nicotine, insulin, and food. Conversely, somatostatin and prostaglandin E_2 are potent endogenous inhibitors of gastric acid secretion. McIntosh[36] suggested that while several substances stimulate gastric acid secretion when administered to human volunteers or laboratory animals, they may not act directly at the parietal cell to stimulate acid secretion. Rather, he proposed, these substances might stimulate the local release of histamine which then acts as the common final mediator of acid secretion. This hypothesis was supported by the observation by several groups that histidine decarboxylase activity in the gastric mucosa was increased significantly by feeding, vagal stimulation, or administration of gastrin.[37-40] The hypothesis was further supported by the observation that two H_2 receptor antagonists, metiamide and cimetidine, substantially reduced gastric acid secretion stimulated by histamine, gastrin, caffeine, insulin, food, or sham feeding;[41] however, several *in vitro* studies using isolated parietal cells have now demonstrated clearly that there are distinct receptors for acetylcholine, gastrin, and histamine. The actions of acetylcholine can be inhibited by anticholinergic agents, while H_2 antagonists will block parietal cell activation by histamine. Neither of these classes of receptor antagonists inhibited gastrin-induced parietal cell activation. Specific receptors or binding sites for gastrin were demonstrated by binding of a radiolabeled gastrin analog on the parietal cell.[42] Because there are potentiating interactions between histamine, gastrin, and cholinergic agents *in vivo*, specific receptor antagonists such as cimetidine can cause an apparent antagonism of the other receptors. This may be related to the apparent ability of some mediators to cause histamine release from mast and/or enterochromaffin cells, and also because these mediators may act synergistically with histamine to stimulate acid secretion.[43] To further

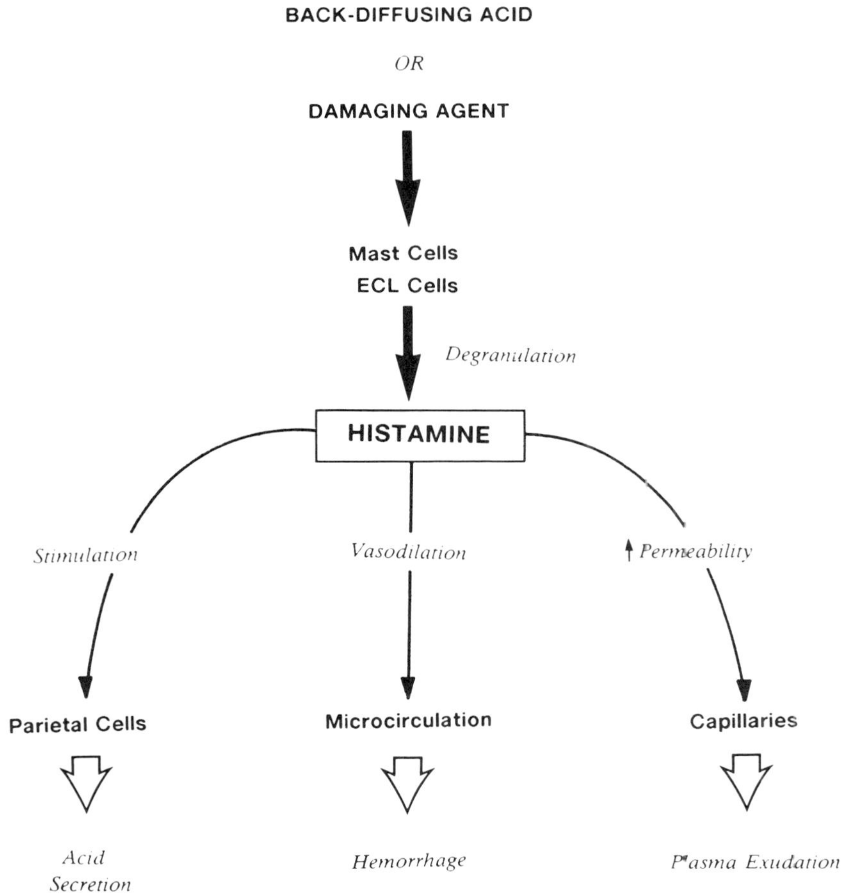

FIGURE 3. Schematic diagram illustrating the interactions involving histamine in the pathogenesis of ulceration of the gastric or duodenal mucosa. Histamine is stored in mast cells and, in some species, in ECL. Once released, histamine acts on parietal cells, causing an increase in acid secretion, and acts on the mucosal vasculature, causing vasodilation and increased capillary permeability. Acid may cause rupturing of microvessels, resulting in hemorrhage.

complicate the matter, substances which have inhibitory actions on parietal cells, such as somatostatin, can be released by gastrin and perhaps other mediators.[43] The mechanisms by which histamine, gastrin, and acetylcholine stimulate the parietal cell are distinct (Figure 4). Histamine, but not gastrin or acetylcholine, stimulates the parietal cell via a cyclic AMP (cAMP)-mediated process. Thus, acid secretion can be stimulated by phosphodiesterase inhibitors[44] and by cAMP analogs.[45] Prostaglandins E_2 and I_2 can inhibit histamine-induced gastric acid secretion, probably by interfering with adenylate cyclase.[46] Gastrin and acetylcholine appear to act on the parietal cell via a calcium-mediated mechanism.[43] These differing intracellular mechanisms may offer an explanation for the potentiating interactions of these mediators of acid secretion.

Interestingly, histamine H_1 receptors may also be involved in the regulation of gastric acid secretion in some species. In the cat and rabbit, there is some evidence that activation of H_1 receptors has an inhibitory effect on acid secretion, since histamine-stimulated acid secretion is higher in the presence of an H_1 antagonist or following stimulation with a specific H_2 agonist, such as 4-methyl-histamine.[45] There is also some evidence that H_1 antagonists can block acid secretion in the dog stomach;[47] however, this has not been found to be the case in man, mouse,

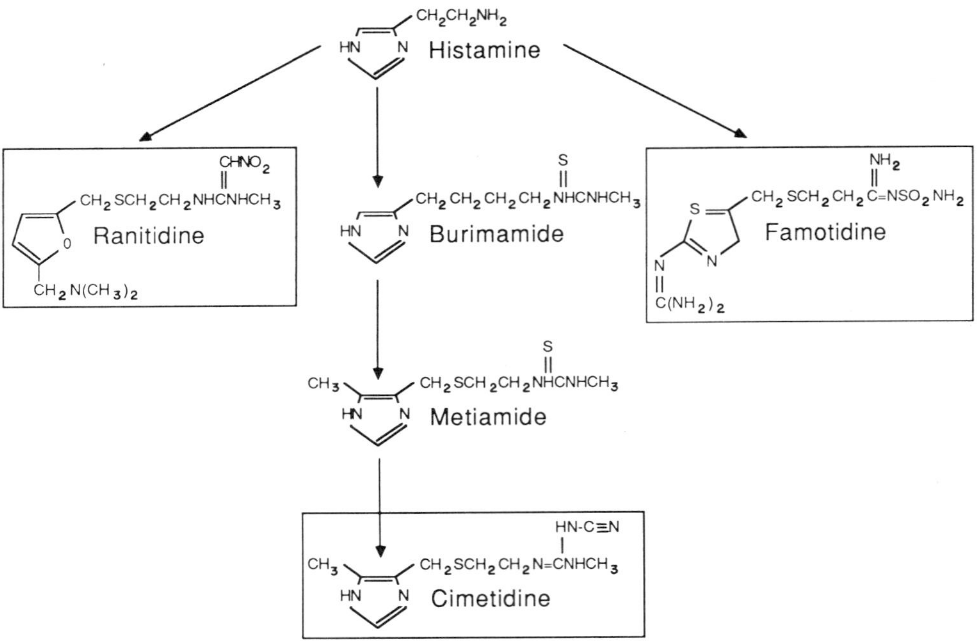

FIGURE 4. Schematic diagram illustrating the chemical structures of histamine and several histamine H_2 receptor antagonists. The structures outlined by boxes are antagonists presently marketed for the treatment of peptic ulcer and other acid-related diseases of the upper gastrointestinal tract.

rat, or guinea pig. Soll[48] reported that H_1 receptor antagonists could inhibit histamine-stimulated acid secretion from isolated parietal cells, but only when used at extremely high concentrations.

B. MUCOSAL BLOOD FLOW

The vascular activity of histamine was first described by Dale and Laidlaw,[2] who found that histamine increased cardiac contractility and in most species, produced systemic hypotension. Histamine was found to constrict the large blood vessels in some species, but in other species dilatation occurred. In the majority of the species examined the most notable vasculature effect of histamine was the production of generalized dilatation of the peripheral capillary beds, which is thought to be responsible for the drop in systemic blood pressure. Dale and Laidlaw[49] also discovered that histamine increased the vascular permeability of small blood vessels. This resulted in edema, decreased body temperature, and increased hematocrit and blood viscosity. In both their 1910 and 1919 publications, Dale and Laidlaw stressed that the vascular actions, as well as most of the other physiological activities, of histamine are both species- and organ-dependent.

In the following sections, the vascular actions of histamine are reviewed. The specific effects of histamine on the gastric and mesenteric vasculature and how these effects may influence gastrointestinal damage are also discussed.

1. General Aspects

In 1929, Dale[50] reviewed the species-dependent variability of the actions of histamine on the peripheral vasculature. He reported that histamine generally induced vasoconstriction in rodents and slight arteriolar constriction in cats. In dog, monkey, and man, however, histamine induced marked arteriolar dilatation.

In the early 1970s, aided by the advent of H_2 receptor antagonists, it became apparent that histamine can play a dual role in the mediation of vasculature contractility. This dual role has also been found to be species- and organ-specific. It has been reported in rabbit, rat, cat, calf, man, chicken, guinea pig, and dog.[4,51]

Black et al.[35,52] found that in cat and dog, the histamine-induced drop in systemic blood pressure was only partially blocked by H_1 antagonists and was unaffected by H_2 antagonists; however, a combination of both H_1 and H_2 antagonists completely inhibited the histamine-induced drop in systemic blood pressure.

Since these studies, many investigators have demonstrated the distribution and actions of H_1 and H_2 receptors in various species and in various organs. Using a radiolabeled microsphere technique, Johnston and Owen[53] found that histamine and histamine antagonists did not affect all of the vascular beds of the cat in the same manner. They reported that neither mepyramine (an H_1 antagonist) nor metiamide (an H_2 antagonist) could prevent the histamine-stimulated decrease in systemic blood pressure, but when administered together, the fall in blood pressure was completely abolished. In the cat stomach, mepyramine did not affect histamine-induced vasodilation, but metiamide effectively prevented it. Furthermore, mepyramine only slightly reduced histamine-induced coronary vasodilation, while metiamide substantially reduced it. The simultaneous administration of both mepyramine and metiamide abolished the coronary vasodilation. Johnston and Owen[54] also reported that similar findings could be demonstrated when the selective H_1 receptor agonist 2-(2-aminoethyl) pyridine and the selective H_2 receptor agonist 4-methylhistamine were used.

Contrary to the findings of Johnston and Owen,[53,54] Eyre and Wells[55] found that in the blood vessels of the calf H_1 receptors mediated vasodilation whereas H_2 receptors mediated vasoconstriction. In contrast to these findings, numerous investigators have found that in rabbit, H_1 receptor stimulation produces vasoconstriction,while H_2 receptor stimulation induces vasodilation of various blood vessels (see Reference 51 for a more detailed review of this subject).

In summary, H_1 and H_2 histamine receptors are found in several vascular beds of numerous species. The population of H_1 and H_2 receptors varies from species to species and from organ to organ. Such variation sheds light on why Dale and Laidlaw[2,49,50] found that the action of histamine was both organ- and species-dependent. For a summary of H_1 and H_2 vasculature effects in various organs and in various species, see Table 1.

2. Measurement Techniques

Since numerous techniques have been utilized for the measurement of gastric blood flow, some of which may be influenced by the secretory state of the mucosa, a brief review of the most commonly used methods is presented below. One of the first procedures used to determine gastric blood flow was the aminopyrine clearance technique described by Jacobson et al.[56] and Cowely et al.[57] In short, large doses of aminopyrine are given intravenously, the serum and gastric juice aminopyrine levels analyzed spectrophotometrically, and the rate of blood flow calculated on the principle that the amount of aminopyrine leaking into the gastric lumen will be proportional to the rate of mucosal blood flow. The validity of this technique has been questioned since aminopyrine was found to stimulate acid secretion and thereby could increase mucosal blood flow.[58] Due to the large doses of aminopyrine that were required for this procedure and the finding that aminopyrine causes bone marrow toxicity, this technique could not be used in human studies.

By radiolabeling aminopyrine with ^{14}C, only trace amounts are required for the quantification of gastric blood flow. Hence, this technique can be used effectively and safely in human studies. ^{14}C-aniline and ^{99}technetium (^{99}Tc) have also been used in clearance studies. ^{14}C-aniline clearance has been found to be comparable to ^{14}C-aminopyrine clearance in several studies using various species, but it should be noted that aniline has a greater tendency to bind to plasma proteins than aminopyrine (for a comprehensive review of this subject, see Reference 58). A clear advantage of the use of aniline over aminopyrine is that aniline does not affect gastric acid secretion.

TABLE 1
Effects of Activation of Histamine H_1 and H_2 Receptors on Vascular Tone in Various Vascular Beds

Vascular bed	Species	Activated receptor H_1	Activated receptor H_2	Ref.
Gastric (submucosal arterioles)	Rat, cat	Dilatation	Dilatation	65
Gastric (total)	Cat	Dilatation	Dilatation	125
	Rat	Dilatation	Dilatation	68, 69
	Rabbit	Constriction	Dilatation	68
	Dog	Dilatation	Dilatation	126
Mesenteric	Cat, rat	Dilatation	Dilatation	64
	Dog	Dilatation	Dilatation	82
Systemic circulation	Cat, dog	Dilatation	Dilatation	127, 128
	Calf	Dilatation	Constriction	129
Aorta	Rabbit	Constriction	Dilatation	130
Temporal artery	Man	NA	Dilatation	131
Ear artery	Rabbit	Constriction	Dilatation	131
Pulmonary artery	Guinea pig	Constriction	NA	132
Pulmonary vein	Calf	Constriction	NA	129
Hepatic vein	Calf	Constriction	NA	133
	Dog	Constriction	NA	134

NA = no noted action.

In the radiolabeled microsphere technique, a known quantity of radiolabeled microspheres is injected into the left ventricle. When the microspheres reach a capillary bed, they become trapped in the vessels that have a smaller diameter than the microspheres used. The gastric blood flow can then be calculated by comparing the radioactivity of the tissue sample, with the radioactivity of a blood sample and the cardiac output.

There have been numerous arguments in the literature over which of the gastric blood flow measurement techniques yields the most accurate results. There are advantages and disadvantages with both the clearance and the microsphere technique. The microsphere technique requires the sacrifice of the test animal, whereas the aminopyrine/aniline clearance technique does not. A further disadvantage of the microsphere technique is that it is much more expensive than the aminopyrine technique. In a study by Archibald et al.,[59] in which these techniques were assessed, it was concluded that comparable results were obtained when acid secretion was stimulated by histamine; however, the aminopyrine technique measured only a small fraction of the blood flow in the nonsecreting stomach.[58] The *in vivo* microscopic technique of Guth and his associates is discussed in a later section.

3. Gastric Vasculature

Menguy was one of the first to report the action of histamine on the gastric vasculature. He found that bolus intravenous administration of a large dose of histamine caused immediate hypotension, followed by marked vasoconstriction and decreased gastric blood flow. This vasoconstrictive response was thought to be due to histamine-induced mediator release. Peter et al.[61] and Jacobson[62] found that systemic administration of small amounts of histamine produced vasodilation and increased gastric blood flow. These investigators also found that the same response could be induced by small, local administrations of histamine that did not affect the systemic vasculature.

Following the development of H_2 antagonists, there was a rush to determine which histamine receptors were involved in the mediation of gastric vascular contractility. Main and Whittle,[63] using the ^{14}C-aniline clearance technique, found that H_1 agonists stimulated vasodilation and increased gastric blood flow. The H_2 receptor agonist, 4-methylhistamine, was found to increase mucosal blood flow and stimulate acid secretion. Main and Whittle[63] felt that this rise in mucosal blood flow was due to the increase in acid secretion, as the response was inhibited by antisecretory prostaglandins and H_2 receptor antagonists. In short, this study concluded that both H_1 and H_2 receptors were found in the gastric vasculature of the rat and that H_2 receptors were primarily responsible for acid secretion, whereas H_1 receptors were involved in vasodilation.

Rees et al.[24] suggested that both H_1 and H_2 receptors were involved in mediation of gastric vascular tone. This was supported by their finding that both H_1 and H_2 receptors had to be blocked in order to prevent the pathophysiological changes associated with bile-induced damage. Using the radiolabeled microsphere technique in the cat, Johnston and Owen[53] found that the H_2 antagonist, metiamide, abolished histamine-induced gastric vasodilation, whereas the H_1 antagonist mepyramine did not affect it. In a similar study, Johnston and Owen[54] reported that the H_1 receptor agonist 2-(2-aminoethyl)pyridine caused vasodilation in the heart, kidneys, and both the small and large intestines, but not in the stomach. Conversely, the H_2 receptor agonist 4-methylhistamine induced vasodilation in the stomach, heart, skeletal muscle, and in the large and small intestines.

Guth and Smith[64] were the first to show that both the H_1 and H_2 receptors were involved in the mediation of histamine-induced vasodilation of the gastric vasculature in the cat and the rat. Their *in vivo* microscopic technique involves transillumination of the gastric mucosa with a high intensity light placed in the lumen of the stomach. The submucosal blood vessels can then be visualized through a small region of the gastric wall where the serosa and muscle layer have been dissected away. This technique allows for direct observation and measurement of the submucosal arterioles in both the corpus and the antrum.[58]

In a follow-up of their 1978 work, Guth et al.[65] reported that histamine, applied topically, induced a dose-dependent increase in the gastric submucosal arteriolar diameter in the rat. Both H_1 (mepyramine) and H_2 (metiamide) antagonists prevented this vasodilation. Interestingly, they found regional differences in the ability of the H_1 and H_2 antagonists to inhibit histamine-induced gastric vasodilation. In the corpus, the H_1 and H_2 antagonists were equally potent in inhibiting vasodilation. In the antrum, H_1 antagonists caused a much greater inhibition than the H_2 antagonists. This regional distribution could also be displayed using the H_1 agonists aminoethyl thiazole and aminoethyl pyridine and the H_2 agonist dimaprit.

Following the studies of Guth and associates,[64,65] numerous investigators reported that both H_1 and H_2 receptors mediated histamine-induced gastric vasodilation. These reports investigated this phenomenon in various species including dog[66,67] and rat.[68,69] In the rabbit, however, H_1 receptor stimulation caused vasoconstriction and H_2 stimulation elicited vasodilation.[68]

Since the initial studies involving the actions of histamine on the gastric vasculature,[61,62] the relationships between histamine stimulation of acid secretion and increased gastric blood flow have been questioned. All of the stimuli that are known to induce gastric acid secretion have also been found to increase gastric blood flow;[63,70] however, it is not known whether or not compounds other than histamine stimulate gastric acid secretion by inducing local histamine release.[45] H_2 antagonists have been found not to affect the resting gastric blood flow in the rat,[30,71] cat,[72] or dog.[73] Main and Whittle[63] also found that resting gastric blood flow in the rat was not affected by prostaglandin inhibition of gastric acid secretion.

There have been numerous studies citing effects of histamine antagonists on vascular changes associated with ulceration. For instance, cimetidine was shown to reduce the fall in gastric blood flow associated with hemorrhagic shock in miniature swine,[74] but not in rats.[30] Metiamide has been found to reduce restraint stress-induced gastric ischemia in the rat.[75] Cho and Ogle[76-78] reported that blockade of either H_1 or H_2 receptors antagonized stress-induced increases in gastric mucosal blood flow in rats and that there was an additive antiulcer activity when both H_1 and H_2 antagonists were administered concurrently. Lau and Ogle[79] found that H_2 receptor blockade antagonized reserpine-induced ulceration and the associated vascular changes in the rat stomach. Reserpine-induced gastric damage is thought to be due to the microcirculatory changes caused by release of histamine from mast cells. Lau and Ogle[79] also found that inhibition of reserpine-induced ulceration by H_2 antagonists was not solely due to acid inhibition, further supporting the role of H_2 receptors in the mediation of vascular changes in gastric damage.

In summary, it is evident that H_1 and H_2 receptors are present in the gastric vasculature and that in most species both H_1 and H_2 receptor stimulation leads to vasodilation and increased gastric blood flow. Such vasodilation can be blocked or mimicked with specific receptor antagonists or agonists, respectively. The role of histamine in the regulation of gastric vascular tone is not entirely dependent on its regulatory role in acid secretion. Finally, in numerous animal models histamine causes gastric damage at least in part through effects on the gastric microvasculature. These vascular changes and the resulting gastric damage can often be inhibited by both H_1 and H_2 antagonists. Thus, further study of the role of histamine in the mediation of gastric vasculature contractility may lead to clearer understanding of the mechanisms involved in the maintenance of the normal gastric vascular tone, as well as in the development and resolution of gastric damage.

4. Mesenteric Vasculature

Histamine increases the mesenteric blood flow in the cat and rat[64,80] and the dog.[81-83] In the cat, stimulation with specific H_1 or H_2 agonists caused vasodilation in the small and large intestines.[54] Furthermore, pretreatment with either mepyramine or metiamide blocked histamine-induced intestinal vasodilation.[53] Contrary to these findings, Guth and Smith[84] and Flynn and Owen[80] found that histamine-induced vasodilation in the intestine was reduced by mepyramine and other H_1 antagonists, but that metiamide did not affect the response to histamine unless it was given concomitantly with mepyramine.

Pawlik et al.[82] and Miller et al.[83] have further characterized the independent roles of H_1 and H_2 receptors in the mesenteric vasodilatory response to histamine in the dog. They found that although both H_1 and H_2 receptors mediated vasodilation, they had differing roles in the overall vasodilatory response. H_1 receptors were found to mediate the initial, transient increase in intestinal blood flow. On the other hand, H_2 receptors mediated a stable vasodilatory response which persisted for as long as the histamine was administered.[85]

C. VASCULAR PERMEABILITY

1. Background

In their pioneering studies, Dale and Laidlaw[2,49,50] found that histamine increased vascular permeability, and when administered intravenously, produced symptoms characteristic of shock induced by trauma or anaphylactoid reactions. It was noted that histamine increased vascular permeability resulting in a decrease in blood volume and an increase in hemoconcentration. The ability of histamine to cause vasodilation and to increase vascular permeability can be demonstrated by the "triple response" produced by injecting histamine intradermally. Histamine injection produces a localized red spot surrounding the injection site due to its direct vasodilatory actions on the microvasculature. A bright red flush or flare then develops around the initial red spot, which is due to vasodilation induced by a histamine-mediated axon reflex.[1] A wheal then develops due to edema caused by histamine-stimulated increases in vascular permeability.[86,87]

Majno and Palade[88] employed light and electron microscopic techniques to investigate where plasma protein leakage occurred. They found that histamine caused contraction of the vascular endothelial cells, resulting in gaps between cells and exposing the basal lamina. The gaps formed from this contractile response are large enough to allow the passage of fluids, plasma proteins, platelets, white cells, and red cells. The increased vascular permeability caused by the separation of endothelial cells is not simply due to histamine induced vasodilation, but is also due to the direct histamine stimulated contractile response of the endothelial cells. The increased capillary membrane permeability induced by histamine is mainly due to the action of histamine on the postcapillary venules.[89] Altura and Halevy[90] added that the increase in the flow of fluid from the capillaries in response to histamine may be due to increased transcapillary vesicular transport.

Histamine increases vascular permeability in most tissues and in most species examined. Irrespective of the tissue or species studied, H_1 antagonists were found to inhibit or completely abolish histamine-stimulated increases in vascular permeability.

2. Effects in the Gastrointestinal Tract

Various techniques have been employed to study the effects of histamine on vascular permeability in the gastrointestinal tract. The most common techniques are determination of radiolabeled plasma protein leakage, measurement of plasma to lymph plasma-protein concentration ratios, and the *in vivo* fluorescence microscopic technique of Guth and Moler.[91]

Wood and Davenport,[92] using an isolated segment of the greater curvature of the dog stomach, found that histamine increased vascular permeability and plasma protein loss into the lumen as measured by ^{131}I-albumin and ^{125}I-fibrinogen. They also found that pyrilamine (H_1 antagonist) and cimetidine inhibited histamine-stimulated increases in vascular permeability.

The *in vivo* fluorescence microscopic technique has been used in several species and in various tissues, but it was Guth and Moler[91] who adapted it for the study of the gastric microvasculature. This technique is similar to that used in the analysis of gastric vascular contractility which has been described previously in this chapter. In brief, it involves monitoring (via a specially adapted television camera) the leakage of fluorescein isothiocyanate-labeled bovine serum albumin from the vasculature.

Nagata and Guth[93] found that topically applied histamine increased the microvascular permeability in the muscularis externa of the rat. Through the use of H_1 and H_2 receptor agonists and antagonists, this effect was found to be mediated by H_1 receptors. It was also noted that histamine did not affect the permeability of the submucosal or superficial mucosal vessels. Since both H_1 and H_2 receptors are present in the submucosal microvasculature of the rat, it was questioned whether the H_1 and H_2 receptors were incapable of mediating changes in vascular permeability in the submucosa or whether vascular permeability could not be increased in this region of the rat stomach. Nagata and Guth[93] found that the permeability of the submucosal microvasculature could be increased (i.e., with bradykinin) and, therefore, it was concluded that the H_1 and H_2 receptors in this region were not involved in the regulation of vascular permeability.

In a subsequent study, Nagata and Guth[94] found that the doses of topically applied histamine required to increase vascular permeability were much greater than those required to increase acid secretion. They found that 10^{-2} *M* histamine was the threshold dose required for increasing vascular permeability, but that this concentration caused maximal acid secretion.

The action of histamine in the mediation of vascular permeability has also been studied in the mesenteric vasculature. Guth and Hirabayashi[95] found that histamine also increased vascular permeability in the muscularis externa of the small bowel of the rat via an H_1 receptor-mediated mechanism. In the cat, histamine increased the vascular permeability of the mesenteric microvasculature. Furthermore, such an effect was potently inhibited by H_1 antagonists.[96] Fox et al.[97] also found that histamine increased the permeability of the mesenteric microvasculature.

Histamine-induced changes in vascular permeability play a role in most inflammatory diseases by affecting the amount of edema in a region, as well as by affecting the ability of inflammatory cells to cross from the vasculature into the interstitium. Knicker and Cochrane[98] suggested that histamine-induced increases in vascular permeability may be involved in the initiation of immune complex disease. They found that colloidal carbon and antigen-antibody complexes were deposited in vessels during a state of increased permeability and that pretreatment with H_1 antagonists altered the deposition of immune complexes such that the development of lesions was reduced or completely inhibited (for a review, see Reference 89). Histamine also has numerous immunological actions which can be either detrimental or beneficial in a disease state. It should also be noted that histamine can cause an increase in lymph flow, as well as an increase in the protein content of lymph. These actions of histamine on the lymphatic system have been found to be inhibited by H_1 antagonists.[99]

In summary, histamine causes increases in vascular permeability in most tissues. These permeability changes have been found to be H_1 receptor-mediated; however, in some systems the H_2 receptor may have a minor role in the mediation of histamine-stimulated increases invascular permeability. By affecting vascular permeability, histamine plays an important role in the process of inflammation (edema formation, leukocyte margination), and therefore may be an important mediator in inflammatory diseases in the gastrointestinal tract.

V. CLINICAL BENEFIT OF TREATMENT WITH H_2 ANTAGONISTS

A. DUODENAL ULCER

The discovery of histamine H_2 receptors and the subsequent development of specific receptor antagonists (see Figure 4) has undoubtedly been the greatest advance in the treatment of duodenal ulcer. The rationale behind the use of H_2 antagonists for duodenal ulcer therapy is the reduction of gastric acidity. The ability to significantly accelerate healing by inhibiting gastric acid secretion or raising gastric pH had earlier been demonstrated by the efficacy of vagotomy and antacid therapy.

Examination of the data from several clinical trials of H_2 antagonists demonstrates that inhibition of basal acid secretion, particularly nocturnal, may be more important in ulcer healing than the ability of an agent to inhibit stimulated acid secretion. This is particularly true for food-stimulated acid secretion, since food itself tends to buffer acid. Thus, most patients find that pain dissipates shortly after eating a meal. Unfortunately, most dosing regimens have been based on the ability of the agent to inhibit stimulated acid secretion. The role of nocturnal acid secretion in the etiology of duodenal ulcer was identified as early as 1943. Dragstedt and Owens[100] reported that duodenal ulcer patients had markedly elevated levels of gastric acid secretion at night, likely reflecting increased vagal tone.

The hypothesis that inhibition of nocturnal acid secretion is the key to ulcer healing with H_2 antagonists is strongly supported by the data collected by Hunt et al.[101] and Howden et al.[102] from several clinical trials with various compounds (see Figure 5). Hunt and colleagues[101] reported a very good correlation between inhibition of nocturnal acid secretion and healing rate. Interestingly, when data from trials of other antiulcer drugs (non-H_2 antagonists) are plotted, they fall very close to the regression line. This may be expected for omeprazole, an H^+/K^+ ATPase inhibitor, since its primary mode of action is thought to be through inhibition of acid secretion; however, data from clinical trials with prostaglandin analogs also fell onto this regression line, suggesting that the healing achieved with these agents could be attributed entirely to their inhibitory effects on acid secretion, and not at all to their reported cytoprotective actions.

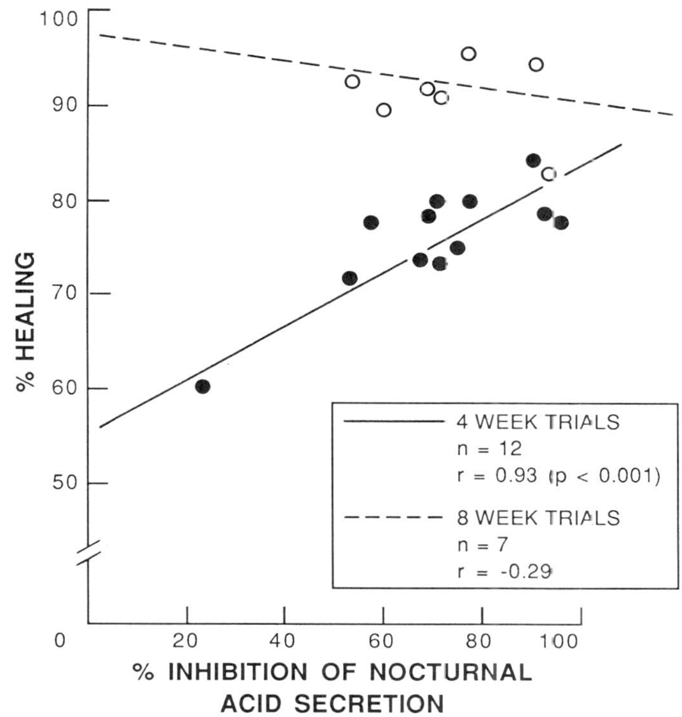

FIGURE 5. Relationship between duodenal ulcer healing after 4 (closed circles) and 8 (open circles) weeks of therapy with various H_2 antagonists and inhibition of nocturnal acid secretion. Each dot represents the mean values from clinical trials in the same dosing regimen with either cimetidine, ranitidine, or famotidine. In total, 124 separate trials with 12 different dosing regimens are included. These trials involved a total of 8375 patients. This graph was constructed using data from Hunt et al.[101] Note that a significant correlation exists between healing and acid suppression after 4 weeks of treatment; however, when treatment is continued for 8 weeks, such a relationship is no longer evident.

Of the numerous clinical trials from which Hunt et al.[101] and Howden et al.[102] collected their data, the highest healing rates achieved (4 and 8 weeks) were observed in trials in which single nighttime doses of cimetidine or ranitidine were given. They noted that a single nocturnal dose of these compounds also has the advantage of not interfering with daytime acid secretion, thereby retaining the protective effect of acid secretion against bacterial overgrowth (see Section E below).

B. GASTRIC ULCER

Several lines of evidence suggest that acid plays much less of a role in the etiology of gastric ulcer than it does in duodenal ulcer. For instance, there is no clear-cut relationship between hypersecretion of acid and gastric ulcer; in fact, most gastric ulcer patients secrete normal or less than normal levels of acid.[103] Whereas duodenal ulcers can be readily produced in laboratory animals via injection of secretagogues, gastric ulcers cannot be induced in this way. Further evidence that inhibition of acid secretion might not be so important in the treatment of gastic ulcer is the observation that omeprazole healed duodenal, but not gastric ulcer faster than ranitidine.[104]

Despite the apparent absence of an "acid etiology" for gastric ulcer, treatment with potent antisecretory agents, such as H_2 antagonists, can produce significant healing. Healing rates at

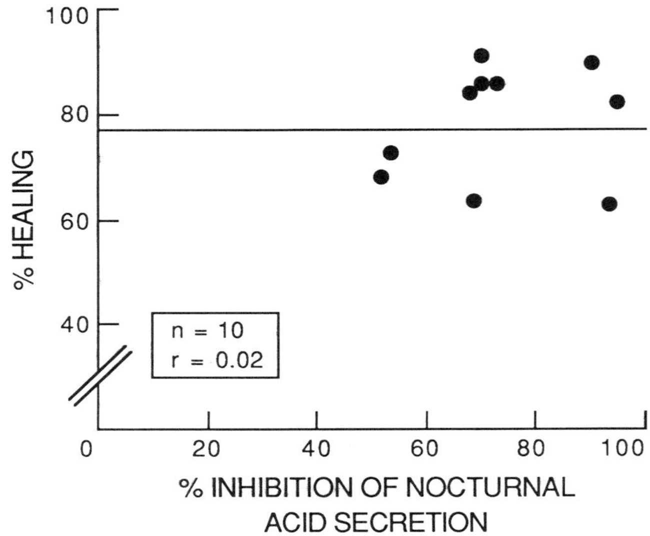

FIGURE 6. Lack of a significant linear relationship between gastric ulcer healing after 6 and 8 weeks of therapy with various H_2 antagonists and inhibition of nocturnal acid secretion. Each dot represents the mean values from clinical trials in which various dosing regimens with either cimetidine, ranitidine, or famotidine were tested. In total, data from 43 trials in which 10 different dosing regimens were used are included. These trials involved a total of almost 3500 patients. This graph was constructed using data from Hunt et al.[101]

4 to 6 weeks tend to fall about 10% lower than those observed in duodenal ulcer patients;[101] however, with continued treatment for 12 weeks, healing rates rise to as high as 90%.

Another difference between duodenal ulcer and gastric ulcer is that there is no relationship between healing of gastric ulcer with H_2 antagonists and their inhibition of nocturnal or 24-h acid secretion[101] (Figure 6). The mechanism of the healing action of H_2 antagonists in gastric ulcer is therefore not clear. It is interesting that similar results were found in animal studies in which H_2 antagonists protected against acute gastric ulceration in the presence of luminal acid (see Section III).

C. ZOLLINGER-ELLISON SYNDROME

Zollinger-Ellison syndrome is a condition associated with hypergastrinemia and usually hypersecretion of gastric acid (for a review of the clinical features of Zollinger-Ellison syndrome, see Reference 105). This condition is caused by the release of gastrin from tumors usually found in the pancreas (non-β–cell tumors) or, to a lesser extent, in the duodenum. Almost all (90 to 95%) of the patients with such gastrinomas develop peptic ulcer; however, the symptoms of peptic ulcer in these patients are much more severe than with common peptic ulcer. These ulcers also appear to be less responsive to the traditional therapies for peptic ulcer. For instance, treatment with antacids and anticholinergic drugs has been disappointing. As outlined earlier in this chapter, H_2 antagonists can partially suppress gastrin-stimulated acid secretion. Thus, with the advent of H_2 antagonists, an effective alternative to surgery in the treatment of Zollinger-Ellison syndrome has been achieved.

The application of H_2 antagonists for the treatment of Zollinger-Ellison syndrome was first noted when metiamide was found to dramatically reduce ulcer pain and to promote healing.[106,107]

Cimetidine has been shown to markedly inhibit gastric acid secretion, reduce the incidence of diarrhea and the severity of pain as well as to promote healing in most Zollinger-Ellison patients.[108-110] It is not clear by what mechanism the H_2 antagonists produce their beneficial actions. Higher doses of cimetidine are required for healing of Zollinger-Ellison-associated peptic ulcer than with common peptic ulcer. In fact, the dose of H_2 antagonist is titrated to reduce gastric acid secretion to less than 10 to 15 mmol/h, a level at which duodenal ulcer will not occur.[101] H_2 antagonists do not appear to reduce the circulating levels of gastrin in Zollinger-Ellison patients, although there was one report of such an action in two of three patients treated with metiamide.[106] Treatment with H_2 antagonists must be continued indefinitely, as even a brief interruption of therapy can result in recurrence. Because of the higher doses of cimetidine which are necessary for efficacy in the treatment of Zollinger-Ellison, a relatively high incidence of side effects has been reported.[111] Such side effects associated with the use of cimetidine have resulted in ranitidine becoming a popular alternative for treatment of Zollinger-Ellison syndrome. Ranitidine is eight times as potent as cimetidine at inhibiting gastric acid secretion,[107] while having a lower incidence of side effects.

In summary, while histamine has not been directly implicated in the pathogenesis of Zollinger-Ellison syndrome, the therapeutic benefits of treatment with histamine H_2 receptor antagonists suggests a role for histamine as a mediator of the peptic ulceration which frequently accompanies this syndrome.

D. REFLUX ESOPHAGITIS

Inflammation of the esophagus can occur when gastric or duodenal contents escape into the esophagus without being associated with belching or vomiting. This condition, known as reflux esophagitis, is often associated with hiatus hernia. Reflux occurs when the lower esophageal sphincter (LES) relaxes inappropriately. In fact, reflux itself can lower LES tone, thus promoting a vicious cycle of events. The clinical manifestations of reflux esophagitis include heartburn, regurgitation, odynophagia (painful swallowing), dysphagia, hemorrhage and several pulmonary symptoms, such as wheezing and hoarseness.[112]

Treatment of reflux esophagitis is aimed at maintaining appropriate LES tone or at reducing intragastric pH. Thus, histamine H_2 receptor antagonists have been successfully employed, sometimes given concomitantly with antacids, for the treatment of reflux esophagitis.[113-116] Use of H_2 antagonists for the treatment of this disease must be continuous. It would appear that the beneficial effects observed with H_2 antagonist therapy are related to their inhibitory actions on acid secretion, since these agents have no significant effect on LES pressure.

E. ADVERSE EFFECTS OF H_2 ANTAGONIST THERAPY

In order to understand the adverse effects of H_2 antagonist therapy, it is first necessary to understand the role of acid in normal gastrointestinal physiology. Aside from providing an optimal pH for the action of pepsin, gastric acid plays a very important bacteriocidal role, thereby protecting the lower gastrointestinal tract from infection. Indeed, there is an inverse relationship between bacterial counts in the stomach and duodenum and the level of gastric acid secretion.[117] Hypochlorhydria and achlorhydria predispose to, and increase the severity of, bacterial and certain parasitic enteric infections.[118] Therefore, prolonged administration of H_2 antagonists could predispose the patient to enteric infection. One consequence of an increased incidence of enteric infection would be increased incidence of diarrhea. In a postmarketing surveillance study which reviewed 9288 cimetidine takers and compared them to an appropriate control population, a significant (5-fold) increase in the incidence of diarrhea was observed in the cimetidine takers. There was no indication of the mechanism of this action of cimetidine, but bacterial infection was suspected.[119] In addition to this large surveillance study, there has also been a case report of severe diarrhea due to small intestinal colonization in cimetidine takers.[120]

As well as an increased risk of diarrhea when bacterial count is raised, there may also be an increased risk of gastric cancer. The intragastric concentration of nitrate-reducing bacteria has been found to be increased in cimetidine takers. This may be important since the N-nitroso compounds which they produce have been demonstrated to be carcinogenic in some animals and these compounds have been implicated in the increased risk of gastric cancer associated with pernicious anemia.[121] Furthermore, as gastric pH rises, there is no longer a negative feedback via antral pH-sensitive receptors to inhibit gastrin release, therefore hypergastrinemia can occur. One long-term consequence of hypergastrinemia, such as that associated with Zollinger-Ellison syndrome or pernicious anemia, is the development of discrete, benign carcinoid tumors in the stomach;[101] however, there have been no long-term studies on H_2 antagonists in which a significant predisposition to gastric cancer has been reported. Such risks of H_2 antagonist therapy may be of little consequence, since most gastric or duodenal ulcer patients are on a course of H_2 antagonist therapy for periods which do not usually exceed 8 weeks; however, longer term treatment with H_2 antagonists has been proposed, since many ulcers return within 1 year of cessation of treatment. The strategy of continuing treatment of patients with low doses of H_2 antagonists is supported by the observations that approximately one third of relapses are symptomless and may progress to perforation before being detected.[122,123]

A further complication associated with the use of cimetidine is its interaction with cytochrome P_{450}, thus prolonging metabolism of some other drugs (e.g., diazepam); however, this is an adverse effect unrelated to the H_2 receptor antagonist activity of cimetidine. Ranitidine and famotidine do not interfere with cytochrome P_{450}.

There are a number of minor adverse effects of each of the H_2 antagonists now on the market. These effects are for the most part unrelated to antagonism of histamine receptors, however, so they are not discussed in this chapter.

VI. SUMMARY AND FUTURE PERSPECTIVES

There is little doubt that histamine is an extremely important mediator of gastrointestinal physiology and pathophysiology.

The physiological roles of histamine include regulation of gastric acid secretion and modulation of gastrointestinal microvascular tone. The high rates of healing obtained with H_2 antagonists in duodenal and gastric ulcer patients indicates the importance of histamine pathophysiologically. The pro-inflammatory actions of histamine suggest that this compound may play a role in inflammatory diseases in the gastrointestinal tract, such as Crohn's disease and ulcerative colitis.

Despite the exhaustive research into the physiology and pharmacology of histamine during the 20th century, there is still a great deal to be learned about the role of this mediator. For instance, the mechanism for the beneficial effects of H_2 antagonists in the treatment of gastric ulcer is not clearly understood. Present evidence would suggest that these beneficial effects are unrelated to inhibition of gastric acid secretion. Another area in which the role of histamine has only recently began to become evident is in the modulation of the immune system. Considering the involvement of the gastrointestinal immune response in diseases such as inflammatory bowel disease, a greater understanding of any modulation by histamine may be extremely important. One of the major breakthroughs in histamine pharmacology, and in the treatment of peptic ulcer disease, was the characterization of H_1 and H_2 receptors. Recently, a third distinct histamine receptor (an H_3 receptor) was described in various regions of the rat brain.[124] The actions mediated via this receptor are unknown, but will certainly be an interesting and active avenue for future research.

REFERENCES

1. **Douglas, W. W.,** Histamine and 5-hydroxytryptamine (serotonin) and their antagonists, in *The Pharmacological Basis of Therapeutics,* 7th ed., Goodman, L. S. and Gilman, A., Eds., Macmillan, New York, 1985, 605.
2. **Dale, H. H. and Laidlaw, P. P.,** The physiological action of β-imidazolylethylamine, *J. Physiol. (London),* 41, 318, 1910.
3. **Best, C. H., Dale, H. H., Dudley, H. W., and Thorpe, W. V.,** The nature of the vasodilator constituents of certain tissue extracts, *J. Physiol. (London),* 62, 397, 1927.
4. **Beaven, M. A.,** Histamine: its role in physiological and pathological processes, *Monographs in Allergy,* Vol. 13, S. Karger, Basel, 1978, 112.
5. **Soll, A. H., Lewin, K. J., and Beaven, M. A.,** Isolation of histamine-containing cells from gastric mucosa: biochemical and morphological differences from mast cells, *Gastroenterology,* 80, 717, 1981.
6. **Lichtenstein, L. M. and Osler, A. G.,** Studies on the mechanisms of hypersensitivity phenomenon. IX. Histamine release from human leukocytes by ragweed pollen, *J. Exp. Med.,* 120, 507, 1964.
7. **Gurll, N. J. and Damianos, A. J.,** Histamine in gastric mucosal injury, in *Basic Mechanisms of Gastrointestinal Mucosal Cell Injury and Protection,* Harmon, J.W., Ed., Williams & Wilkins, Baltimore, 1981, 179.
8. **Heatley, R. V.,** The gastrointestinal mast cell, *Scand. J. Gastroenterol.,* 18, 449, 1983.
9. **Rees, W. D. W., Rhodes, J., Williams, B. C., Owen, E., and Newcombe, R. G.,** Effect of mast cell degranulation on gastric mucosal damage produced by sodium taurocholate in the rat, *Gastroenterology,* 74, 492, 1978.
10. **Davenport, H. W.,** Salicylate damage to the gastric mucosal barrier, *New Engl. J. Med.,* 276, 1307, 1967.
11. **Johnson, L. R. and Overholt, B. F.,** Release of histamine into gastric venous blood following injury by acetic or salicylic acid, *Gastroenterology,* 52, 505, 1967.
12. **Davenport, H. W.,** Back diffusion of acid through the gastric mucosa and its physiological consequences, in *Progress in Gastroenterology,* Vol. 2, Glass, G. J., Ed, Grune & Stratton, New York, 1970, 42.
13. **Tepperman, B. L. and Soper, B. D.,** Relationship of hydrogen ion back-diffusion to histamine liberation from canine oxyntic mucosa, *Can. J. Physiol. Pharmacol.,* 58, 188, 1980.
14. **Robert, A., Nezamis, J. E., and Stowe, D. F.,** Drug-induced gastric (steroid) and duodenal (secretagogues) ulcers, in *Experimental Ulcer,* Gheorghiu, T., Ed., Gerhard Witzstrock, Baden-Baden, 1975, 22.
15. **Watt, J.,** The mechanisms of histamine ulceration in the guinea pig, *Gastroenterology,* 37, 741, 1959.
16. **Takeuchi, K., Ishihara, Y., Kunimi, H., and Okabe, S.,** Effects of FPL-52694, a new mast cell stabilizer, on gastric secretion and various acute gastric lesions in rats, *Agents Actions* 14, 637, 1984.
17. **Hansen, D. G., Aures, D., and Grossman, M. I.,** Histamine augments gastric ulceration produced by intravenous aspirin in cats, *Gastroenterology,* 74, 540, 1978.
18. **Guth, P. H. and Hall, P.,** Microcirculatory and mast cell changes in restraint induced ulcer, *Gastroenterology,* 50, 562, 1966.
19. **Ritchie, W. P., Breen, J. J., and Grigg, D. I.,** Prevention of stress ulcer by reducing gastric tissue histamine, *Surgery,* 62, 596, 1967.
20. **Ritchie, W. P., Breen, J. J., Grigg, D. I., and Wangensteen, O.,** Effect of decreased levels of endogenous gastric tissue histamine on acid secretion and stress ulcer formation in the rat, *Gut,* 8, 32, 1967.
21. **Levine, R. G. and Senay, E. C.,** Histamine in the pathogenesis of stress ulcers in the rat, *Am. J Physiol.,* 214, 892, 1968.
22. **Tran, T. A. and Gregg, R. V.,** Transmittal of restraint-induced gastric ulcers by parabiosis in rat, *Gastroenterology,* 66, 63, 1974.
23. **Moody, F. G., Cheung, L. Y., Simons, M. A., and Zalewsky, C.,** Stress and the acute gastric mucosal lesion, *Am. J. Dig. Dis.,* 21, 148, 1976.
24. **Rees, W. D. W., Rhodes, J., Wheeler, M. H., et al.,** The role of histamine receptors in the pathophysiology of gastric mucosal damage, *Gastroenterology,* 72, 67, 1977.
25. **Gurll, N. J., Zinner, M. J., and Callahan, W.,** Effect of histamine H_2 antagonism by metiamide on the response of the canine gastric mucosa to acid and bile salt, *Gastroenterology,* 73, 255, 1977.
26. **Cheung, L. Y. and Porterfield, G.,** Is histamine a mediator in bile-induced mucosal injury?, *J. Surg. Res.,* 24, 272, 1978.
27. **O'Brien, P. E. and Carter, D. C.,** Effect of gastric secretory inhibitors on the gastric mucosal barrier, *Gut,* 16, 437, 1975.
28. **Bommelaer, G. and Guth, P. H.,** Protection by histamine receptor antagonists and prostaglandin against gastric mucosal barrier disruption in the rat, *Gastroenterology,* 77, 303, 1979.
29. **Guth, P. H., Aures, D., and Paulsen, G.,** Topical aspirin plus HCl gastric lesions in the rat: cytoprotective effect of prostaglandins, cimetidine, and probanthine, *Gastroenterology,* 76, 88, 1979.

30. **Owen, D. A. A., Parsons, M. E., Farrington, H. E., and Blakemore, R.,** Reduction by cimetidine of acute gastric hemorrhage caused by reinfusion of blood after exposure to exogenous acid during gastric ischemia in rats, *Gastroenterology,* 77, 979, 1979.
31. **Safaie-Shirazi, S., Foster, L. D., and Hardy, B. M.,** The effect of metiamide, an H_2-receptor antagonist, in the prevention of experimental stress ulcers, *Gastroenterology,* 71, 421, 1976.
32. **Okabe, S., Takeuchi, K., Urushidani, T., and Takagi, K.,** Effects of cimetidine, a histamine H_2-receptor antagonist, on various experimental gastric and duodenal ulcers, *Am. J. Dig. Dis.,* 22, 677, 1977.
33. **Schwarz, K.,** Ueber penetrierende magen — und jejunal — geschwüre, *Beitr. II Klin. Chir.,* 67, 96, 1910.
34. **Popielski, L.,** β-Imidazoläthylamin und die organextrakte ersterteil: β-imidazolyläthylamin als mächtiger erreger der magendrüsen, *Pfluegers Arch. Ges. Physiol.,* 178, 214, 1920.
35. **Black, J. W., Duncan, W. A. M., Durant, C. J., Ganellin, C. R., and Parsons, E. M.,** Definition and antagonism of histamine H_2-receptors, *Nature,* 236, 385, 1972.
36. **McIntosh, F. C.,** Histamine as a normal stimulant of gastric secretion, *Q. J. Exp. Physiol.,* 28, 87, 1938.
37. **Aures, D., Hakanson, R., and Schauer, A.,** Histidine decarboxylase and DOPA decarboxylase in the rat stomach, *Eur. J. Pharmacol.,* 3, 217, 1968.
38. **Hakanson, R., Lilja, G., and Owman, C.,** Properties of a new system of amine-storing cells in the gastric mucosa of the rat, *Eur. J. Pharmacol.,* 1, 188, 1967.
39. **Synder, S. H. and Epps, L.,** Regulation of histidine decarboxylase in rat stomach by gastrin: the effect of inhibitors of protein synthesis, *Mol. Pharmacol.,* 4, 187, 1968.
40. **Kahlson, G. and Rosegren, E.,** New approaches to the physiology of histamine, *Physiol. Rev.,* 48, 155, 1968.
41. **Soll, A. H. and Walsh, J. H.,** Regulation of gastric acid secretion, *Ann. Rev. Physiol.,* 41, 35, 1979.
42. **Soll, A. H., Amirian, D. A., Thomas, L. P., Reedy, T. J., and Elashoff, J. D.,** Gastrin receptors on isolated canine parietal cell, *J. Clin. Invest.,* 74, 1434, 1984.
43. **Soll, A. H.,** Mechanisms of action of antisecretory drugs. Studies on isolated fundic mucosal cells, *Scand. J. Gastroenterol,* 21(Suppl. 125), 1, 1986.
44. **Puurunen, J., Lucke, C., and Schwabe, U.,** Effect of phosphodiesterase inhibitor 4-(3-cyclopentyloxy-4-methoxyphenyl)-pyrrolidone (ZK63711) on gastric secretion and mucosal cyclic AMP, *Naunyn-Schmiedeberg's Arch. Pharmacol.,* 304, 69, 1978.
45. **Hirschowitz, B. I.,** An update on histamine receptors and gastrointestinal tract, *Dig. Dis. Sci.,* 30, 998, 1985.
46. **Soll, A. H. and Whittle, B. J. R.,** Interactions between prostaglandins and cyclic AMP in the gastric mucosa, *Prostaglandins,* 21(Suppl.), 39, 1981.
47. **Tepperman, B. L., Tague, L. L., and Jacobson, E. D.,** Inhibition of canine gastric acid secretion by H_1 receptor antagonist to histamine, *Dig. Dis. Sci.,* 23, 801, 1978.
48. **Soll, A. H.,** Secretagogue stimulatiom of ^{14}C-aminopyrine accumulation of isolated canine parietal cells, *Am. J. Physiol.,* 238, G366, 1980.
49. **Dale, H. H. and Laidlaw, P. P.,** Histamine shock, *J. Physiol. (London),* 52, 355, 1919.
50. **Dale, H. H.,** Some chemical factors in the control of the circulation, *Lancet,* 216, 1179, 1929.
51. **Chand, N. and Eyre, P.,** Classification and biological distribution of histamine receptor subtypes, *Agents Actions,* 5, 277, 1975.
52. **Black, J. W., Owen, D. A. A., and Parsons, E. M.,** An analysis of the depressor responses to histamine in the cat and dog: involvement of both H_1 and H_2 receptors, *Br. J. Pharmacol.,* 54, 319, 1975.
53. **Johnston, B. M. and Owen, D. A. A.,** Histamine and histamine antagonists and regional blood flow, *Eur. J. Pharmacol.,* 44, 355, 1977.
54. **Johnston, B. M. and Owen, D. A. A.,** Tissue blood flow and distribution of cardiac output in cats changes caused by intravenous infusion of histamine and histamine receptor agonists, *Br. J. Pharmacol.,* 60, 173, 1977.
55. **Eyre, P. and Wells, P. W.,** Histamine H_2 receptors modulate systemic anaphylaxis a dual cardiovascular action of histamine in calf, *Br. J. Pharmacol.,* 49, 364, 1973.
56. **Jacobson, E. D., Eisenberg M. M., and Swan, K. F.,** Effect of histamine on gastric blood flow in conscious dogs, *Gastroenterology,* 51, 466, 1966.
57. **Cowely, D. J., Code, C. F., and Fiasse, R.,** Gastric mucosal blood flow during secretory inhibition by gastrin pentapeptide and gastron, *Gastroentorology,* 56, 659, 1969.
58. **Guth, P. H. and Ballard, K. W.,** Physiology of gastric circulation. in *Physiology of Gastrointestinal Tract,* Johnson, L. R., Ed., Raven Press, New York, 1981, 709.
59. **Archibald, L. H., Moody, F. G., and Simons, M. A.,** Comparison of gastric mucosal blood flow as determined by aminopyrine clearance and -labelled microspheres, *Gastroenterology,* 69, 630, 1975.
60. **Menguy, R.,** Effects of histamine on gastric blood flow, *Am. J. Dig. Dis.,* 7, 383, 1962.
61. **Peter, E. T., Nocoloff, D. M., Sosin, H., Walter, A. I., and Wangesteen, O. H.,** Relationship between gastric blood flow and secretion, *Fed. Proc.,* 21, 264, 1962.
62. **Jacobson, E. D.,** Effects of histamine, acetylcholine and norepinephrine on gastric vascular resistance, *Am. J. Physiol.,* 204, 1013, 1963.

63. **Main, I. H. M. and Whittle, B. J. R.,** A study of the vascular and acid secretory response of the rat gastric mucosa to histamine, *J. Physiol.,* 257, 407, 1976.
64. **Guth, P. H. and Smith, H.,** Histamine receptors in mesenteric circulation of the cat and rat, *Am. J. Physiol.,* 234, E370, 1978.
65. **Guth, P. H., Moler, T. L., and Smith, E.,** H_1 and H_2 histamine receptor in rat gastric submucosal arterioles, *Microvasc. Res.,* 19, 320, 1980.
66. **Charbon, G. A., Brouwers, A. A., and Sala, A.,** Histamine H_1- and H_2-receptors in the gastrointestinal circulation, *Arch. Pharmacol.,* 312, 123, 1980.
67. **Meiners, D. J., Deshpande, Y. G., and Kaminski, D. L.,** The role of histamine in control of gastric mucosal blood flow in dogs, *J. Surg. Res.,* 32, 608, 1982.
68. **Salvatti, P. and Whittle, B. J. R.,** Vascular responses of the isolated perfused stomach of rabbit and rat to histamine, *Eur. J. Pharmacol.,* 89, 63, 1983.
69. **Koo, A.,** *In vivo* characterization of histamine H_1- and H_2-receptors in the rat stomach microcirculation, *Br. J. Pharmacol.,* 78, 181, 1983.
70. **Guth, P. H. and Smith, E.,** The effects of gastrointestinal hormones on the gastric microcirculation, *Gastroenterology,* 71, 435, 1976.
71. **Main, I. H. M. and Whittle, B. J. R.,** The effects of E and A prostaglandins on gastric mucosal blood flow and acid secretion in the rat, *Br. J. Pharmacol.,* 49, 428, 1973.
72. **Harris, D. W., Smy, J. R., Reed, J. D. , and Venables, C. W.,** The effects of burimamide and metiamide on basal gastric function of the cat, *Br. J. Pharmacol.,* 53, 293, 1975.
73. **Delaney, J. P., Micheal, H. M., and Bond, J.,** Cimetidine on gastric blood flow, *Surgery,* 84, 190, 1978.
74. **Levine, B. A., Schwesinger, W. H., Sirinek, K. R., et al.,** Cimetidine prevents reduction in gastric mucosal blood flow during shock, *Surgery,* 84, 113, 1978.
75. **Schwille, P. O., Lang, G., and Hofmann, P.,** Rat gastric secretion and mucosal blood flow during restraint stress — effect of a low dose of metiamide, *Res. Exp. Med.,* 171, 205, 1977.
76. **Cho, C. H. and Ogle, C. W.,** The effects of zinc sulfate on vagal-induced mast cell changes and ulcers in the rat stomach, *Eur. J. Pharmacol.,* 43, 315, 1977.
77. **Cho, C. H. and Ogle, C. W.,** Histamine H_1 and H_2 receptor mediated gastric microcirculatory effects in the aetiology of stress ulceration in the rat stomach, *Experientia,* 34, 1294, 1978.
78. **Cho, C. H. and Ogle, C. W.,** Cholinergic mediated gastric mast cell degranulation with subsequent histamine H_1 and H_2 receptor activition in stress ulceration in rats, *Eur. J. Pharmacol.,* 55, 23, 1979.
79. **Lau, H. K. and Ogle, C. W.,** An evaluation of the influence of increases gastric acid in the arteriology of reserpine induced ulcers in rat stomachs, *Pharm. Res. Commun.,* 2, 253, 1979.
80. **Flynn, S. B. and Owen, D. A. A.,** Histamine receptors in the peripheral vascular beds in the cat, *Br. J. Pharmacol.,* 5, 181, 1975.
81. **Pawlik, W., Shepherd, A. P., and Jacobson, E. D.,** Effects of vasoactive agents on intestinal oxygen consumption and blood flow in dogs, *J. Clin. Invest.,* 56, 484, 1975.
82. **Pawlik, W., Tague, L. L., Tepperman, B. L., Miller, T. A., and Jacobson, E. D.,** Histamine H_1- and H_2-receptor vasodilation of canine intestinal circulation, *Am. J. Physiol.,* 233, E219, 1977.
83. **Miller, T. A., Tepperman, B. L., Taque, L. L., Pawlik, W., and Jacobson, E. D.,** Characteristics of H2 receptor blockage in the canine mesenteric circulation, *J. Surg. Res.,* 27, 119, 1979.
84. **Guth, P. H. and Smith, E.,** H_1 and H_2 histamine receptors in the cat mesenteric circulation, *Microvasc. Res.,* 11, 119, 1976.
85. **Tepperman, B. L. and Jacobson, E. D.,** Mesenteric circulation, in *Physiology of the Gastrointestinal Tract,* Johnson, L. R., Ed., Raven Press, New York, 1981, 1317.
86. **Lewis, T. and Grant, R. T.,** Vascular reactions of the skin to injury. The liberation of a histamine-like substance in injured skin, *Heart,* 11, 209, 1924.
87. **Lewis, T.,** *The Blood Vessels of the Human Skin and Their Responses,* Shaw & Son, London, 1927.
88. **Majno, G. and Palade, G. E.,** Studies on inflammation; effects of histamine and serotonin on vascular permeability an electron microscope study, *J Biophys. Biochem. Cytol.,* 11, 571, 1961.
89. **Busse, W. W.,** Histamine: mediator and modulator in inflammation, in, *Handbook of Inflammation,* Vol. 1, Glynn, L. E., Houck, J. C., and Weismann, G., Eds., Elsevier/North-Holland, Amsterdam, 1979, 1.
90. **Altura, B. M. and Halevy, S.,** Cardiovascular actions of histamine in Histamine II anti-histamine chemistry, metabolism and physiological and pharmacological actions, in *Handbuch der Experimentellen Pharmakologie,* Vol. 18, Rocha e Silva, V., Ed., Springer-Verlag, Berlin, 1978, 1.
91. **Guth, P. H. and Moler, T. L.,** *In vivo* fluorescence microscopy of the gastric microcirculation, *Gastroenterology,* 76, 1147, 1979.
92. **Wood, J. G. and Davenport, H. W.,** Measurement of canine gastric vascular permeability to plasma proteins in the normal and protein losing states, *Gastroenterology,* 82, 725, 1982.

93. **Nagata, H. and Guth, P. H.,** Effect of histamine on microvascular permeability in the rat stomach, *Am. J. Physiol.,* 245, G201, 1983.
94. **Nagata, H. and Guth, P. H.,** Effect of topical histamine on mucosal microvascular permeability and acid secretion in the rat stomach, *Am. J. Physiol.,* 246, 654, 1984.
95. **Guth, P. H. and Hirabayashi, K.,** The effect of histamine on the microvascular permeability in the muscularis externa of the rat small intestine, *Microvasc. Res.,* 25, 322, 1983.
96. **Mortillaro, A., Granger, N. A., Kvietys, P. R., Rutili, G., and Taylor, A. E.,** Effects of histamine and histamine antagonists on the of intestinal capillary permeability, *Am. J. Physiol.,* 240(5), G381, 1981.
97. **Fox, J., Galey, F., and Wayland, H.,** Action of histamine on the mesenteric microvasculature, *Microvasc. Res.,* 19, 108, 1980.
98. **Knicker, W. T. and Cochrane, C. G.,** The localization of circulating immune complexes in experimental serum sickness, *J. Exp. Med.,* 127, 119, 1968.
99. **Lewis, G. P. and Winsey, N. J. P.,** The action of pharmacologically active substances on the flow and composition of the cat hindlimb lymph, *Br. J. Pharmacol.,* 40, 446, 1970.
100. **Dragstedt, L. R. and Owens, F. M.,** Supra-diaphragmatic section of the vagus nerves in treatment of duodenal ulcer, *Proc. Soc. Exp. Biol. Med.,* 53, 152, 1943.
101. **Hunt, R. H., Howden, C. W., Jones, D. B., Burget, D. W., and Kerr, G. D.,** The correlation between acid suppression and peptic ulcer healing, *Scand. J. Gastroenterol.,* 21(Suppl. 125), 22, 1986.
102. **Howden, C. W., Jones, D. B., and Hunt, R. H.,** Nocturnal doses of H_2 receptor antagonists for duodenal ulcer, *Lancet,* 1, 647, 1985.
103. **Grossman, M. I., Kirsner, J. B., and Gillespie, I. E.,** Basal and Histalog-stimulated gastric secretion in control subjects and in patients with peptic ulcer or gastric cancer, *Gastroenterology,* 45, 14, 1963.
104. **Classen, M., Damman, H. G., Domschke, W., Hutterman, W., Londong, W., Rehner, M., Simon, B., Witzel, L., and Berger, J.,** Omeprazole heals duodenal but not gastric ulcers more rapidly than ranitidine, *Hepatogastroenterology,* 32, 243, 1985.
105. **McGuigan, J. E.,** The Zollinger-Ellison syndrome, in *Gastrointestinal Disease,* 3rd ed., Sleisenger, M. H. and Fordtran, J. S., Eds., W. B. Saunders, Philadelphia, 1983, 693.
106. **Blair, E. L., Grund, E. R., Miller, M. B., Reed, J. D., Sanders, D. J., Thompson, M. J., and Venables, C. W.,** Metiamide in Zollinger-Ellison syndrome, *Am. J. Dig. Dis.,* 20, 1123, 1975.
107. **Richardson, C. T. and Walsh, J. H.,** The value of a histamine H_2 receptor antagonist in the management of patients with Zollinger-Ellison syndrome, *N. Engl. J. Med.,* 294, 133, 1976.
108. **Burland, W. L. and Simkins, M. A., Eds.,** *Cimetidine: Proc. 2nd Int. Symp. on Histamine H_2 Receptor Antagonists,* Excerpta Medica, Amsterdam, 1977, 392.
109. **Sharp, P. C. and Hawkins, B. W.,** Efficacy and safety of cimetidine long term treatment with cimetidine, in *Cimetidine: Proc. 2nd Int. Symp. on Histamine H_2 Receptor Antagonists,* Burland, W. L. and Simkins, M. A., Eds., Excepta Medica, Amsterdam, 1977, 358.
110. **Bonfils, S., Mignon, M., and Gratton, J.,** Cimetidine treatment of acute and chronic Zollinger-Ellison syndrome, *World J. Surg.,* 3, 597, 1979.
111. **Jansen, R. T., Pandol, S. I., and Martin, J. C.,** Diagnosis and management of Zollinger-Ellison Syndrome, *J. Clin. Gastroenterol.,* 5(Suppl.), 123, 1983.
112. **Pope, C. E.,** Gastroesophageal reflux disease (reflux esophagitis), in *Gastrointestinal Disease,* 3rd ed., Sleisenger, M. H. and Fordtran, J. S., Eds., W. B. Saunders, Philadelphia, 1983, 449.
113. **Behar, J., Brand, D. L., Brown, F. C., Castell, D. O., Cohen, S., Crossley, R. J., Pope, C. E., and Winans, C. S.,** Cimetidine in the treatment of symptomatic gastroesophageal reflux, *Gastroenterology,* 74, 441, 1978.
114. **Powell-Jackson, P., Barkley, H., and Northfield, T. C.,** Effect of cimetidine in symptomatic gastro-oesophageal reflux, *Lancet,* 2, 1068, 1978.
115. **Wesdorp, E., Bartelsman, J., Pape, K., Dekker, W., and Tytgat, G. N.,** Oral cimetidine in reflux esophagitis: a double-blind controlled trial, *Gastroenterology,* 74, 821, 1978.
116. **Fiasse, R., Hanin, C., Lepot, A., Descamps, C., Lamy, F., and Dive, C.,** Controlled trial of cimetidine in reflux esophagitis, *Dig. Dis. Sci.,* 25, 750, 1980.
117. **Gray, J. D. A. and Shiner, M.,** Influence of gastric pH on gastric and jejunal flora, *Gut,* 8, 574, 1967.
118. **Giannella, R. A., Broitman, S. A., and Zamcheck, N.,** Influence of gastric acidity on bacterial and parasitic enteric infections. A perspective, *Ann. Intern. Med.,* 78, 271, 1973.
119. **Colin-Jones, D. G., Langman, M. J. S., Lawson, D. H., and Vessey, M. P.,** Post-marketing surveillance of the safety of cimetidine: twelve-month morbidity report, *Q. J. Med.,* 54, 253, 1985.
120. **Ruddell, W. S. J. and Losowsky, M. S.,** Severe diarrhoea due to small intestinal colonisation during cimetidine treatment, *Br. Med. J.,* 281, 273, 1980.
121. **Ruddell, W. S. J., Bone, E. S., Mill, M. J., and Walters, C. L.,** Pathogenesis of gastric cancer in pernicious anaemia, *Lancet,* 1, 521, 1978.
122. **Cargill, J. M., Peden, N., Saunders, J. H. B., and Wormsley, K. G.,** Very long-term treatment of peptic ulcer with cimetidine, *Lancet,* 2, 1113, 1978.

123. **Marks, I. N., Wright, J. P., Lucke, W., and Girdwood, A. H.,** Relapse rates after initial healing with sucralfate and cimetidine, *Scand. J. Gastroenterol.,* 17, 429, 1982.
124. **Arrang, J.-M., Garbang, M., Lancelot, J.-C., Lecomte, J.-M., Pollard, H., Robba, M., Schunack, W., and Schwartz, J.-C.,** Highly potent and selective ligands for histamine H_3-receptors, *Nature,* 327, 117, 1987.
125. **Harvey, C. A. and Owen, D. A. A.,** Time dependence of the interaction between histamine and histamine receptor antagonists in the cardiovascular system, *Br. J. Pharmacol.,* 68, 187, 1980.
126. **Gerber, J. G. and Nies, A. S.,** Canine gastric mucosal vasodilation with prostaglandins and histamine analogs, *Dig. Dis. Sci.,* 27, 870, 1982.
127. **Parsons, M. E. and Owen, D. A. A.,** Receptors involved in the cardiovascular responses to histamine, in *International Symposium on Histamine H_2-Receptor Antagonists,* Wood, C. J. and Simkins, M. A., Eds., Smith, Kline & French Laboratories, London, 1973, 127.
128. **Powell, J. R. and Brody, M. J.,** Identification of two vascular histamine receptors in the dog, in *International Symposium on Histamine H_2-Receptor Antagonists,* Wood, C. J. and Simkins, M. A., Eds., Smith, Kline & French Laboratories, London, 1973, 137.
129. **Eyre, P.,** Pharmacology of bovine pulmonary vein anaphylaxis *in vitro, Br. J. Pharmacol.,* 43, 302, 1971.
130. **Ercan, Z. S. and Tiker, R. K.,** Histamine receptors in isolated rat stomach fundus and rabbit aortic strips, *Pharmacology,* 15, 118, 1977.
131. **Glover, W. E., Carroll, P. R., and Latt, N.,** Histamine receptors in human temporal and rabbit ear arteries, in *International Symposium on Histamine H_2-Receptor Antagonists,* Wood, C. J. and Simkins, M. A., Eds., Smith, Kline & French Laboratories, London, 1973, 169.
132. **Okpako, D. T.,** A dual action of histamine on guinea pig lung vessels, *Br. J. Pharmacol.,* 45, 311, 1972.
133. **Holroyde, M. C. and Eyre, P.,** Reactivity of isolated bovine mesenteric and hepatic veins to vasoactive agents and specific antigen, *Eur. J. Pharmacol.,* 30, 36, 1975.
134. **Richardson, P. D. I. and Withrington, P. G.,** A comparison of the effect of bradykinin, 5-hydroxytryptamine and histamine on the hepatic arterial and portal venous vascular beds of the dog: histamine H_1 and H_2 receptor populations, *Br. J. Pharmacol.,* 60, 123, 1977.

Chapter 3

PEPSINS

A. Allen, D. A. Hutton, A. J. Leonard, J. P. Pearson, and L. A. Sellers

TABLE OF CONTENTS

I. TYPES OF PEPSINS AND PEPSIN STRUCTURE

Pepsins are proteinases which are active below pH 5 and are secreted in the gastric juice of vertebrates. They belong to the group of aspartate proteinases and have an active site consisting of a deep cleft containing two aspartic acid residues within hydrogen bonding distance of each other.[1] Pepsins are endopeptidases with a relatively broad specificity but with a preference for peptide bonds between hydrophobic amino acids, particularly phenylalanine and tyrosine.[2] Pepsins are more active on denatured protein and the acid conditions of the gastric juice will facilitate their activity in this respect. Pepsins are secreted extracellularly in a precursor form, pepsinogen, which is rapidly and autocatalytically converted to an active enzyme under acid conditions.[3] Pepsins are irreversibly denatured at pH values above 7.2, while pepsinogen is resistant to denaturation at values up to pH 10.[4] Pepsins are distinct from other aspartate proteinases such as cathepsin D, an intracellular acid proteinase present in lysosomes.[5] Unlike pepsin, cathepsin D is not irreversibly inactivated above pH 7 nor is it secreted as an inactive precursor.

Eight zones of proteolytic activity have been identified in human gastric juice and acidified extracts of gastric mucosa by agar gel electrophoresis[6] (Figure 1). Seven of these proteinase zones, pepsins 1, 2, 3, 3a, 4, 5, and 6, were irreversibly inactivated by alkali, while the remaining zone 7 was not. Pepsin 3 is always the most abundant of the pepsins present in human gastric juice, usually followed by pepsin 5.[7] The others are present in much smaller quantities, the exception being pepsin 1, which makes a variable contribution to peptic activity. Pepsin 1 can account for up to 26.9% of the total pepsin activity in pentagastrin stimulated gastric juice from peptic ulcer patients.[8] Pepsin 5, pyloric pepsin, and gastricsin are the same enzyme and homologous with porcine pepsin C.[7] Proteinase zone 7 almost certainly corresponds to the slow-moving proteinase identified immunologically by Samloff[9,10] which is also not irreversibly inactivated at neutral pH. Since this slow-moving protease is likely to be a tissue cathepsin more characteristic of the mucosa than the secreted luminal pepsins, it will not be discussed further.

There are some significant differences in size and composition between the pepsins isolated from gastric juice by ion exchange chromatography.[7,11] Pepsin 1 is the largest with a molecular weight of 43,810[11] and has been shown on polyacrylamide gel electrophoresis (PAGE) to be associated with a faster moving component of 48,000.[7] Pepsins 2, 3, and 5 have molecular weights of 39,950, 37,150, and 31,620, respectively, demonstrating a relationship between increasing electrophoretic mobility and increasing molecular weight.[11] Pepsin 1 has one or possibly two phosphate groups per molecule[7] and is associated with carbohydrate. Treatment with hyaluronidase changes the electrophoretic mobility of pepsin 1, suggesting the presence of hyaluronic acid.[12] More recently, proteoglycan has been separated from purified pepsin 1 by equilibrium centrifugation in the high salt conditions of a cesium chloride density gradient containing 4 *M* guanidinium chloride.[13] Pepsin 1, fractionated by ion exchange chromatography, contained up to 50% carbohydrate composed of hexosamines, neutral sugars, sialic acid, and uronic acid.[13]

Pepsins differ in their pH optima and relative proteolytic activities with a given substrate. Pepsins 1, 2, 3, and 5 have optima of pH 1.9, 2.1, 2.4 to 2.8, and 2.0 to 3.6, respectively, using bovine hemoglobin substrate.[11] Pepsin 3 has relatively more proteolytic activity with hemoglobin substrate than pepsin 1 but the reverse is true with an ovalbumin substrate.[14] With collagen as a substrate pepsin 1 has an optima of pH 3.0 and 5 times the activity of pepsin 3 which has no optima between pH 1.2 and 4.0.[15] Both pepsin types 1 and 3 attack the telopeptide cross-links which join together the collagen α_1 and α_2 chains but they do not act as collagenases in that the chains themselves remain intact. Particularly interesting is the increased mucolytic activity shown by pepsin 1 relatively to pepsin 3[16] and discussed in relation to peptic ulcer disease later. It is possible that the proteoglycan component associated with pepsin 1 but not pepsin 3 may contribute to such differences in activity.

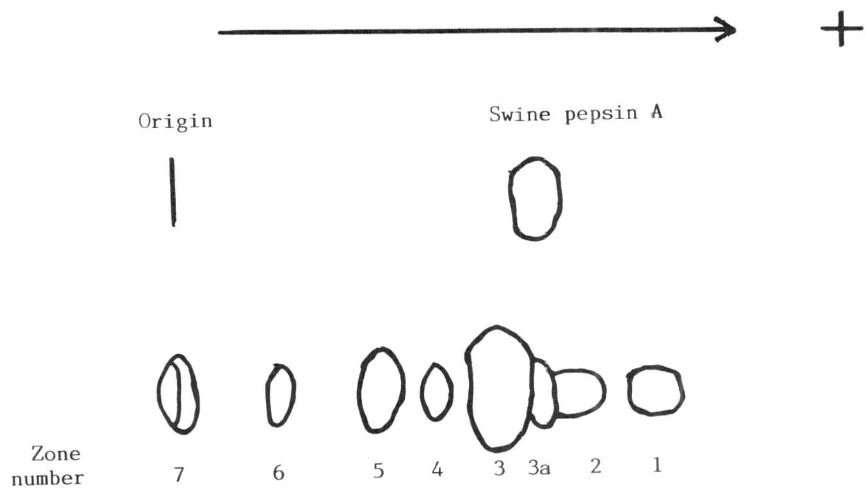

FIGURE 1. Electrophoresis of human gastric juice on agar gels, at pH 5.0. The zones of proteolytic activity appear white against a stained background. Zones of pepsin activity are numbered after Etherington and Taylor.[6]

Two immunological groups of pepsinogens, PGI and PGII, have been isolated and on activation produce pepsin A and pepsin C, respectively.[9,17] PGI and PGII have different activities with artificial substrates, for example, PGI hydrolyses the substrate tyrosyl phenylalanine more rapidly than PGII, while the reverse is true for other dipeptides such as tyrosyl alanine or tyrosyl threonine. The two pepsinogen groups have different tissue origins. PGI is secreted by oxyntic glands of the fundic mucosa whereas PGII is secreted by the pyloric glands of the antrum, the proximal duodenum, and the oxyntic glands. These two groups can be further separated into five pepsinogens for PGI and two for PGII on the basis of electrophoretic mobility toward the anode on agar gels. PGI contains pepsinogens 1 through 5 (1 has the fastest mobility and therefore is the most acidic). PGII contains the two slowest moving pepsinogens, 6 and 7.[9] Presumably each pepsinogen gives rise to a specific pepsin, however, the picture is complicated, and it has been suggested that a single pepsinogen can produce more than one pepsin and conversely two pepsinogens can produce a single pepsin.[18]

Recently, it has been shown using monoclonal antibodies that PGI can be subdivided into α- and β-PGI.[19] The two major α-PGI pepsinogens are 3 and 5 and the major β-PGI pepsinogen is 4. These correspond to the major pepsinogen genes PGA3, PGA4, and PGA5. Apart from the immunological differences PGI and PGII display other differences. PGI has a molecular weight of 43,500 ± 700 and PGII 40,500 ± 900.[20] The pepsins produced have molecular weights of 34,100 for pepsin "I" (pepsins A) and 31,400 for pepsin "II" (pepsins C).[21] The pH optima and the activity of the two groups of pepsins using hemoglobin as a substrate also differ.[10,20] PGI pepsins have optimal activity at pH 1.5 to 2.0 and PGII at pH 3.2, while PGII pepsins have 1.7 times the specific activity of PGI. It is not absolutely clear which of the pepsins isolated from gastric juice[6] correspond to these pepsinogens but pepsins 1, 2, 3, 3a, and 4 almost certainly correspond to PGI (Table 1). Pepsin 5 is homologous to pepsin C and belongs to the immunological group PGII and pepsin 6 also presumably belong to this group although this has not yet been confirmed.

II. ACTIVATION OF PEPSINOGENS TO PEPSIN

Pepsinogen is spontaneously converted to pepsin below pH 5 and the mechanism of this process has been elucidated in detail for porcine pepsinogen.[22] When activated, pepsinogen loses two peptides which together constitute the proenzyme segment of 44 amino acids located at the

TABLE 1
Classification of Human Gastric Proteases

Pepsinogens in mucosal tissue				
Immunological groups	**Pepsinogens present**[9]	**Tissue origin**	**Activated pepsin**	**Pepsins in gastric juice**[15]
PGI	1, 2, 3, 4, 5	Oxyntic glands	Pepsin A	1, 2, 3, 3a, 4
PGII	6 & 7		Pepsin C	
		Pyloric glands	(gastricsin)	5, 6
		Oxyntic glands		
		Proximal		
duodenum				
5 low moving	SMP proteinase		Pepsin B	7

Note: Numbers in both columns refer to the electrophoretic mobility of the proteins on agar gels; 1 is the fastest moving.

N-terminal end of the zymogen peptide chain. Pepsinogen conformation is stabilized by electrostatic interactions between basic amino acids on the proenzyme segment and carboxyl groups on the enzyme.[23] Below pH 5 the carboxyl groups become protonated, abolishing the stabilizing electrostatic interactions, and a conformational change occurs which results in the hydrolysis of the peptide bond between leucine 16P and isoleucine 17P at the active site of the enzyme. This cleavage produces an enzymatically active pseudopepsin molecule and releases a 16 amino acid peptide from the N-terminus.[24,25] Pseudopepsin is further converted into active pepsin, by either intermolecular cleavage by another pseudopepsin or fully activated pepsin molecule, with cleavage of a leucine (44P):isoleucine[1] bond and release of a 28 amino acid peptide from the N-terminus. Both the 16 and 28 amino acid peptides are usually degraded to smaller peptides.[26] The activation of human pepsinogen is by a similar mechanism except that the proenzyme fragment removed is 47, not 44 amino acids long.[27]

III. THE MOLECULAR BIOLOGY OF PEPSINOGENS

Elucidation of the structure of the pepsinogen genes by recombinant DNA technology provides a definitive approach to understanding the patterns and regulation of biosynthesis of the secreted zymogens and their characteristic polymorphic variation. The human pepsinogen gene has been isolated with the aid of a cDNA probe from pig pepsinogen m-RNA.[28,29] It consists of 9.4 kb pairs comprising of 9 exons and 8 introns of various length. The predicted amino acid sequence is 373 residues, 82% of which is homologous with pig pepsinogen. The newly translated human pepsinogen contains a signal peptide of 15 amino acids cleaved off during intracellular processing. This signal peptide and part of the peptide cleaved off on activation of the pepsinogen are coded for in exon 1. The pepsinogen gene has two homologous sequences, each with an active site, located in exons 3, 4, 6, and 7: with exons 3,7 and exons 4,6 the same. Three different genes, localized in chromosome region 11q 13, code for human pepsinogen A.[30,31] These genes code for secreted pepsinogens 3, 4, and 5. The two other pepsinogens present in the pepsinogen A group (pepsinogens 1 and 2, Table 1) are thought to arise by intracellular posttranslational modification of the three primary gene products.

As many as 18 different pepsinogen phenotypes have been demonstrated in man, distinguished from each other by the relative amounts of the different pepsinogens expressed.[32] It has been suggested that this phenotypic variation is a reflection of the expression of different chromosomal haplotypes containing varying numbers of the three pepsinogen A genes.[33] At least two of the human pepsinogen A genes are closely linked and this with their similarity in structure could give rise to unequal crossover or homologous recombination; this would account for the halotype variation in the copy number of pepsinogen A genes.[34] A full understanding of the genetic basis of the phenotypic variation of secreted pepsins could be important in early diagnosis of gastric cancer. Thus, a significant association has been shown between phenotypes that have increased expression of the pepsinogen 5 gene and gastric cancer.[35] This same region of human chromosome also shows several nonrandom rearrangements associated with leukemia, myeloma and lymphoma, and the pepsinogen A gene may prove to be a useful marker in the early detection of these cancers.[36]

IV. ASSAY OF PEPSIN ACTIVITY

The conventional assay of pepsin activity depends on distinguishing hydrolyzed protein from nonhydrolyzed protein by precipitation of the latter with trichloroacetic acid (TCA). The hydrolyzed peptide remains in solution and is estimated by a standard colorimetric assay for protein. The original method of Anson and Mirsky[37] used hemoglobin for a substrate and subsequent modifications of the method have used plasma and serum,[38] radioactive iodinated albumin,[39] and cesin.[40] Alternative assays for pepsin employing similar approaches include pepsin solubilization of an insoluble protein powder labeled with Remazobrilliant blue;[41] nephelometric estimation of undigested bovine serum albumin (BSA) precipitated with sulfosalicylic acid[42] and peptic digestion of an albumin bromophenol blue substrate.[43]

A sensitive and more accurate method for estimating proteolytic activity is by measuring trinitrophenylated derivatives of new N-terminal groups which form on peptide bond hydrolysis.[44] The sensitivity of the assay is improved by blocking preexisting amino groups on the protein producing substrates such as dimethyl cesin[45] and succinyl albumin.[46] Using succinyl albumin substrate, this method has been adopted to measure pepsin activity in samples of gastric juice.[47] The method which measures N-terminal formation has advantages over previous methods in that it directly assays peptide bond hydrolysis rather than the qualitative size and conformational changes necessary to prevent precipitation of the protein from solution by TCA. The N-terminal assay is an order of magnitude more sensitive and can be used to detect 0.1 μg pepsin.

The mucolytic or mucus dissolving activity of pepsin has been assayed by measuring the drop in viscosity of a mucus glycoprotein solution on peptic hydrolysis.[16] A typical specific viscosity for a 5 mg ml^{-1} solution of purified polymeric pig gastric mucus glycoprotein is about 2 and this will decrease to about 0.5 following exhaustive degradation by pepsin to the digested glycoprotein units. The N-terminal assay has also been used to measure pepsin mucolytic activity.[47,48]

Both pepsins[6] and pepsinogens[49] have been separated by electrophoresis on an agar gel support. The pepsins are identified on the gel by incubating the gel at acid pH in a protein substrate solution and staining the undigested protein remaining on the gel. The pepsin spots appear white against a stained background. This method has been used to semiquantify the relative amounts of pepsin types 1 through 7 in gastric juice from patients with peptic ulcer disease.[8] A modification of this method for quantifying pepsin types in gastric juice samples was to identify pepsins on a small strip of the agar gel following electrophoresis, section the gel accordingly, elute the pepsins, and estimate them quantitatively by the sensitive N-terminal assay.[4]

Radioimmunoassays have been developed to measure serum levels of the two major, immunologically distinct, classes of pepsinogens PGI and PGII.[20,50] This technique, which is sensitive to nanogram quantities of the zymogens, has been used extensively to assay the relative pepsinogen levels in patients with peptic ulcer, atrophic gastritis, and gastric cancer.[10,35]

Recently, the immunological assay of the pepsinogen classes in serum has been developed as an enzyme-linked immunosorbent assay (ELISA).[51,52] Estimation of pepsins in gastric juice by rocket immunoelectrophoresis has been described using antibodies raised against the chromatographically purified enzymes.[53]

V. INHIBITORS OF PEPSINS

Pepstatins, pentapeptides produced by various actinonmyces, are substrate analog inhibitors of gastric juice proteinases.[54] Other aspartic proteinases are inhibited by pepstatins which have been shown by X-ray crystallography to bind at the cleft of the active site of the enzyme.[55] Pepsins 1 and 3 are both effectively inhibited by pepstatin but not pepsin 5.[7]

Carbenoxolone sodium decreases peptic activity in human gastric juice.[56] A suspension of carbenoxolone sodium at pH 4 inhibits isolated pig pepsin A and human pepsins 1, 3, and 5.[57] The ratio of carbenoxolone to pepsin for 50% inhibition is high and it has been proposed that the carbenoxolone does not bind directly to the enzyme active site but hinders access of the peptide substrate.[7]

Whole hepatic canine bile and individual conjugated or unconjugated bile salts inhibit pepsin hydrolysis of hemoglobin and synthetic APDT.[58,59] This inhibition of pepsin by bile salts is noncompetitive and may include nonspecific protein denaturation due to detergent effects.

Sucralfate, a basic aluminum salt of sucrose octasulfate has been shown to inhibit pepsin hydrolysis by binding electrostatically and noncompetitively inhibiting formation of an enzyme substrate complex.[60] Mucolysis of pig gastric mucin by pepsin has also been shown to be inhibited by sucralfate, although this was described as competitive.[48] A variety of larger negatively charged polymers have been shown to inhibit pepsin activity; these include amylopectin, a highly sulfated pentapolysaccharide;[60] polyacrylates,[61] connective tissue proteoglycans, and carrageenans.[62] The mechanism of inhibition of these negatively charged polyanions is to bind to the pepsin and its substrates and prevent their interactions.

VI. THE STRUCTURE OF THE GASTRODUODENAL MUCUS BARRIER

The primary gastroduodenal mucus secretion is a water insoluble gel adherent to the mucosal surfaces. It can be readily observed *in situ* on unfixed mucosal sections as a thin layer of translucent gel between the mucosal surface and luminal bathing solution.[63,64] The adherent mucus layer over the gastric and duodenal mucosal surfaces is always seen to be continuous, varying in thickness from 50 to 450 μm, median 180 μm for human antral stomach, and 10 to 300 μm, median 80 μm for rat stomach and duodenum. Physical studies on isolated mucus *in vitro* show it to be a gel formed by noncovalent interactions between large molecular-sized mucus glycoproteins or mucins.[65] It is resistant to mechanical disruption but it will flow over a relatively long time scale (about 1 h) and reseal if sectioned, a property enabling it to form a continuous protective cover over the mucosal surface. Mucus gel is not solubilized by exposure to a wide pH range (pH 1 to 8), to bile, or hypertonic solutions (2 *M* NaCl); however mucus gel is dissolved by proteolytic enzymes, e.g., pepsin, or by thiol-reducing agents, e.g., *N*-acetylcysteine and mercaptoethanol.[65,66]

For the adherent mucus gel to provide a fully effective protective barrier against the gastric juice, it is important that its cover over the mucosa is continuous. Such continuity is always evident on unfixed sections of undamaged gastroduodenal mucosa.[63,67,68] The adherent mucus gel is 95% water and studies show that the extracellular mucus layer is dehydrated and distorted during histological fixation or routine preparative procedures for the electron microscope.[64,67,69,70] To observe the continuity of the adherent mucus layer on undamaged mucosa, it is necessary to use unfixed mucosal sections,[63] prior fixation of the mucus gel with antibodies,[69]

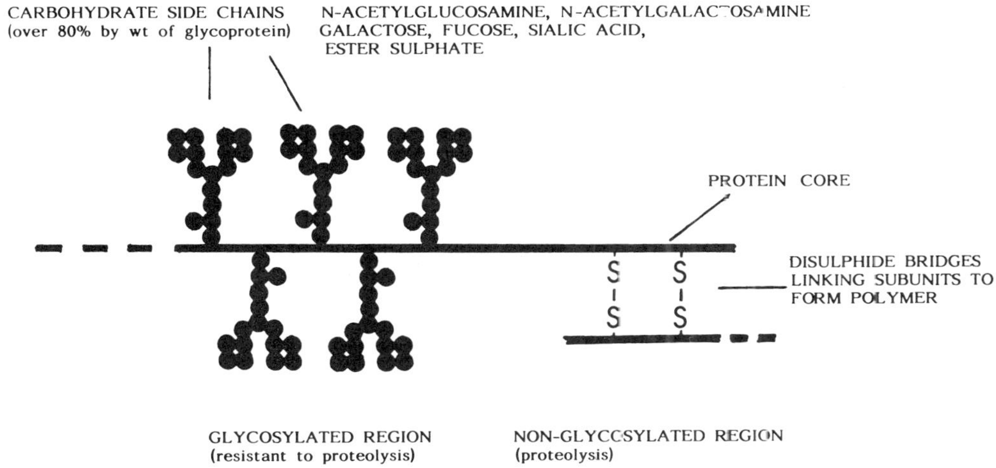

FIGURE 2. A diagrammatic representation of the structure of gastroduodenal mucins.

or by freeze fixation.[70] The adherent mucus gel layer is physically distinct from the soluble mucus in the lumen.[63] The viscous soluble mucus is unlikely to provide a significant barrier to the gastric juice with which it is freely mixed. Soluble mucus contains degraded mucus from pepsin hydrolysis of the surface mucus gel.

The principal gel-forming constituents of mucus secretions are large molecular weight mucins. Mixed with mucus secretions are other gastrointestinal secretions (e.g., enzymes and secretory immuno-globulin), microorganisms, sloughed-off cells, and ingested food at various stages of digestion.[71,72] Such nonmucus components, both lipid and protein, have been implicated in the properties of mucus secretions;[73,74] however the full rheological properties of the native secretion can be reproduced by concentration of the purified mucin alone.[65] The structure and properties of gastrointestinal mucins have been reviewed in detail;[71,72,75] here only structural features relevant to pepsin mucolysis are described.

Native gastroduodenal mucus has a polymeric structure formed from glycoprotein subunits (mol wt 5×10^5) joined by disulfide bridges.[66,71,75] Each subunit consists of a central protein core to which are attached numerous closely packed carbohydrate chains (Figure 2). These oligosaccharide side chains are complex (up to 19 sugars in length) in gastric mucin[77,78] and carry a negative charge due to ester sulfate and sialic acid. The protein core of each glycoprotein subunit consists of glycosylated regions where carbohydrate side chains are attached and nonglycosylated regions, which are essentially free of carbohydrate. The glycosylated regions are rich in the amino acids, serine, threonine, and proline; the nonglycosylated regions, rich in cysteine, are the sites of the disulfide bridges which link the subunits together to form a polymeric structure.[79,80] The size of the gastrointestinal polymeric mucins is at least 2×10^6 and probably of the order of 8 to 10×10^6. The tightly packed sheath of carbohydrate chains protects the glycosylated region of the protein core from proteolytic attack. The exposed nonglycosylated protein core of the polymeric glycoprotein is readily attacked by proteolytic enzymes (e.g., pepsin) to produce degraded, highly glycosylated, glycoprotein units of substantially smaller molecular size (approximately 5×10^5). These degraded glycoprotein units which have lost 30 to 50% of the protein core without detectable loss of carbohydrate are resistant to further digestion. The polymeric structure of the mucin is essential for gel formation, the reduced subunits or proteolytically degraded glycoprotein subunits do not form a gel.[65,65] Thus, at the molecular level, the mucolytic action of pepsin on mucus gel is the result of hydrolysis of the nonglycosylated protein core where the intersubunit disulfide links are located, and this in turn destroys the polymeric gel-forming structure to produce soluble degraded glycoprotein.

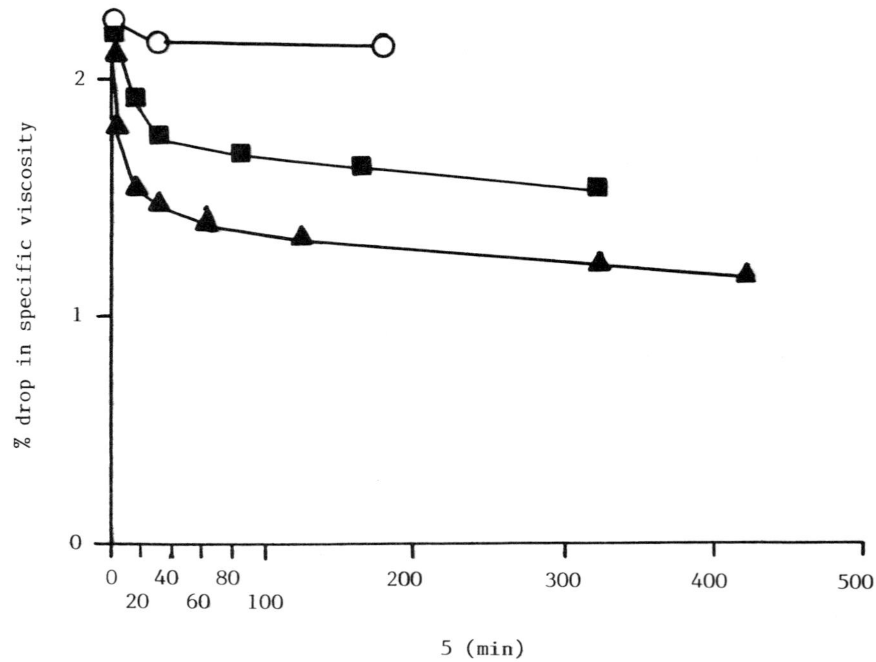

FIGURE 3. Assay of mucolytic activity of human pepsins using gastric mucus glycoprotein substrate at pH 2.5, 37°C. Pepsin 1 (▲), pepsin 3 (■), control: glycoprotein in the absence of added pepsin (O).[16]

It has long been recognized that pepsin and other proteolytic enzymes dissolve mucus secretions. Peptic autolysis of gastric mucosa has been used for decades as a preparation method of blood group substances which are degraded mucus glycoproteins.[81] The hydrolysis by pepsin of the highly viscous polymeric mucin to degraded low viscosity glycoprotein units can be followed by measuring solution viscosity[16] (Figure 3). Using this viscosity assay for pepsin mucolysis, pepsin 1 has been shown to have substantially increased activity relative to pepsin 3 (Figure 4). For equivalent amounts of proteolytic activity (using hemoglobin substrate) pepsin 1 has about twice the rate of mucolysis than pepsin 3 at the optimum pH 2.[16] More striking, however, were the results for higher pH values (4 to 5) when pepsin 1 showed substantial mucolytic activity in contrast to pepsin 3, which essentially was inactive above pH 4. The reason for the increased susceptibility of the mucus protein core to pepsin 1 is unknown but apart from the significance of these results in relation to peptic ulcer disease, discussed below. These studies demonstrate the importance of using the endogenous substrates when measuring pepsin activities. A simple method for assaying the relative amounts of polymeric and degraded mucin in a preparation is by gel-filtration on Sepharose 2B. Thus, on hydrolysis of human gastric, pig gastric or duodenal mucus gel, and isolated mucins there is a progressive decrease in the amount of excluded polymeric mucin and a parallel increase in included pepsin degraded mucin.[16,82]

VII. THE GASTRODUODENAL MUCUS BARRIER AND PROTECTION AGAINST PEPSIN *IN VIVO*

Gastroduodenal mucus gel is a selective permeability barrier allowing small ions and molecules to diffuse through its matrix, but not large molecular weight proteins.[83,84] Therefore, a continuous layer of mucus gel over the mucosal surface will act as a diffusion barrier to pepsins in the lumen preventing their digestion of the underlying epithelium[16,64] (Figure 5). Pepsin in the

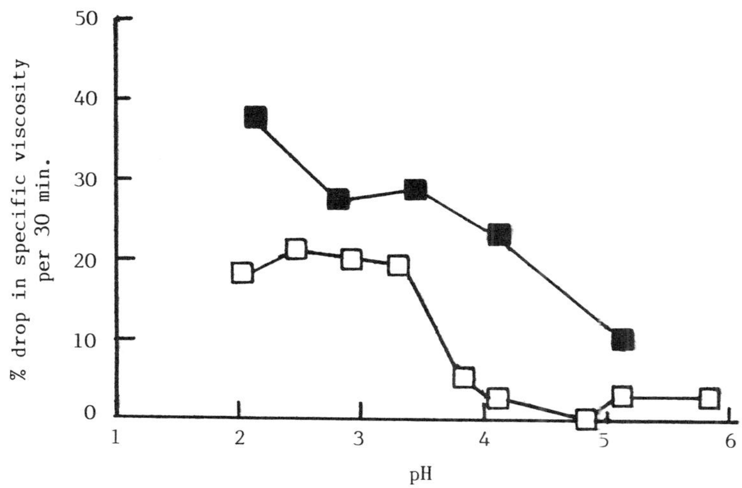

FIGURE 4. pH profile of human pepsin 1 (■) and 3 (□) digestion of gastric mucus. Samples of pepsin 1 and 3 had the same amount of proteolytic activity at pH 2.2 using a succinyl albumin substrate. Mucolytic activity was assessed by measuring the percentage fall in specific viscosity (V_{sp}) over 30 min at 37°C.[16]

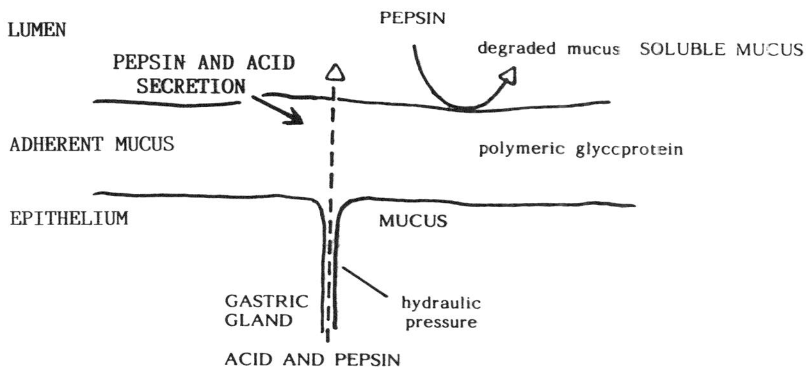

FIGURE 5. A diagrammatic representation of the gastroduodenal mucus barrier to pepsins.[64]

gastric juice will, however, dissolve the adherent mucus gel barrier at its luminal aspect to produce soluble degraded mucin. Since a continuous layer of adherent mucus gel is observed over the normal mucosa, it can be deduced that a dynamic balance exists at the mucosal surface where secretion of new mucus gel by the mucosa replaces that lost by erosion of mucus into the lumen by peptic hydrolysis augmented by mechanical shear.

Direct evidence for the peptic hydrolysis of the mucus barrier *in vivo* comes from studeis in man and in animal models. In gastric washouts from duodenal ulcer patients following insulin stimulation there is an approximate threefold stimulation in pepsin activity, and this is accompanied by a parallel threefold increase in the content of degraded mucin glycoprotein.[85] In vagotomized patients this rise in both pepsin and degraded mucin content of gastric washouts was absent following insulin stimulation. Pepsin erosion of the adherent mucus barrier has been demonstrated by its instillation into the lumen of a ligated rat stomach *in vivo*.[64,86] Instillation of acid pH 2.2 alone for 1 h into a rat stomach does not result in any observable damage to the continuous adherent mucus gel layer or the underlying epithelium and results in a small steady release of glycoprotein (100 μg h^{-1}). Instillation of pepsin (2 mg ml^{-1}) pH 2.2 resulted in a dramatic fivefold increase in the amount of glycoprotein present in the luminal juice compared to the pH 2.2 acid controls. The adherent mucus layer following pepsin treatment, under these conditions, changes from a continuous, translucent layer to one which is granular in appearance with areas of discontinuity. Evidence that pepsin has penetrated the mucus layer and is digesting the epithelium is seen histologically by focal lesions and bleeding into the lumen. Such experiments provide evidence that under normal circumstances the adherent mucus gel provides a protective barrier against digestion of the epithelium by luminal pepsin.

The gastric glands that secrete acid and pepsin do not possess an adherent mucus barrier. During secretion, acid at concentrations below pH 1 are attained in the lumen of the gastric gland and under such conditions, newly secreted pepsinogen will rapidly be converted autocatalytically to pepsin. The apical membranes of these glands must be resistant to their own secretions. This has been demonstrated with monolayers of pepsinogen secreting canine chief cells which can adequately resist acidification to pH 2;[87] however, the epithelial layer *in vivo* is sensitive to luminal pepsin if the enzyme penetrates the mucus barrier as shown in the rat ligated stomach model discussed above.[86] How newly secreted pepsin and acid in the gastric gland gain access into the gastric lumen through the apparently continuous cover of mucus over the mouth of the gland is uncertain. A reasonable hypothesis is that the volume of pepsin and acid secretion creates a hydraulic pressure which physically pushes the secretion through the overlying mucus gel into the lumen. Current methods for observing the mucus gel are not sufficiently sensitive to show if intermittent holes occur in the mucus gel cover over the entrance of the gastric glands during secretion.

VIII. PEPSIN AND MUCOSAL DAMAGE: ANIMAL MODELS

Mucosal damaging agents may be divided into two groups: (1) the endogenous aggressors acid, pepsin, and bile which are secreted naturally into the gastroduodenal lumen and (2) exogenous damaging agents such as alcohol, nonsteroidal anti-inflammatory drugs (NSAID), etc., administered by man to himself or experimental animals.[64] Natural gastroduodenal defense mechanisms have presumably evolved against acid, pepsin, or bile and the mucosal response to these agents may well not be the same as that following exposure to exogenous damaging agents. It would follow that peptic ulceration results from a chronic impairment of these natural mucosal defense mechanisms against the natural aggressors.

The presence of low pH in the gastroduodenal lumen is accepted as an essential part of the pathological ulceration process; however there is a substantial amount of evidence in animal models that the presence of pepsin rather than acid per se can be the ulcerogenic agent. Early studies showed the cat or dog jejunum, while resistant to 0.1 *M* HCl perfusion, was readily ulcerated and in some cases perforated, when pepsin 1 to 2 mg ml^{-1} was added.[88,89] An increased incidence of gastric ulceration in rats was observed when pepsin 1 mg ml^{-1} was added to acid (pH 1.3) perfusates under pressure.[90] Acid (0.5 *M* HCl) perfusion alone did not damage rat stomach or duodenum, but addition of pepsin was seen to produce lesions, although gastric juice perfusion was more effective still.[91] Administration of pepsin pH 2 induced acute esophagitis in rats which was prevented by the pepsin inhibitor amylopectin.[92] Pepsin, but not acid pH 2, *in vitro* has been shown to cause a breakdown in mucosal resistance of frog gastric and esophageal mucosa.[93,94]

From its location the adherent mucus barrier must be the first line of gastroduodenal mucosal defense against the gastric juice. This mucus barrier supports surface neutralization of acid by gastroduodenal mucosal bicarbonate and the establishment of the surface pH gradients.[95-98] As discussed above, the mucus barrier normally provides an effective diffusion barrier to pepsin; however, models such as the rat ligated stomach model demonstrate that excess pepsin (2 mg ml^{-1}) in the lumen will progressively erode the adherent mucus layer more rapidly than it can be replaced, resulting in epithelial erosion.[64,86] Distinct differences are seen between the mucosal response to pepsin damage and that following ethanol damage. Thus, the adherent mucus barrier offers little if any protection against ethanol which rapidly penetrates through it to cause necrosis and exfoliation of the underlying epithelium. This is followed by re-epithelialization[99-101] protected by a thick fibrin-based gelatinous coat and neutralizing plasma exudate.[99,100,102] Following pepsin damage, no re-epithelialization or formation of a thick protective fibrin-based gel cover such as that characteristic of repair following acute ethanol damage are apparent.[103] This thick gelatinous coat, protecting the re-epithelializing rat gastric mucosa following ethanol damage, once formed, is destroyed by high concentrations (500 mg ml^{-1}) of pepsin or *N*-acetylcysteine (0.5%) with inhibition of epithelial repair.[104]

IX. PEPSINS IN PEPTIC ULCER DISEASE

Patients with duodenal ulcer (DU) disease as a group have, on average, a 1.5 to 2 times greater pepsin and acid outputs compared to nonsymptomatic controls.[105] Pepsin output in DU patients is greater for both basal and stimulated secretions[106,107] as well as in biopsies from their gastric antrum.[108] It has also been reported that pepsin secretion is higher in active DU patients than those with inactive or healed DU.[109-111] The pH of the duodenum is often lower in DU patients compared to controls with a minimum pH for most of the latter falling in the range pH 1.5 to 4.0.[106,112,113] Patients with gastric ulcer[64] in contrast to DU patients have both pepsin and acid outputs in the same range as nonsymptomatic controls. Considerable work has been done on serum pepsinogens in relation to peptic ulcer disease and levels are generally higher in DU patients and particularly recurrent ulcer patients prior to surgery;[10,20,50] however, measurement of serum pepsinogen levels is of limited value for clinical diagnosis and their precise relationship to the levels of pepsins in gastric juice has yet to be elucidated.

Particularly interesting in view of the increased mucolytic activity of pepsin 1 are the changes in the amounts of this enzyme in peptic ulcer disease. Pepsin 3 is the major pepsin in man, and pepsin 1 accounts for only 3.6% of total pepsin activity in nonulcer controls; however, in gastric and duodenal ulcer patients, pepsin 1 accounts for 23 and 16.5%, respectively, of the total pepsin activity present.[114-116] This ulcer-associated pepsin, pepsin 1, has been shown not only to digest mucus more readily than pepsin 3, but at the optimum pH 2.0 (2-fold greater activity) it is active at higher pH values where the difference is even more exaggerated (at pH 4 there is a 6-fold greater activity).[13] Similarly, gastric juice from duodenal ulcer patients digests mucus more readily than that from nonsymptomatic controls both at the optimum pH of 2 and markedly at higher pH values, e.g., pH 4. While the pH of the stomach is below pH 4 for much of the time, the pH of the duodenal lumen is usually above this value.[113,117] Thus, the raised concentration of pepsin 1 in the gastric juice of peptic ulcer patients would be expected to increase breakdown of the mucus barrier under conditions likely to pertain in the higher pH conditions of the duodenal bulb as well as at the lower pH conditions of the stomach.

Changes in the structure of the adherent mucus gel layer that would be predicted to impair its protective efficacy have been shown to occur in peptic ulcer disease. Analysis of mucus glycoprotein from gastrectomy specimens shows 67, 50, and 35% polymeric glycoprotein occurs in the adherent gel lining the gastric mucosa of nonulcerated, duodenal ulcer, and gastric ulcer patients, respectively.[118] These groups were statistically different from one another and in fact there was no overlap in the patients' samples for gastric ulcer and those from normal, nonulcerated mucosa. Structural studies on gastrointestinal mucus (already discussed) have shown that gel-formation is absolutely dependent on the polymeric structure of the component glycoproteins. There is a direct correlation between the relative amount of polymeric glycoprotein to lower molecular size subunit and the strength and overall stability of the gel sample as measured by rheological methods.[119] Thus, it would appear that a very much structurally weaker adherent mucus barrier covers the gastric mucosa of gastric ulcer and to a lesser extent duodenal ulcer patients than compared to the normal adherent gel. An interesting study in a rat animal model has been reported where a natural variation occurs in the percentage of glycoprotein that is in the polymeric form in nonulcerated rats.[120] After inducing chronic gastric ulceration with aspirin, a strong inverse correlation was observed between the severity of ulceration and the amount of mucin that was polymerized prior to ulceration. This preexistent potential weakness in the mucus barrier of individual rats can be related to the susceptibility of the stomach to chronic ulceration. Further evidence for a disrupted gastric mucus layer in peptic ulcer patients comes from the observation of unfixed sections of gastric mucosa.[121] In nonulcerated stomachs, a layer of translucent gel with a median thickness of 180 μm is observed, while in duodenal ulcer patients there is a significant decrease to a median of 120 μm. Adherent mucus over the antral mucosal surface of gastric ulcer patients is markedly more heterogenous than that from nonulcerated stomachs due to mixing of mucus with cellular material, making accurate thickness readings impossible. The reason for the disruption of the mucus barrier is unknown, but in part could reflect increased peptic degradation due to raised pepsin 1 levels in these patients. There are other possible explanations for the breakdown of the adherent mucus barrier in peptic ulcer patients including increased release of lysosomal proteases or colonization by proteinase secreting Campylobacter.

X. SUMMARY

Pepsins and acid are the natural aggressors secreted in the gastric juice. The dictum no acid-no ulcer has long been accepted, but it may well be that no pepsin-no ulcer equally applies. Luminal pepsin at concentrations high enough to erode through the mucus gel barrier will cause exfoliation of the epithelial layer and vascular damage. This pepsin-induced mucosal damage occurs at pH 2, whereas acid (pH 2) alone does not affect the mucosal barrier. Under normal circumstances the mucus barrier would appear to be the primary mucosal defense against pepsin with secretion of new mucus adequately replacing that lost from erosion by pepsin and mechanical abrasion. In peptic ulcer disease this adherent mucus gel barrier is impaired in a manner compatible with increased peptic erosion.

The secretory pattern of pepsinogens and their relation to the pepsins in the gastric juice is complex. Studies of pepsins in gastric juice in relation to peptic ulcer disease have lagged behind those on acid. What is clear, however, is that there are changes in the secreted pepsins as well as in the serum and mucosal pepsinogens in peptic ulcer disease. In particular there is a rise in pepsin 1 relative to the major pepsin 3 in peptic ulcer disease. Moreover, pepsin 1 has increased mucolytic activity particularly at the higher pH values (pH 4 and above) occurring in the duodenal bulb. Pepsin 1 also has increased collagenolytic activity which may further augment its aggressive potential. More studies are necessary to demonstrate quantitatively the correlation between increased pepsin aggression and peptic ulcer disease. To do this, improved methods for quantitating pepsin types in gastric juice need to be developed.

Future successful therapeutic developments in peptic ulcer disease could well be directed to selective inhibition of pepsins generally, or even at pepsin 1, together with a strengthening of the mucus barrier against peptic erosion. Such therapy would allow an acid environment to be maintained in the stomach, yet at the same time reduce aggression against the natural mucosal defenses. Current antiulcer drugs, i.e., H_2 blockers, antacids, and polyanions may well, in part, be successful due to their inhibition of pepsin activity both in the stomach and duodenal lumen.

REFERENCES

1. **Andreeva, N. S., Gustchina, A. E., Fedorow, A. A., et al.,** X-ray crystallographic studies of pepsin, *Adv. Exp. Med. Biol.,* 95, 23, 1977.
2. **Powers, J. C., Harley, A. D., and Myers, D. V.,** Subsite specificity of porcine pepsin, *Adv. Exp. Med. Biol.,* 95, 141, 1977.
3. **Ryle, A. P.,** The porcine pepsins and pepsinogens, *Methods Enzymol.,* 19, 316, 1970.
4. **Hersey, S. J.,** Pepsinogen secretion, in *Physiology of the Gastrointestinal Tract,* Johnson, L. R., Ed., Raven Press, New York, 1987, 947.
5. **Barrett, A. J.,** in *Proteinases in Mammalian Cells and Tissues,* Barrett, A. J., Ed., Elsevier/North Holland, Amsterdam, 1977, 209.
6. **Etherington, D. J. and Taylor, W. H.,** Nomenclature of the pepsins, *Nature,* 216, 279, 1967.
7. **Taylor, W. H.,** Biochemistry and pathological physiology of pepsin 1, *Adv Clin. Enzymol.,* 2, 79, 1982.
8. **Walker, V. and Taylor, W. H.,** Pepsin 1 secretion in chronic peptic ulceration, *Gut,* 21, 766, 1980.
9. **Samloff, I. M.,** Pepsinogens, pepsins and pepsin inhibitors, *Gastroenterology,* 60, 586, 1979.
10. **Samloff, I. M.,** Peptic ulcer disease. An update, in *Pepsinogens in Peptic Ulcer Disease,* Biomedical Information, New York, 1979.
11. **Roberts, N. B. and Taylor, W. H.,** A comparison of the properties of pure human pepsins 1, 2, 3, and 5, *Biochem. J.,* 128, 103, 1972.
12. **Ryle, A. P. and Foltman, B.,** Human pepsins 1 and 2 (fast pepsins). Heterogeneity and carbohydrate content, in *Aspartic Proteinases and Their Inhibitors,* Kostka, V., Ed., Walter de Gruyter, Berlin, 1985, 97.
13. **Pearson, J. P., Allen, A., Roberts, N. B., and Taylor, W. H.,** The carbohydrate component of human pepsin 1, *Clin. Sci.,* 72 (Suppl. 16), 33P, 1987.
14. **Walker, V. and Taylor, W. H.,** Ovalbumin digestion by human pepsins 1, 3 and 5, *Biochem. J.,* 176, 429, 1978.
15. **Etherington, D. J. and Taylor, W. H.,** The collagen degrading activity of purified human pepsins 1 and 3, *Clin. Sci.,* 58, 30, 1980.
16. **Pearson, J. P., Ward, R., Allen, A., Roberts, N. B., and Taylor, W. H.,** Mucus degradation by pepsin: comparison of mucolytic activity of human pepsin 1 and pepsin 3 — implications in peptic ulceration, *Gut,* 27, 243, 1986.
17. **Hirschowitz, B. H.,** Pepsinogen, *Grad. Med. J.,* 60, 743, 1984.
18. **Tang, J. and Tang, K. I.,** Purification and properties of a zymogen from human gastric mucosa, *J. Biol. Chem.,* 238, 606, 1963.
19. **Taggert, R. T. and Samloff, I. M.,** Immunochemical, electrophoretic and genetic heterogeneity of pepsinogen I, *Gastroenterology,* 92, 143, 1987.
20. **Samloff, I. M.,** Pepsinogens I & II. Purification from gastric mucosa and radioimmunoassay in serum, *Gastroenterology,* 82, 26, 1982.
21. **Mills, J. N.** and **Tang, J.,** Molecular weight and amino acid composition of human gastricsin and pepsin, *J. Biol. Chem.,* 242, 3093, 1967.
22. **James, N. G. and Sielecki, A. R.,** Molecular structure of an aspartic proteinase zymogen, porcine, pepsinogen, at 1.8Å resolution, *Nature,* 319, 33, 1986.
23. **Perlmann, G. E.,** The optical rotatory properties of pepsinogen, *J. Mol. Biol.,* 6, 452, 1963.
24. **Dykes, C. W. and Kay, J.,** Conversion of pepsinogen into pepsin is not a one-step process, *Biochem. J.,* 153, 141, 1976.
25. **Kay, J. and Dykes, C. W.,** in *Acid Proteases, Structure, Function and Biology,* Tang, J., Ed., Plenum Press, New York, 1977.
26. **Dunn, B. M., Deyrup, C., Moesching, W. G., Gilbert, W. A., Nolan, R. J., and Trach, L.,** Inhibition of pepsin by zymogen activation fragments, *J. Biol. Chem.,* 253, 7269, 1978.
27. **Kageyama, T. and Takahashi, K.,** Isolation of an activation intermediate and determination of the amino acid sequence of the activation segment of pepsinogen A, *Biochem, J.,* 88, 571, 1980.
28. **Sogawa, K., Ichihara, Y., Takahashi, K., Fujii-Kuriyama, Y., and Mummatsu, M.,** Molecular cloning of complementary DNA to swine pepsinogen mRNA, *J. Biol. Chem.,* 256, 12561, 1981.
29. **Sogawa, K., Fujii-Kuriyama, Y., Nizukami, Y., Ichiham, Y., and Takahashi, K.,** Primary structure of human pepsinogen gene, *J. Biol. Chem.,* 258, 5306, 1983.
30. **Taggart, R. T., Mohandas, T. K., Shaws, T. B., and Bell, G. I.,** Variable numbers of pepsinogen genes are located in the centromenic region of human chromosome II and determine the high frequency electrophoretic polymorphisin, *Proc. Natl. Acad. Sci. U.S.A.,* 82, 6240, 1985.
31. **Nakai, H., Byers, M. G., Shaws, T. B., and Taggart, R. T.,** Assignment of the pepsinogen gene complex (PGA) to human chromosome region 11q 13 by *in situ* hybridization, *Cytogen. Cell Genet.,* 43, 215, 1986.

32. **Franks, R. R., Pronk, J. C., Pals, J. C., Defize, J., Westervell, B. D., Meuivissen, S. G. M., Kreuning, J., and Eriksson, A. W.,** Genetics of urinary pepsinogen. A new hypothesis, *Human Genet.*, 65, 385, 1984.
33. **Taggart, R. T., Samloff, I. M., Roffel, L. J., Graham, A., Cass, C., Petersen, G. M., Rotter, J. I., Skolnick, M. H., Schwartz, C., and Bell, G. I.,** Relationships between the human pepsinogen DNA and protein polymorphisms, *Am. J. Human Genet.*, 38, 848, 1986.
34. **Hayano, T., Sogawa, K., Ichipara, Y., Fujii-Kuriyama, Y., and Takahashi, K.,** Close linkage of human chromosomal pepsinogen A genes, *Biochem, Biophys. Res. Commun.*, 138, 289, 1986.
35. **Westervell, B. D., Pals, G., Defize, J., Pronk, J. C., Frants, R. R., Ooms, E. C. M., Kreuning, J., Eriksson, A. W., and Meuwissen, J. G. M.,** Pepsinogen A polymorphism in gastric mucosa and urine, with special reference to patients with gastric cancer, *Clin. Genet.*, 30, 202, 1986.
36. **Berger, R., Bloomfield, C. D., and Sutherland, G. R.,** Report of the committee on chromosome rearrangement in neoplasia and on fragile sites, 8th International Workshop on human gene mapping, *Cytogenet. Cell Genet.*, 40, 490, 1985.
37. **Anson, M. L. and Mirsky, A. E.,** The estimation of pepsin with hemoglobin, *J. Gen. Physiol.*, 16, 59, 1932.
38. **Hunt, J. N.,** A new method for estimating peptic activity in gastric contents, *Biochem. J.*, 42, 104, 1948.
39. **Klotz, A. P. and Duvall, M. R.,** The laboratory determination of pepsin in gastric juice with radioactive-iodinated albumin, *J. Lab. Clin. Med.*, 50, 753, 1957.
40. **Ford, T. F., Hermon-Taylor, J., and Grant, D. A. W.,** A sensitive fluorometric assay for the simultaneous estimation of pepsin and pepsinogen in gastric mucosa. *Clin. Chim. Acta,* 126, 17, 1982.
41. **Rinderknecht, H., Geokas, M. C., Silverman, P., et al.,** A new ultrasensitive method for the determination of proteolytic activity, *Clin. Chim. Acta,* 21, 197, 1968.
42. **Gerring, E. L. and Allen, E. A.,** A nephelometric pepsin method, *Clin. Chim. Acta,* 24, 437, 1969.
43. **Gray, S. P. and Billings, J. A.,** Kinetic assay of human pepsin with albumin-bromophenol blue as substrate, *Clin. Chim. Acta,* 29/3, 447, 1983.
44. **Lin, Y., Means, G. E., and Feeney, R. E.,** The action of proteolytic enzymes on *N,N*-dimethyl proteins, *J. Biol. Chem.*, 244, 789, 1969.
45. **Mikuni-Takagaki, Y. and Hotta, K.,** Application of trinitrophenylation for the measurement of a-amino residues resulting from peptic digestion, *Biochim. Biophys. Acta,* 481, 631, 1977.
46. **Furihata, C., Senma, T., Saito, D., Matushima, J., and Sugimura, T.,** A new fluorescent microscopy method for pepsin using succinyl albumin, *Anal. Biochem.*, 84, 479, 1978.
47. **Hutton, D. A., Allen, A., Pearson, J. P., Ward, R., and Venables, C. W.,** Separation of pepsins in human gastric juice: analysis of proteolytic and mucolytic activity. *Biochem. Soc. Trans.,* 14, 735, 1986.
48. **Slomiany, B. L., Laszewicz, W., and Slomiany, A.,** *In vitro* inhibition of peptic degradation of porcine gastric mucus glycoprotein by sucralfate, *Scand. J. Gastroenterol.*, 20, 857, 1985.
49. **Samloff, I. M.,** Slow moving protease and the seven pepsinogens. Electrophoretic demonstration of the existence of eight proteolytic fractions in human gastric mucosa, *Gastroenterology,* 57(6), 659, 1969.
50. **Samloff, I. M., Liebman, W. M., and Panitch, N. Y.,** Serum group 1 pepsinogen by radioimmunoassay in control subjects and patients with peptic ulcer, *Gastroenterology,* 69(1), 83, 1975.
51. **Huang, S. C., Miki, K., Hirano, K., Hayashi, Y., Furihata, C., Shimizu, A., Ichinose, M., Oka, H., Matsushima, T., and Takahashi, K.,** Enzyme-linked immunosorbent assay of serum pepsinogen 1, *Clin. Chim. Acta,* 162, 85, 1987.
52. **Pals, G., Rasanen, V., Meuwissen, S. G. M., Frants, R. R., Kostense, P. J., and Eriksson, A. W.,** Enzyme-linked immunosorbent assay and radioimmunoassay of serum pepsinogen A, *Scand. J. Clin. Lab. Invest.*, 47, 29, 1987.
53. **Axelsson, C. K., Axelsson, N. H., Szecsi, P. B., and Foltmann, B.,** Determination of pepsin (EC 3.4 23.1) and gastricsin (EC 3.4 23.3) in gastric juice by rocket immunoelectrophoresis, *Clin. Chim. Acta,* 129, 323, 1983.
54. **Aoyagi, T. and Umezawa, H.,** Structure and activities of protease inhibitors of microbial origin, in *Proteases and Biological Control,* Vol. 2, Reich, E., Rifkin, D. B., and Shaw, E., Eds., Cold Spring Harbor Laboratory, Cold Spring Harbor, New York, 1975, 429.
55. **Subramanian, E., Swan, I. D. A., Liu, M., Davies, D. R., Jenkins, J. A., Tickle, I. J., and Blundell, T. L.,** Homology among acid proteases: comparison of crystal structures at 3H resolution from *Rhizopus chinensis* and *Endothia parasitica, Proc. Natl. Acad. Sci. U. S. A.*, 74, 556, 1977.
56. **Berstad, A.,** Inhibition of peptic activity in man by carbenoxolone sodium, *Scand. J. Gastroenterol.*, 7, 129, 1972.
57. **Roberts, N. B. and Taylor, W. H.,** The inactivation by carbenoxolone of individual human pepsinogens and pepsins, *Clin. Sci. Mol. Med.*, 45, 213, 1973.
58. **Tompkins, B. K., Chow, J. F., and Clarke, J. S.,** Reduction of pepsin activity by bile, *Am. J. Surg.*, 124, 207, 1972.
59. **Toshijumi, E. and Tompkins, R. K.,** Further studies on the inhibition of pepsin by bile salts, *Am. J. Surg.*, 203, 8, 1986.

60. **Samloff, I. M.,** Inhibition of pepsin aggression by sucralfate. The view from the ulcer crater, *Scand. J. Gastroenterol.,* 18(Suppl. 83), 7, 1983.
61. **Foster, S. N. E., Allen, A., and Pearson, J. P.,** A mechanism for the mucosal protective action of polyacrylates on the gastric mucus barrier, *Gut,* 26(10), A1109, 1985.
62. **Baillie, A. J. and Anderson, W.,** Macroanionic inhibition of peptic activity by high and low molecular weight macroanions, *Nature,* 218, 770, 1968.
63. **Kerss, S., Allen, A., and Garner, A.,** A simple method for measuring thickness of the mucus gel layer adherent to rat, frog and human gastric mucosa: influence of feeding, prostaglandin, *N*-acetylcysteine and other agents, *Clin. Sci.,* 63, 187, 1982.
64. **Allen, A., Hutton, D. A., Leonard, A. J., Pearson, J. P., and Sellers, L. A.,** The role of mucus in protection of the gastroduodenal mucosa, *Scand. J. Gastroenterol.,* 21(Suppl. 125), 71, 1986.
65. **Bell, A. E., Sellers, L. A., Allen, A., Cunliffe, W. J., Morris, E. R., and Ross-Murphy, S. B.,** Properties of gastric and duodenal mucus: effect of proteolysis, disulfide reduction, bile, acid, ethanol and hypertonicity on mucus gel structure, *Gastroenterology,* 88, 269, 1985.
66. **Allen, A.,** Structure of gastrointestinal mucus glycoproteins and the viscous and gel-forming properties of mucus, *Br. Med. Bull.,* 34, 28, 1978.
67. **McQueen, S., Allen, A., and Garner, A.,** Measurements of gastric and duodenal mucus gel thickness, in *Mechanisms of Mucosal Protection in the Upper Gastrointestinal Tract,* Allen, A., Flemstrom, G., Garner, A., Silen, W., and Turnburg, L. A., Eds., Raven Press, New York, 1984, 215.
68. **Sellers, L. A., Carroll, N. J. H., and Allen, A.,** Misoprostil-induced increases in adherent gastric mucus thickness and luminal mucus output, *Dig. Dis. Sci.,* 31, 91S, 1986.
69. **Rozee, K. R., Cooper, D., Lam, K., and Costerton, J. W.,** Microbial flora of the mouse ileium mucus layer and epithelial surface, *Appl. Environ. Microbiol.,* 1451, 1982.
70. **Sakata, T. and Englehart, W. V.,** Luminal mucin in the large intestine of mice, rats and guinea pigs, *Cell Tissue Res.,* 219, 629, 1981.
71. **Allen, A.,** Structure and function of gastrointestinal mucus, in *Physiology of the Gastrointestinal Tract,* 1st ed., Johnson, L. R. and Associates, Eds., Raven Press, New York, 1981, 617.
72. **Neutra, M. R. and Forstner, J. F.,** Gastrointestinal mucus: synthesis, secretion, function, in *Physiology of the Gastrointestinal Tract,* 2nd ed., Johnson, L. R., Ed., Raven Press, New York, 1987, 975.
73. **Clamp, J. R. and Creeth, J. M.,** Some non-mucin components of mucus and their possible biological roles, in *Mucus and Mucosa,* Ciba Foundation Symposium No. 109, Pitman, London, 1984, 121.
74. **Sarosiek, J., Slomiany, A., Takagi, A., and Slomiany, B. L.,** Hydrogen ion diffusion in dog gastric mucus glycoprotein: effect of associated lipids and covalently bound fatty acids, *Biochem. Biophys. Res. Commun.,* 118, 523, 1984.
75. **Allen, A.,** Gastrointestinal mucus, in *Handbook of Physiology.*
76. **Snary, D., Allen, A., and Pain, R. H.,** Conformational changes in gastric mucoproteins induced by caesium chloride and guanidinium chloride, *Biochem. Biophys. Res. Commun.,* 40, 844, 851, 1970.
77. **Slomiany, B. L. and Meyer, K.,** Isolation and structural studies of sulphated glycoproteins of hog gastric mucosa, *J. Biol. Chem.,* 247, 5062, 1972.
78. **Slomiany, B. L., Zdebska, E., and Slomiany, A.,** Structural characterization of neutral oligosaccharides of human H^+Le^{b+} gastric mucin, *J. Biol. Chem.,* 259, 2863, 1984.
79. **Pearson, J. P., Allen, A., and Parry, S.,** A 70,000 molecular weight glycoprotein isolated from purified pig gastric mucus glycoprotein by reduction of disulphide bridges and its implication in the polymeric structure, *Biochem. J.,* 197, 155, 1981.
80. **Scawen, M. and Allen, A.,** The action of proteolytic enzymes on the glycoprotein from pig gastric mucus, *Biochem. J.,* 163, 363, 1977.
81. **Kabat, A.,** *Blood Group Substances,* Academic Press, New York, 1956.
82. **Pearson, J. P., Allen, A., and Venables, C. W.,** Gastric mucus: isolation and polymeric structure of the undegraded glycoprotein: its breakdown by pepsin, *Gastroenterology,* 78, 709, 1981.
83. **Allen, A.,** The structure and function of gastrointestinal mucus, in *Basic Mechanisms of Gastrointestinal Mucosal Protection,* Harmon, J. W., Ed., Williams & Wilkins, Baltimore, 1981, 351.
84. **Williams, S. E. and Turnberg, L. A.,** Retardation of acid diffusion by pig gastric mucus: a potential role in mucosal protection, *Gastroenterology,* 79, 299, 1980.
85. **Younan, F., Pearson, J. P., and Allen, A.,** Gastric mucus degradation *in vivo* in peptic ulcer patients and the effects of vagotomy, in *Mucus in Health and Disease II,* Chantler, E. N., Elder, J. B., and Elstein, M., Eds., Plenum Press, New York, 1982, 235.
86. **Leonard, A. and Allen, A.,** Gastric mucosal damage by pepsin, *Gut,* 27, A1236, 1986.
87. **Sanders, M. J., Ayalon, A., Roll, M., and Soll, A. H.,** The apical surface of canine chief cell monolayers resists H^+ back diffusion, *Nature,* 313, 82, 1985.

88. **Schiffrin, M. J. and Warren, A. A.,** Some factors concerned in the production of experimental ulceration of the G-I tract in cats, *Am. J. Dig. Dis.*, 9, 205, 1942.
89. **Driver, R. L., Chappell, R. H., and Carmichael, E. B.,** Effect of concentration of pepsin and the differential susceptibility of jejunal segments in experimental jejunal ulcers in the dog, *Am. J. Dig. Dis.*, 9, 205, 1942.
90. **Alphin, R. S., Vokac, V. A., Gregory, R. L., et al.,** Role of intragastric pressure, pH and pepsin in gastric ulceration in the rat, *Gastroenterology*, 73, 495, 1977.
91. **Joffe, S. N., Roberts, N. B., Taylor, W. H., and Baron, J. H.,** Exogenous and endogenous acid and pepsins in the pathogenesis of duodenal ulcers in the rat, *Dig. Dis. Sci.*, 25, 837, 1980.
92. **Goldberg, H. I., Dodds, W. J., Gee, S., et al.,** Role of acid and pepsin in acute experimental esophagitis, *Gastroenterology*, 56, 223, 1969.
93. **Kivilaakso, E., Fromm, D., and Silen, W.,** Effect of bile salts and related compounds on isolated esophageal mucosa, *Surgery*, 87, 280, 1980.
94. **Kivilaakso, E., et al.,** In frog gastric mucosa *in vitro*, acid does not result in ulceration until pepsin (400 μg ml^{-1}) is added to the solution, *Gastroenterology*, 77, 31, 1978.
95. **Allen, A. and Garner, A.,** Gastric mucus and bicarbonate secretion and their possible role in mucosal protection, *Gut*, 21, 249, 1980.
96. **Flemstrom, G. and Garner, A.,** Gastroduodenal HCO_3 transport: characteristics and proposed role in acidity regulation and mucosal protection, *Am. J. Physiol.*, 242, G183, 1982.
97. **Ross, I. N., Bahari, H. M. M.,** and **Turnberg, L. A.,** The pH gradient across mucus adherent to rat fundic mucosa *in vivo* and the effect of potential damaging agents, *Gastroenterology*, 81, 713, 1981.
98. **Kivilaakso, E. and Flemstrom, G.,** Surface pH gradient in gastroduodenal mucosa, *Scand. J. Gastroenterol.*, 19, 50, 1984.
99. **Morris, G. P. and Wallace, J. L.,** The roles of ethanol and of acid in the production of gastric mucosal erosions in rats, *Virchows Arch. (Cell Pathol.)*, 38, 23, 1981.
100. **Lacy, E. R.,** Gastric mucosal resistance to a repeated ethanol insult, *Scand. J. Gastroenterol.*, 20(Suppl. 10), 63, 1985.
101. **Silen, W. and Ito, S.,** Mechanisms for rapid re-epithelialisation of the gastric mucosal surface, *Ann. Rev. Physiol.*, 47, 217, 1985.
102. **Sellers, L. A., Allen, A., and Bennett, M. K.,** Formation of a fibrin based gelatinous coat over repairing rat gastric epithelium following acute ethanol damage: interaction with adherent mucus, *Gut*, 28, 839, 1987.
103. **Allen, A., Bennett, M. K., Leonard, A. J., and Sellers, L. A.,** Pepsin and ethanol damage: two different mechanisms of response by the rat gastric mucosa, *J. Physiol.*, 391, 69, 1987.
104. **Wallace, J. L. and Whittle, B. J. R.,** Role of mucus in the repair of gastric epithelial damage in the rat. Inhibition of epithelial recovery by mucolytic agents, *Gastroenterology*, 91, 603, 1986.
105. **Hirschowitz, B. J.,** Apparent and intrinsic sensitivity to pentagastrin of acid and pepsin secretion in peptic ulcer, *Gastroenterology*, 86, 43, 1984.
106. **Rhodes, J. and Prestwich, C. J.,** Acidity at different sites in the proximal duodenum of normal subjects and patients with duodenal ulcer, *Gut*, 7, 509, 1966.
107. **Murthy, S. N. S., Dinoso, V. P., Jr., Clearfield, H. R., and Chey, W. Y.,** Serial pH changes in the duodenal bulb during smoking, *Gastroenterology*, 75, 1, 1978.
108. **Mikii, K., Ichinose, M., Furihata, C., et al.,** Potential peptic activity of pepsinogen of human gastroduodenal mucosa determined by fluorescent microassay method using succinyl albumin, *Clin. Chim. Acta*, 121, 337, 1982.
109. **Venables, C. W.,** The value of a combined pentagastrin/insulin test in studies of stomach ulceration, *Gut*, 10, 1053, 1969.
110. **Elder, J. B. and Smith, I. S.,** Gastric-acid output, pepsin output and lean body mass in normal and duodenal-ulcer subjects, *Lancet*, 1, 1000, 1975.
111. **Achord, J. L.,** Gastric pepsin and acid secretion in patients with acute and healed duodenal ulcer, *Gastroenterology*, 81, 15, 1981.
112. **Archambault, A. P., Rovelstad, R. A., and Carlson, H. C.,** *In situ* pH of duodenal bulb contents in normal and duodenal ulcer subjects, *Gastroenterology*, 52, 940, 1967.
113. **Rhodes, J., Apsimon, H. T., and Lawrie, J. J.,** pH of the contents of the duodenal bulb in relation to duodenal ulcer, *Gut*, 7, 502, 1966.
114. **Taylor, W. H.,** Pepsins of patients with peptic ulcer, *Nature*, 227, 76, 1970.
115. **Walker, V. and Taylor, W. H.,** Pepsin 1 secretion in chronic peptic ulceration, *Gut*, 21, 766, 1980.
116. **Roberts, N. B., Sheers, R., and Taylor, W. H.,** Pepsin 1 secretion in normal human subjects, *Clin. Sci.*, 61, 37, 1981.
117. **Lennard-Jones, J. E. and Balouris, N.,** Effect of different foods on the acidity of the gastric contents in patients with duodenal ulcer, *Gut*, 6, 113, 1965.

118. **Younan, F., Pearson, J. P., Allen, A., and Venables, C. W.,** Changes in the structure of the mucus gel on the mucosal surface of the stomach in association with peptic ulcer disease, *Gastroenterology,* 82, 827, 1982.
119. **Sellers, L. A. and Allen, A.,** Mechanical characterization and properties of gastrointestinal mucus gels, *Biorheology,* 24, 615, 1987.
120. **Bagshaw, P. F., Munster, D. J., and Wilson, J. G.,** Molecular weight of gastric mucus glycoprotein is a determinant of the degree of subsequent aspirin induced chronic gastric ulceration in the rat, *Gut,* 28, 287, 1987.
121. **Allen, A., Ward, R., Cunliffe, W. J., Hutton, D. A., Pearson, J. P., and Venables, C. W.,** Changes in adherent mucus gel and pepsinolysis in peptic ulcer patients, *Dig. Dis. Sci.,* 30, 365, 1985.

Chapter 4

NEURAL FACTORS AND GASTRIC MUCOSAL DEFENSE

Brant E. Victor and Thomas A. Miller

TABLE OF CONTENTS

I. INTRODUCTION

The stomach is innervated by both extrinsic and intrinsic nerves. The entire extrinsic gastric nerve supply is derived from the autonomic nervous system. Components of the *extrinsic system* consist of the parasympathetic fibers of the vagus nerves and sympathetic fibers arising from the visceral splanchnic nerves. The *intrinsic* enteric nervous *system* within the gastric wall is an extensive network of fibers composed of varying types of nerves that can function independently of the central nervous system, and is intimately related with the extrinsic system of afferent and efferent nerves. Although the intrinsic system appears to play an important role in effecting responses mediated by the extrinsic system, the two systems are clearly distinct.[1] One example of the autonomy of the intrinsic enteric neurons from that of the extrinsic nerves is the fact that gastric motility undergoes few long-term alterations after vagal and splanchnic denervation.

The importance of neural factors in maintaining gastric mucosal integrity and effecting defense mechanisms when the epithelium is exposed to various noxious insults is only partially understood. It is the purpose of this chapter to review data relevant to these considerations. Since the intrinsic nervous system has not been selectively studied with regards to induction, prevention, or modulation of experimentally induced mucosal injury, the subsequent discussion will focus primarily upon the extrinsic nervous system and the role that it may play in mucosal defense.

II. ANATOMY OF GASTRIC INNERVATION

A. VAGUS NERVES: PARASYMPATHETIC INNERVATION

The anatomy of the human, dog, cat, and rat vagus nerves is similar, although some specific differences exist which will be duly noted. In the human stomach, the vagus nerves consist of both afferent and efferent fibers. Afferent visceral sensory fibers receive stimuli from receptors within the stomach, relaying these stimuli to the central nervous system (CNS). From the CNS, long preganglionic efferent, visceral motor nerves relay information, arising from central modulation of the afferent stimuli or as the efferent link of a vagovagal reflex arc, to the intrinsic enteric postganglionic neurons for eventual excitation or inhibition of the target cells. These vagal efferent fibers arise from the dorsomedial nucleus (DMN) of the vagus located bilaterally in the floor of the fourth ventricle in the medulla oblongata. The vast majority of preganglionic nerves originating in the DMN are believed to project to the stomach based on studies demonstrating such relationships in rats.[2,3] In addition to the DMN, the ambiguous complex has also been found to contain some vagal neurons.[1,4] Further, there are higher levels of CNS input into the DMN which modulate vagal output, including input from the limbic system and hypothalamus.[5,6] From the cell bodies in the DMN, the long parasympathetic preganglionic efferent axons (comprising approximately 20% of the vagal nerve fibers) then pass through the jugular foramen and travel in the neck within the carotid sheaths being closely associated with the carotid arteries and internal jugular veins.

The vagal efferent fibers destined for the stomach usually remain within the left and right vagal trunks proper until they pass posterior to the left and right mainstem bronchi, respectively. At this level the nerves disperse, forming a plexus around the esophagus (with some fibers cross-mixing) only to amalgamate at the level of the diaphragm, usually forming discrete anterior and posterior vagal trunks. During development of the human embryo, the stomach undergoes a 90° rotation such that the closely associated left vagus becomes anteriorly positioned and the right vagus lies posteriorly (nemonic "LARP"). It should be noted that there are often single or multiple branches off the vagal trunks at the diaphragmatic level exterior to, or within the wall of, the esophagus.[7] Once through the esophageal hiatus, the anterior vagal trunk descends to the level of the gastric cardia where the hepatic branch or branches arise which travel in the lesser omentum and then form the hepatic plexus; from this plexus fibers are sent to the liver and biliary tree, as well as to the pylorus. The remainder of the anterior vagal nerve courses along the lesser curvature as the "anterior nerve of Latarjet" giving off approximately five to ten main branches that innervate the anterior wall of the stomach, extending inferiorly to the antrum. The majority of fibers in the posterior vagal trunk branch off, at about the same level as the hepatic branch of the anterior vagus, to join the celiac plexus for eventual innervation of the small intestine, proximal colon, and pancreas. In cats, vagal fibers also project as far as the rectum.[8] The remaining posterior gastric vagal nerve (i.e., posterior nerve of Latarjet) also follows the lesser curvature and with its five to six main branches innervates the posterior gastric wall.

Both the anterior and posterior gastric vagal nerves can be followed to their penetrance into the outer longitudinal muscle layer. The terminals of the preganglionic fibers typically synapse with cell bodies in the myenteric (Auerbach's) and submucosal (Meissner's) plexuses. These plexuses form part of the intrinsic enteric nervous system. The short postganglionic axons from cell bodies in the plexuses innervate cells in the mucosa (predominantly parietal cells in the fundus and antral gastrin cells), muscular layers, and blood vessel smooth muscle. There are considerably more intrinsic postganglionic fibers than extrinsic preganglionic fibers so that few extrinsic impulses can effect a magnified intrinsic gastric response.

The majority (approximately 80% or more) of fibers within the vagus nerves are unmyelinated visceral afferent nerve axons,[9] although this varies somewhat between species. From gastric stretch or chemoreceptors, afferent vagal nerves to the CNS have their cell bodies in the nodose ganglia located at or just inferior to the jugular foramen. The sensory projections continue to the medulla oblongata to form the tractus solitarius from which many fibers will terminate in the nucleus of the tractus solitarius (primarily), or to the area postrema, or to the DMN giving anatomic credence for a direct vagovagal reflex.[2,10]

B. SPLANCHNIC NERVES: SYMPATHETIC INNERVATION

The cell bodies of the splanchnic nerves to the stomach arise bilaterally in the intermediolateral cell column of the fifth or sixth to ninth thoracic (T5 or T6-T9) segments of the spinal cord. As opposed to the vagus nerves, the axons of these neurons are mostly myelinated. Preganglionic fibers pass through the ventral roots to form the white communicating rami of the thoracic nerves. From there, they pass through the sympathetic trunk ganglia (which are paired structures coursing on the right and left lateral sides of the vertebral column), the fibers from T5-T9 coalescing to form the right and left greater splanchnic nerves. It is to be noted, however, that these nerves can often vary in their thoracic spinal origin.[11] Once formed, the greater splanchnic nerves descend along the anterior or anterolateral surface of the vertebral column penetrating the muscular portion of the diaphragm to synapse with postganglionic adrenergic nerve cell bodies in the celiac ganglia located on the sides of the celiac axis. After fibers from the celiac ganglia contribute to the formation of the celiac plexus (overlying the abdominal aorta in proximity to the origins of the celiac and superior mesenteric arteries), they proceed to the stomach in association with branches of the celiac artery, with vagal nerve branches, or as discrete nerves at the level of the abdominal esophagus and proximal stomach. The splanchnic terminals richly innervate the gastric blood vessels and intramural ganglia with some, but much fewer, terminals residing in the muscle layers or mucosa.[12,13]

In addition to the efferent sympathetic fibers described above, the celiac ganglia and plexus also contain sensory afferent fibers originating in the stomach, duodenum, and pancreas. These fibers convey gastric sensations, such as pain, from gastric receptors through the celiac plexus and ganglia without synapsing on other nerves. Impulses then ascend in the afferent fibers in the greater splanchnic nerve, travel through the sympathetic trunks, and enter the appropriate thoracic spinal nerves through the white communicating rami to the cell bodies of these long axonal nerves in the dorsal root ganglia. From there, the fibers pass into the spinal cord gray matter whereupon they finally make their first synapse. Generally, one of two visceral sensory pathways then become evident: a simple visceral reflex arc or a pathway destined for higher CNS levels of consciousness. In a simple visceral reflex arc, fibers entering the spinal cord synapse upon short interneurons in the gray matter which then secondarily synapse on preganglionic efferent neurons in the lateral horn gray matter (intermediolateral nucleus of the spinal cord). The efferent pathway as described above completes the involuntary reflex arc.

The visceral afferent fibers carrying impulses which will become consciously manifest ascend to the reticular formation in the medulla and midbrain or to the thalamic nuclei after having crossed the spinal cord via the anterior commissure. Consciousness of the noxious stimuli is achieved once these impulses are relayed to the cerebral cortex (postcentral gyrus) from the thalamus. It is important to note that the brain receives visceral pain impulses (usually from intense stretching or tension in the gastroduodenal wall, but also from anoxia, inflammation, and various noxious agents and metabolites) from both sides of the body. These afferent nerves also converge upon cutaneous nerves in the same spinal cord level and brain pathways. These circumstances explain why gastric and duodenal ulcer disease is typically felt in the midepigastric region.

C. NEURAL TRANSMISSION

Acetylcholine is considered to be the predominant neurotransmitter at the synaptic junctions between pre- and postganglionic vagal nerves, at vagal nerve terminals and at the junction between preganglionic splanchnic nerves and the celiac ganglia. Most postganglionic splanchnic nerve cells upon appropriate stimulation release norepinephrine, and to a much lesser extent, dopamine. Presently, this scheme is an oversimplification as a significant proportion of autonomic fibers to the gut are now considered peptidergic instead of the classical adrenergic or cholinergic designations.[14,15] In addition, it has been demonstrated by histoimmunofluorescent techniques that adrenergic vagal efferent fibers also exist in rats, cats, and dogs.[16] That the full physiologic significance of these more recently discovered peptidergic neurons and adrenergic vagal fibers has yet to be elucidated precludes an understanding of possible pathologic roles. Thus, this discussion will primarily focus on the more "classical" roles of the cholinergic and adrenergic nerves in mucosal physiology and pathophysiology.

III. ROLE OF NEURAL FACTORS IN GASTRIC FUNCTION

A. GASTRIC SECRETION

1. Hydrochloric Acid

The most widely studied of gastric neural functions is that of the vagus and its effects upon acid secretion. Perhaps one reason for this is based on the importance of luminal acid in both human and experimental gastroduodenal ulcer production. Although most humans that develop ulcers of the stomach and duodenum are not hypersecretors of acid,[17] the dictum put forth by Schwarz of "no acid-no ulcer"[18] generally holds true.

Vagal innervation is necessary for the basal (interdigestive) secretion of acid as well as the cephalic phase of acid secretion. It is also important in modulating the gastric phase of acid production in response to a meal. In contrast, the vagi appear to be nonessential for the intestinal phase of gastric acid secretion. The three main endogenous agents stimulating parietal cell secretion of hydrochloric acid (HCl) are acetylcholine (Ach), gastrin, and histamine, each of which can be directly or indirectly influenced by the vagus nerves. Ach released at vagal and/or intrinsic nerve terminals within the oxyntic region of the stomach directly stimulates HCl secretion from parietal cells, whereas release of this secretagogue within the antral and pyloric regions of the stomach stimulates G-cells in turn to release gastrin into the bloodstream, subsequently leading to acid secretion. Ach also acts synergistically with gastrin and histamine to potentiate the acid secretory response in oxyntic mucosa.[19] Although a number of other peptides with varying functions have also been identified within vagal neurons (both centrally and peripherally) by immunohistochemical techniques,[20] their effects upon cells in the gastric mucosa have yet to be clearly defined.

During the interdigestive period, basal secretion is regulated primarily by a tonic vagal excitation upon parietal cells and G-cells, although very important differences in the amount of basal acid secretion exist among various species.[21] For instance, dogs are low (<1% of maximal acid output), humans are intermediate (approximately 1% of maximal acid output), and rats and rabbits are high (20 to 25% of maximal acid output) basal secretors.[22] This vagal influence on basal acid secretion is supported by studies in which vagotomy and anticholinergic drugs have been shown to markedly decrease basal acid production in rats, dogs, and humans.[23-26]

In considering the cephalic and gastric phases of postprandial or stimulated acid secretion, it is convenient to think of them as separate entities; however, it should be kept in mind that this arrangement is artificial and done solely for the sake of simplicity. In the "normal" stimulated physiologic state, these phases occur for all practical purposes simultaneously.

The initial stimuli producing vagal excitatory effects on the stomach during the cephalic phase include the thought, sight, smell, taste, chewing, and swallowing of food. Although it is not certain how vagal centers are activated by these stimuli, it is clear that efferent vagal fibers are the common output tract relaying impulses from these centers to the stomach for stimulation of acid secretion. In humans, vagally mediated direct muscarinic cholinergic stimulation of the parietal cells by acetylcholine is the mechanism responsible for the majority of acid secretion during this phase. The importance of the cephalic phase is exemplified by sham feeding which results in near-maximal rates of acid secretion in dogs[27,28] and from 40 to greater than 50% of maximal acid output to exogenous pentagastrin in humans.[29-31] One study even achieved sham-fed acid secretion up to 85% of peak acid output to large doses of pentagastrin.[32] Vagotomy abolishes this sham-feeding response in both dogs[33] and humans.[34] Atropine also suppresses the acid response to sham feeding in dogs[27] and humans.[35] Benzilonium, a muscarinic, anticholinergic agent as well, markedly attenuates acid secretion in humans; however, a small acid response is still obtained following such drug administration,[35] suggesting that a second agent may be partially responsible for direct vagal activation of parietal cells (in addition to Ach).

The vagi are the sole known mediators of the cephalic phase, their action being predominantly, but not exclusively, that of direct stimulation of acid release from parietal cells. They also stimulate G-cell release of gastrin in the antrum. In dogs, vagally mediated gastrin release is required for the complete stimulation of cephalic phase acid secretion, whereas in humans it may be contributory,[36] but does not appear essential to this acid response.[30,37] Nevertheless, vagally mediated gastrin release has been demonstrated in humans during this phase.[38] The mediator of human gastrin release in this phase of acid secretion is uncertain, but does not appear to be Ach, as demonstrated by the fact that atropine actually augments gastrin release.[38]

The two factors responsible for acid production during the gastric phase are a potent chemical stimulation of gastrin release by primarily peptides and amino acids within the gastric lumen,[39] which is neurally independent, and atropine sensitive cholinergic reflexes in response to gastric distension. Distension of the human stomach with saline stimulated acid secretion up to 24% of the maximal acid secretory response to histamine.[30] Balloon distension of the fundus produced graded elevations of acid output up to 50% of maximal.[40] In dogs, gastric saline distension produced progressive increases in acid output, plateauing at 40% of the maximal stimulation to exogenous gastrin.[41] Atropine abolished and proximal gastric vagotomy suppressed (although not completely) the acid response to distension in humans.[42] These observations indicate that both long vagovagal and short intramural atropine-sensitive cholinergic reflexes exist. The long vagovagal reflex is characterized by mechanoreceptor stimulation to distension in the gastric wall, with impulses relayed cephalad via afferent vagal sensory fibers to the vagal nuclei. From there, efferent signals travel down the vagi to the parietal cells. Gastrin release in response to fundic distension in the human is insignificant. There is also evidence for local, short reflexes mediating acid secretion in response to distension. These reflexes, referred to as the oxyntopyloric and pyloro-oxyntic reflexes, are mediated by intrinsic gastric neurons and are atropine sensitive as well.

The effects of the sympathetic nervous system on gastric acid output have been of interest for over 80 years.[43] Despite numerous research efforts over the ensuing years to the present day, there does not yet exist a clear, uniform opinion of its role. The reasons for this are not difficult to comprehend when it is realized that the splanchnic nerves, as well as exogenously administered catecholamines produce complex actions within the mucosa, blood vessels, and musculature of the stomach, and these physiologic actions can be interdependent. This complexity is further increased as one attempts to correlate observations noted in different animal models under various experimental conditions in response to differing types of sympathetic nerve stimulation (or denervation), or routes of administration and dosages of sympathomimetics and sympatholytics. Finally, consideration must be given to direct and reflex effects of these conditions upon the cardiovascular system that may occur which may further impact the stomach. Therefore, the generally accepted role of the sympathetic nerves will be presented, keeping in mind that there usually can be found conflicting observations in the literature.

Splanchnic nerve stimulation typically results in a decrease in gastric acid output. This is not a simple cause-and-effect relationship, however. It is well accepted that norepinephrine administration or sympathetic nerve stimulation reduces gastric mucosal blood flow.[44,45] In addition, it has been demonstrated that the sympathetically induced decrease in mucosal blood flow is followed by a reduction in gastric acid secretion.[46] These results suggest that vasoconstriction (and hence lowered mucosal blood flow) secondary to sympathetic nerve activity is the mechanism responsible for gastric acid secretion inhibition.[47] Further evidence in support of this concept is derived from work on anesthetized cats.[48] Sympathetic nerve stimulation in this experimental animal failed to significantly decrease acid secretion in response to vagal stimulation or submaximal doses of pentagastrin provided the resultant rise in systemic blood pressure was not altered and mucosal blood flow was likewise maintained. When blood pressure elevation was prevented, however, acid secretion and mucosal blood flow were significantly altered. Thus, vasoconstriction likely accounts for much of the inhibition of acid secretion.

In more recent experimentation in the dog, it has been noted that acid secretion is directly dependent on gastric blood flow only at low flow rates when oxygen delivery to, and subsequent consumption by, the tissue is severely limited.[49] Gastric acid secretion can vary independently of blood flow when the flow is sufficiently high[49,50] to provide adequate oxygen supplies. Thus, while sympathetic nerve stimulation and catecholamine (alpha and beta) administration do generally result in inhibition of acid secretion, and this inhibition is at least partially dependent on blood flow effects, whether direct inhibitory effects on the parietal cells occur has yet to be determined. Studies suggesting a possible direct inhibitory effect have utilized β-adrenergic agonists which have vasodilatory properties. Some studies have demonstrated inhibition of acid secretion by these agents despite an increasing mucosal blood flow;[51] however, there are other studies displaying contrary results.[52] Employing current technology of parietal cell and gastric gland isolation procedures, more definitive answers regarding direct effects of catecholamines on acid secretion should be forthcoming.

If sympathetic nerve fibers are inhibitory to parietal cell secretion, then gastric splanchnic denervation should expectantly aid in clarification of this issue. Unfortunately, mixed results have been obtained. Surgical sympathetectomy increased gastric acid output in rats[53] and basal and stimulated acid secretion in total pouch preparations in dogs.[54] Chemical sympathetectomy with the false neurotransmitter 6-hydroxydopamine caused an increase in gastric acid secretion in response to submaximal doses of pentagastrin in dogs[55] and an increase in gastric acid output in rats.[53] These results suggest inhibitory actions of sympathetic nerves on gastric acid secretion. In concurrence, antagonistic actions between the excitatory vagus and inhibitory splanchnic fibers have previously been suggested[56] and have been more recently demonstrated in rats;[53] however, contrary to the aforementioned studies, other investigators have observed opposing results, noting no change in gastric acid output in animals undergoing sympathectomy.[57-59] In other studies, splanchnicectomized miniature swine displayed no change in basal acid secretion from preoperative levels; however, peak acid output to pentagastrin stimulation nearly doubled.[60] In still other studies, celiac ganglionectomy in miniature swine resulted in no change in basal or maximally stimulated acid output.[61] Immunosympathectomy likewise failed to increase acid output in pylorus ligated rats.[62]

2. Mucus and Bicarbonate

The role of mucus in gastric mucosal protection remains a controversial issue as discussed elsewhere in this book (Chapters 1 and 3). By itself, mucus most likely offers very little protection against noxious insults. Likewise, bicarbonate production by the stomach, which approaches only 5 to 10% of the capability of the gastric epithelium to secrete acid, is also unlikely to offer significant protection against damaging substances by itself. When coupled together, however, a combined mucus-bicarbonate barrier may be of considerable importance in maintaining gastric mucosal integrity. Thus, bicarbonate secreted into a layer of unstirred mucus with the subsequent development of a standing pH gradient, as has been described,[63,64] would provide for a much more efficient hydrogen ion diffusion barrier. In this context, any role of the nervous system on the secretion of these substances is pertinent in a discussion of mucosal defense.

The influence of the parasympathetic and sympathetic nerves to the stomach on mucus and bicarbonate output are far from completely understood. Vagal cholinergic activity is considered one of several major stimuli for mucus secretion. It has been shown that administration of various cholinergic agents topically,[65,66] intravenously,[67] and especially intraarterially[68] results in increased mucus secretion. Further, direct stimulation of the vagal nerves has been demonstrated to elicit the release of mucus from the gastric mucosa;[69] however, not all studies have been confirmational.[70,71] The sympathetic nerves do not appear to be major direct effectors of mucin biosynthesis and/or its release in the stomach. The obscurity in this area demands further investigation before definitive statements can be made about this relationship.

In addition to its apparent humoral control, neural factors also appear to be of importance in gastric bicarbonate production. The primary neural control of gastric bicarbonate secretion is by cholinergic stimulation, which has yet to be fully characterized. During the vagally mediated cephalic phase of gastric secretion, there is an increase in bicarbonate secretion concomitant with, but independent of, hydrogen ion secretion, which is inhibited by atropine[32] and benzilonium bromide.[72] In addition, direct high strength electrical stimulation or heating of the vagal nerves in cats resulted in increased bicarbonate secretion (it was suggested that substance P was the responsible preganglionic neurotransmitter), which was blocked by atropine.[72] Alkalinization of the sheep antrum was observed after vagal stimulation with insulin-induced hypoglycemia.[73] Cholinergic agents also stimulate gastric bicarbonate secretion in humans,[74] dogs,[75] and guinea pigs,[76] among others. It has been suggested that cholinergic stimulation of alkalinization may be mediated by increases in intracellular cGMP as a second messenger.[75]

Similar to mucus, the role of the sympathetic nervous system in bicarbonate secretion is virtually unknown. In available studies, norepinephrine reportedly decreased bicarbonate secretion in the rabbit antrum[77] and bicarbonate transport in the amphibian antral and fundic mucosa *in vitro* without affecting hydrogen ion secretion.[78] In the rat duodenal mucosa, however, α_1-adrenergic agonists were found to stimulate bicarbonate secretion and this secretion could be inhibited by administration of α_2-adrenergic agonists.[79] These findings suggest that the sympathetic nerves may play a physiologic role in bicarbonate secretion, but research in this area is still in its infancy.

B. PROSTAGLANDIN METABOLISM

Prostaglandins of the E, F, and I types have been found in high concentrations in the mucosa and secretions of the stomach and intestines[80-83] in humans and virtually all experimental animals studied, although species differ with respect to the distribution of particular subtypes in the gastrointestinal tract. These prostaglandins are generally not stored,[84] but are rapidly synthetized and released upon appropriate stimulus and exert their activity at the site where they are produced.[83] Exogenously administered prostaglandins exert many effects on the stomach including inhibition of acid secretion, stimulation of mucus and bicarbonate secretion, mucosal blood flow enhancement, promotion of longitudinal smooth muscle contraction, and perhaps the mediation of a trophic action.[85,86] Taken together, these observations indicate a potentially very important role for these substances in gastrointestinal physiology.

Most of the available information suggests a role for the vagus nerves in endogenous gastric prostaglandin regulation and secretion. Vagal fiber stimulation in an *in vitro* perfused rat whole stomach preparation increased the formation and release of PGE_2 and $PGF_{2\alpha}$ from the serosal side (presumably from smooth muscle membranes).[87] Utilizing a similar model, another study revealed that electrical stimulation of the vagal nerve fibers resulted in increased release of PGE_1.[88] Because of the high luminal levels of this prostaglandin, it was concluded that the mucosa liberated more prostaglandin than the muscle. In another study, the mucosal release of PGE_1 was reduced or abolished by tetrodotoxin or hexamethonium.[88] In yet another study, it was demonstrated that elevation of a PGF_2-like product upon vagal nerve stimulation or Ach infusion occurred, and again prostaglandin from the luminal fractions greatly exceeded those of the serosal fractions.[89] Both atropine and hexamethonium individually inhibited the prostaglandin output when administered concomitantly with the stimulus. Finally, elevated fundic gastric mucosal PGE_2 levels secondary to bile duct ligation in young pigs was reduced by highly selective vagotomy.[90]

It has been further suggested that prostaglandins may mediate their effects through cholinergic pathways in the stomach[91] and other tissues.[89] Indirect evidence for this comes from the observation that prostaglandin-induced alkaline secretion in the dog stomach is abolished with concomitant atropine or tetrodotoxin administration.[92] Discordant views are derived from observations in rats in which no change in gastric PGE_1 occurred chronically postvagotomy (although the levels were measured in full thickness tissue samples),[93] nor were mucosal levels of PGE_2 acutely altered with significance postvagotomy.[94]

The role of the sympathetic nervous system in prostaglandin regulation is even less clearly understood. Sympathetic fiber stimulation failed to change the degree of formation and release of $PGF_{2\alpha}$ from *in vitro* rat stomachs,[87] yet both epinephrine and norepinephrine have been reported to increase prostaglandin synthetase activity.[95] Further studies are clearly required before definite conclusions can be drawn.

C. MUCOSAL BLOOD FLOW

Proposals attempting to explain ways in which adequate mucosal blood flow protects the mucosa from potential ulceration include (1) the maintenance of a sufficient supply of oxygen and energy substrates so that mucosal energy metabolism may effectively proceed, and (2) the maintenance of intraepithelial and intramural acid-base balance (i.e., buffering or removal by other means of influxing hydrogen ion).[85]

The gastric mucosa receives the majority of blood flow to the stomach and the corpus mucosa generally receives more than the antral mucosa.[96,97] These circumstances have important implications in the maintenance of gastric mucosal integrity. The factors primarily regulating blood flow to the gastric mucosa are the secretory (metabolic) state of the stomach (i.e., greater secretory activity demands greater blood flow) and the autonomic neural stimuli.

Vagal stimuli generally result in vasodilation and increased gastric blood flow, and splanchnic stimulation results in vasoconstriction and decreased flow. Electrical vagal stimuli in rats produce a rapid, direct vasodilation of submucosal arterioles (eliciting an increase in mucosal blood flow) independent of acid secretory enhancement.[98] This vasodilation was not affected by a dosage of atropine that inhibited Ach-induced vasodilation indicating an atropine-resistant, noncholinergic vagal effect. The responsible neurotransmitter has yet to be identified. The effect of vagotomy on gastric mucosal blood flow has been studied with regards to early and long-term changes. The initial response to vagotomy is a decrease in gastric mucosal blood flow,[99,100] which has been observed in humans and experimental animals. The chronic response to vagotomy, however, is less clear. One study demonstrated no significant long-term alterations in gastric mucosal blood flow after vagotomy,[101] while another study described depression of flow as long as 3 months postvagotomy.[100]

Stimulation of the sympathetic nerves to the stomach in experimental animals produces a submucosal arteriole vasoconstriction, resulting in a dimunition in mucosal blood flow.[102] The responsible neurotransmitter is primarily norepinephrine, mediating its effects at α-adrenergic receptors. If sympathetic nerve stimulation is prolonged, vessels may "escape" constricting influences, thereby raising mucosal blood flow[103,104] to a new steady state. In further support of the inhibitory influence of sympathetics on mucosal blood flow in the stomach, splanchnic nerve sectioning and celiac ganglionectomy in rats[105] have been demonstrated to promote mucosal blood flow. Although the effects of exogenously administered catecholamines are often complex and nonspecific, evidence exists that intravenous norepinephrine and epinephrine administration to dogs results in an initial reduction in gastric mucosal flow.[44,106,107] This is in keeping with the generally accepted view that catecholamines with predominant α-adrenergic properties stimulate vasoconstriction.

D. MOTILITY

The stomach functions to accommodate food loads, mechanically mix food with gastric secretions, triturate the foodstuffs to smaller particles, and control the rate of delivery of the resultant chyme into the duodenum for further digestion and absorption These processes occur as a result of gastric motility regulated in major part by both vagal and splanchnic nerves, and to a lesser degree by humoral effectors.

Vagal afferent nerve fibers carry information to higher CNS levels from various types of receptors in the alimentary tract, including gastric stretch and chemoreceptors. The involuntary gastric motility responses are directed to the stomach mainly via vagal efferent fibers. The efferent fibers responsible for exciting or relaxing gastric smooth muscle contractions are of two types: (1) low-threshold cholinergic fibers, which, when appropriately stimulated, result in gastric smooth muscle contractions of primarily the antrum and body and (2) high-threshold noncholinergic, nonadrenergic nerve fibers which relax the body and fundus and mediate the efferent link of receptive relaxation and gastric accommodation reflexes. These active reflexes reduce proximal stomach tone in response to sham feeding, esophageal distension, and gastric distension,[108] and are necessary for the prevention of excessively high intragastric pressures. Vagotomy severely impairs these reflexes.[108,109] Truncal vagotomy also results in an initial dyscoordination of antral phasic contractions[110] (which may, however, eventuate in a late adaptive recovery process), and this creates a delayed gastric emptying as the subsequent force of contractions is reduced.[111] Innumerable studies have shown delayed gastric emptying in response to solid meals following truncal vagotomy with increased transit time of liquids, whereas with proximal gastric vagotomy, solid meal emptying is unaffected because of the preserved nervous control of antral contractions.

The primary role of the splanchnic nerves on gastric motility is inhibitory as one might expect from recall of the effects of the well-known mass sympathetic discharge phenomena of the "fight or flight" reaction on the abdominal viscera. Once stimulated, the splanchnic nerves act upon the gastric wall smooth muscle directly and/or indirectly on neurons in Auerbach's plexus to promptly decrease antral peristaltic waves and relax the proximal stomach.[112] The responsible neurons are adrenergic. Sympathectomy results in the opposite effect, i.e., increased tone and peristaltic contractile force enhancing gastric emptying. In addition to the apparent inhibitory effect of splanchnic nerve stimulation, there is also evidence for motor excitatory properties,[113] although more work in this area is required before attributing physiologic significance to this observation.

E. EPITHELIAL PROLIFERATION

The gastric mucosa undergoes continuous exfoliation and renewal. In fact, the surface epithelium is replaced about every 3 to 4 d.[114,115] Considering the noxious milieu to which the epithelium is constantly exposed and the metabolic demands placed on it, its proliferative ability could be crucial in the maintenance of gastric mucosal integrity. Trophic influences of hormones upon the gastric mucosa are well documented. These hormones include gastrin[116,117] and epidermal growth factor.[118] Although neural factors appear to regulate tissue growth in the salivary glands,[119] and perhaps other portions of the digestive tract, a neural role for the mediation of gastric epithelial proliferation has not been well studied. A vagally mediated trophic effect has been implicated in cats undergoing central parasympathetic stimulation[120] and in the rat gastric corpus,[121] but other studies in this latter species have failed to confirm a mucosal trophic role for the vagus nerves.[122,123] It was suggested[124] that the reason for these conflicting observations was that the absence of mucosal atrophy in some studies following bilateral vagotomy was due to the rise and subsequent trophic activity of gastrin in response to both gastric distension and the change in intraluminal pH to a more alkaline environment. To avoid this potential counteracting hormonal effect, unilateral vagotomy was performed in the rat, taking advantage of the fact that each vagal trunk innervates only one side of the stomach. Pyloroplasty was also performed to prevent gastric retention. Utilizing this technique, 8 weeks postvagotomy there was no increase in serum gastrin levels, but atrophy of the oxyntic mucosa of the denervated side of the stomach was observed.[124] This recent study demonstrating a likely role of the vagus nerves in maintenance of the oxyntic mucosal cell mass should entice further research in this area.

The direct role of the splanchnic nerves in epithelial proliferation has been poorly studied; however, stress, which results in sympathetic stimulation, has been shown to alter this process.[125] Additionally, exogenously administered epinephrine or norepinephrine causes some reduction in the rate of gastrointestinal mucosal cell renewal.[126,127] Conversely, guanethidine (a selective "sympathectomizing" agent) reduced the mitotic index and lengthened intestinal cell generation cycle time.[128] Sympathectomy likewise inhibited gastric fundic mucosal epithelial proliferation.[129] It is also plausible that indirectly, through vasoconstrictive effects, the splanchnic nerves could alter epithelial proliferation by decreasing mucosal blood flow and thereby adversely affecting those metabolic processes necessary for mucosal renewal.

IV. THE ROLE OF NEURAL FACTORS IN GASTRIC MUCOSAL DEFENSE

A. PARASYMPATHETIC INNERVATION

As reviewed in the previous section, the vagus nerves play an important role in modulating both basal and stimulated acid secretion in the stomach of man and animals. Since some degree of luminal acidity, albeit at times often small, is required for the development of gastric and duodenal injury under most clinical conditions, and when gastroduodenal damage is induced experimentally, it is not surprising that altering the gastric secretory capacity of the stomach by transsection of the vagus fibers can be beneficial, not only in terms of healing a previously disrupted epithelium, but also in its prevention. In this sense, vagotomy is actually protective and assists the gastric epithelium in its ability to resist the potentially deleterious effects of various noxious stimuli. An example of this is the Shay rat preparation which consistently results in the formation of gastric erosions due to the increase in luminal acidity that occurs over time following the pylorus ligation. By blocking the capacity of the oxyntic mucosa to secrete HCl with a vagotomy, the resultant injurious effects of this increasing acidity are greatly attenuated. Various experimental models of stress that routinely result in gastric damage are also less ulcerogenic if a previous vagotomy has been performed, presumably through a similar mechanism, namely a decrease in luminal acidity.[130] Finally, a number of topical damaging agents, many of which belong to the nonsteroidal anti-inflammatory group of chemical compounds, which require an acid pH to elicit their injurious effects,[131,132] are much more innocuous if vagal innervation has been disrupted.[131,133] Examples of such substances include acetylsalicylic acid (ASA), indomethacin, and phenylbutazone.

Although the protective effects of vagotomy in the experimental circumstances just enumerated seem to be primarily mediated through inhibition of acid secretion that then results in a more alkaline intraluminal pH, evidence is also available indicating that vagotomy and various antimuscarinic agents such as atropine, pirenzipine, and probanthine can prevent mucosal damage induced by an agent like ASA independent of any direct effects on acid secretory activity, as for example when ASA is topically applied to the gastric epithelium in an acidic medium.[94,134-136] Although it has been suggested that slight, but perhaps statistically unnoted, inhibition of endogenous acid secretion by vagotomy or anticholinergic drugs in the gland depths may be responsible for maintaining mucosal integrity against injury under these circumstances,[136] this explanation appears to be highly speculative, particularly when it is realized that the pH of the luminal bathing solution remains unchanged despite these experimental manipulations. A similar protective effect upon interruption of the vagal nerves and anticholinergic administration, independent of effects on acid secretion, has been demonstrated when gastric damage was produced in rats by indomethacin.[137] Thus, it would appear that inhibition of acid secretion is not necessarily the major mechanism responsible for the ability of vagotomy or blockade of the vagus nerve by anticholinergic agents to mediate their protective effects against the nonsteroidal anti-inflammatory drugs (NSAID).

Precisely how vagotomy elicits its protective properties under some experimental conditions independent of its known effects on inhibiting gastric acid production remains to be elucidated. One report suggests that vagotomy may actually enhance resistance of the gastric epithelium to injury through direct effects on gastric mucosal barrier function. In rats in which destructive lesions were made in the lateral hypothalamus, an abrupt increase in parasympathetic activity to the stomach occurred with subsequent development of grossly identifiable gastric mucosal erosions.[138] Interestingly, this parasympathetic activity resulted in an increased "leakiness" of the gastric mucosal barrier (i.e., an increased luminal hydrogen ion loss and sodium gain with a moderate fall in the transmucosal potential difference) that was detectable even before any visible defects of the mucosa were present. Because vagotomy and propantheline prevented such lesion formation, it was suggested that the mechanism of their protective action was through prevention of barrier disruption, even though direct effects on acid secretion by these experimental manipulations could not be entirely excluded.

Another suggested possibility is that vagotomy may enhance endogenous prostaglandin production; thus, through synthesis and release of these fatty acids with their known protective effects, vagal denervation would be beneficial. This possibility seems unlikely, however, since tissue levels of prostaglandins following vagotomy or atropine administration in the rat stomach were shown not to be different from those observed in corresponding control animals.[93,94]

The importance of motility in the development of gastric damage and its prevention by vagotomy was recently examined in an indomethacin-induced gastric damage model.[139] Rats exposed to indomethacin topically were observed to have enhanced smooth muscle contractions in the stomach which were prevented by both vagotomy and atropine, such manipulations also protecting the mucosa from developing erosions in response to this damaging agent. Also note that the protective effects of vagotomy and atropine were shown to be independent of any acid antisecretory effects. Since indomethacin is known to directly affect the central nervous system in such a way that gastric hypermotility occurs,[137,139] and vagal innervation normally stimulates gastric motility, indomethacin may in part induce its damaging effects through cholinergic stimulation which then results in smooth muscle contractions and subsequent damage; by altering this reflex arc, blockade of vagal impulses by atropine or vagotomy itself would then be potentially protective. Along these same lines, phenylbutazone is also known to increase gastric motility[140] (which may be responsible for its damaging effects and the prevention of such damage by vagotomy), and electrical vagal stimulation leads to smooth muscle spasm and the subsequent intragastric pressure increases that occur result in gastric lesion formation.[141] Of additional interest, patients developing gastric ulcers appear to have an increased amplitude and duration of antral muscular contractions compared to corresponding control patients,[142] although this is not an entirely settled issue.[143]

To make matters even more confusing, evidence is also available which indicates that intact vagal innervation, rather than vagal disruption, may be beneficial under certain experimental conditions. In rats exposed to absolute ethanol, the damaging effects of this concentration of alcohol were aggravated if previous vagotomy had been performed.[91] Further, the known protective effects of 16,16-dimethyl PGE_2 in preventing alcohol injury were obviated in vagotomized rats.[91] This adverse effect on protection was noted whether the vagotomy was performed acutely or 7 d previously, thus excluding any acute trauma as being the cause of this finding. When the mucosal damaging agent was 80 m*M* aspirin, the ability of 16,16-dimethyl PGE_2 to prevent gastric injury was equally efficacious whether prior vagotomy had been performed. Of additional note, the central vagal stimulant 2-deoxy-glucose was also noted to be protective against alcohol injury, and this effect was abolished if prior vagotomy had been performed. Finally, the mild irritant, 30% ethanol, likewise lost its capabilities to prevent gastric mucosal injury induced by 100% ethanol (a process known as adaptive cytoprotection)[91] if prior vagotomy had been performed. These studies were interpreted as indicating that aspirin- and ethanol-induced gastric damage were mediated through different mechanisms and that the vagus nerve influences the ability of prostaglandin and mild irritants to prevent alcohol-induced injury.[91]

Other studies have supported these findings. In experiments using a similar rat model, the ability of prostacyclin to prevent alcohol damage was also adversely influenced by surgical vagotomy.[144] Of further note, rats subjected to chronic minimal restraint (metal ring placed subcutaneously in the back of the neck) were more resistant to alcohol-induced gastric damage as long as vagal innervation was intact.[145] This form of adaptive cytoprotection was obliterated if such animals had been subjected to prior vagotomy. Finally, a concentration of 40% ethanol which normally does not damage rat gastric mucosa was shown to be injurious under vagotomized conditions.[146]

How intact vagal innervation mediates the protective effects of prostaglandins and mild irritants or chronic minimal restraint against alcohol damage and vagotomy aggravates the damaging effects of alcohol remain to be determined. Since prostaglandins are known to stimulate mucosal blood flow, enhance epithelial renewal, and stimulate mucous and bicarbonate secretion,[147] it may be that vagal influences are necessary to modulate these potentially protective processes. Of further interest in this regard, chemical ablation by capsaicin of vagal unmyelinated afferent neurons in the rat has been shown to exacerbate gastric mucosal lesions caused by pylorus ligation and acid distention of the stomach as well as a variety of noxious agents including indomethacin, ethanol, and cysteamine.[148] Two possible mechanisms have been suggested to explain this sensory nerve-mediated gastric protection. Szolcsanyi and Bartho[149] have proposed that these afferent neurons of the vagus locally release vasodilator substances within the gastric mucosa that thereby enhance mucosal blood flow. When such sensory pathways become disrupted the relative resultant ischemia allows the mucosa to become more susceptible to injury under a given set of potentially ulcerogenic conditions. The other mechanism proposes a reflex arc between vagal afferent fibers and the sympathetic nervous system that could also ensure and possibly enhance mucosal perfusion and thereby contribute to gastric mucosal protection.[148] Such a reflex arc has been demonstrated anatomically between the vagus nerve and the celiac nerve[150] and may be mediated through β-adrenergic activation since salbutamol, a β-agonist, can reduce the incidence of acute lesion formation in the rat induced by histamine, reserpine, indomethacin, exogenous acid, and stress.[51] Of equal note, prostaglandins have been shown to interact with sympathetic nerves and indomethacin (an inhibitor of prostaglandin synthesis) increases norepinephrine turnover and its release from sympathetic nerve endings.[151] To what extent these experimental observations account for the protective effect of intact vagal innervation must await further study.

It should be obvious from the foregoing discussion that the role of the vagus nerves in mucosal defense is far from understood and will require considerably more clarification. Why vagotomy should be protective against some noxious insults and deleterious against others remains to be determined. As answers to these questions become unraveled, the means by which the stomach normally resists injury should become more clearly defined.

B. SYMPATHETIC INNERVATION

As with the vagal nerves, the physiologic role of sympathetic innervation in the pathogenesis of gastric injury and protection remains unclear. Virtually all of the available data concerning this aspect of the autonomic nervous system have been derived from studies in which mucosal injury has been induced by some form of stress. The preponderance of evidence to date suggests that mucosal ischemia secondary to α-adrenergic-mediated vasoconstriction in response to norepinephrine release at sympathetic terminals is integral in the stress-related erosive process. Surgical sympathetectomy[61,152,153] and administration of sympathetic antagonists[154-156] prevent these erosive lesions presumably by preventing significant blood flow deficits. Furthermore, endogenous norepinephrine appeared to be a major factor inducing cold-restraint stress lesions in studies using normotensive[156,157] and spontaneous hypertensive rats.[157] Clinically, this is supported by the observation that the relative gastric mucosal blood volume in patients suffering from major thermal or head injuries was reduced in those patients demonstrating mucosal lesions compared to those without lesion formation.[158]

Despite these findings which confirm what one might intuitively expect, there are other studies demonstrating diametrically opposite results. For instance, chemical sympathectomy[156,159] has been shown to render the gastric mucosa more susceptible to stress injury. Of further note, α- and β-adrenergic agonists were noted to be protective against cold-restraint stress.[160] Why such discordant findings exist has not been determined and must await further investigation. As already noted in the previous section, salbutamol, a β-adrenergic agonist, can prevent gastric injury that occurs under various vagotomized conditions[51] and lends credence to the existence of a vagal-celiac arc that may play an important role in mucosal defense under normal conditions.[148,150]

The reasons that a decrease in mucosal blood flow is likely to be responsible for the development of gastric damage under stressed conditions were previously noted. Marked "ulceration" of the rabbit gastric mucosa in conjunction with a decrease in intramural pH within the epithelium was observed in a hypovolemic shock model.[161] These observations support the notion that maintenance of blood flow and an efficient subsequent hydrogen ion disposal are important in preventing mucosal damage under such conditions. Likewise, a relative lack of adequate mucosal oxygen supplies was thought to contribute to stress injury in hypotensive rats.[162] A reduction in gastric alkaline secretion by catecholamines may also be implicated to some degree in stress injury.[78] Finally, depressed epithelial proliferation of fundic mucosa, but not antral mucosa, has been observed in rats subject to water immersion restraint stress.[163]

On a biochemical level, adenosine triphosphate (ATP) levels following hemorrhagic shock in rodents were significantly decreased, while AMP levels were markedly increased.[162] Such findings led to the proposal that cell death secondary to a deficit in mucosal energy substrates is the forerunner to the development of gastric lesion formation. In recent years, formation of oxygen-derived free radicals has also been implicated in mediating damage during ischemia and reperfusion following resuscitation in various tissues including the alimentary tract, a circumstance that appears to be greatly enhanced when ATP catabolism exists.[164,165] Also of note in regard to oxygen-derived free radical injury is the ability of sulfhydryl compounds (of which glutathione is the major constituent intracellularly) in preventing such injury, apparently through scavenging hydrogen peroxide, one of the components of the free radicals formed.[166] What role these highly damaging radicals will be shown to play in the pathogenesis of gastric mucosal injury remains to be determined.

Taken together, the thrust of these experimental findings imply that the gastric mucosa does not tolerate the anaerobic state well, and provide an explanation for the injurious effects that occur in response to vasoconstriction during stressful circumstances.

ACKNOWLEDGMENT

This review was supported in part by grant DK25838 from the National Institutes of Health.

REFERENCES

1. **Furness, J. B. and Costa, M.,** Types of nerves in the enteric nervous system, *Neuroscience,* 5, 120, 1980.
2. **Leslie, R., Gwyn, D., and Hopkins, D.,** The central distribution of the cervical vagus nerve and gastric afferent and efferent projections in the rat, *Brain Res. Bull.,* 8, 37, 1982.
3. **Norgren, R. and Smith, G. P.,** The central distribution of vagal subdiaphragmatic branches in the rat, *Neurosci. Abstr.,* 9, 611, 1983.
4. **Shapiro, R. E. and Miselis, R. R.,** The central organization of the vagus nerve innervating the stomach of the rat, *J. Comp. Neurol.,* 238, 473, 1985.
5. **Shiraishi, T.,** Effects of lateral hypothalamic stimulation on medulla oblongata and gastric vagal neural responses, *Brain Res. Bull.,* 5(Suppl. 4), 133, 1980.
6. **Innes, D. L. and Marvin, T. F.,** Gastric mucosal ulceration associated with electrochemical stimulation of the limbic brain, *Brain Res. Bull.,* 5(Suppl. 1), 33, 1980.
7. **Loeweneck H.,** Functional anatomy of the vagus nerves in the upper abdomen, in *Vagotomy: Latest Advances,* Holle, F. and Andersson, S., Eds., Springer-Verlag, New York, 1974, 6.
8. **Satoni, H., Yamamoto, T., Ise, H., and Takatami, H.,** Origins of the parasympathetic fibers to the cat intestine as demonstrated by the horseradish peroxidase method, *Brain Res.,* 151, 571, 1978.
9. **Hillap, N. A.,** Peripheral autonomic mechanisms, in *Handbook of Physiology,* Vol. 2, Sect. 1, Magoun, H. W., Ed., American Physiological Society, Washington, D. C., 1960, 979.
10. **Barber, W. D. and Burks, T. F.,** Brain stem response to phasic gastric distension, *Am. J. Physiol.,* 245, G242, 1983.
11. **Edwards, L. F. and Baker, R. C.,** Variations in the formation of the splanchnic nerves in man, *Anat. Rec.,* 77, 335, 1940.
12. **Furness, J. B. and Costa, M.,** The adrenergic innervation of the gastrointestinal tract, *Ergebn. Physiol. Biol. Chem. Exp. Pharm.,* 69, 1, 1974.
13. **Goyal, R. K.,** Neurology of the gut, in *Gastrointestinal Disease,* Sleisenger, M. H. and Fordtran, J. S., Ed., W. B. Saunders, Philadelphia, 1978, 156.
14. **Gershon, M. D. and Erde, S. M.,** The nervous system of the gut, *Gastroenterology,* 80, 1571, 1981.
15. **Polak, J. M. and Bloom, S. R.,** Neuropeptides of the gut: a newly discovered major control system, *World J. Surg.,* 3, 393, 1979.
16. **Ahlman, B., Larson, G., Bombeck, C., and Nyhus, L.,** Origin of the adrenergic nerve fibers in the subdiaphragmatic vagus in the dog, *Am. J. Surg.,* 137, 116, 1979.
17. **Grossman, M. I., Kirsner, J. B., and Gillespie, I. E.,** Basal and histolog-stimulated gastric secretion in control subjects and in patients with peptic ulcer or gastric cancer, *Gastroenterology,* 45, 14, 1963.
18. **Schwarz, K.,** Ueber penetrierende Magen-und Jejunalgeschwure, *Beitr. Klin. Chir.,* 67, 96, 1910.

19. **Soll, A. H. and Walsh, J. H.,** Regulation of gastric acid secretion, *Annu. Rev. Physiol.,* 41, 35, 1979.
20. **Dockray, G. J.,** Brain-gut peptides, *Viewpoints Dig. Dis.,* 13, 5, 1981.
21. **Mulvihill, S. J., Pappas, T. N., Garcia, R., and Debas, H. T.,** Interspecies variation in acid secretion: a comparative study, *Gastroenterology,* 88, 1511, 1985.
22. **Debas, H. T.,** Peripheral regulation of gastric acid secretion, in *Physiology of the Gastrointestinal Tract,* 2nd ed., Johnson, L. R., Ed., Raven Press, New York, 1987, 931.
23. **Hakanson, R., Hedenbro, J., Liedberg, G., and Vallgren, S.,** Effect of vagotomy on gastric acid secretion in the rat, *Acta Physiol. Scand.,* 115, 135, 1982.
24. **Antia, F., Rosiere, C. E., Robertson, C., and Grossman, M. I.,** Effect of vagotomy on gastric secretion and emptying time in dogs, *Am. J. Physiol.,* 66, 470, 1951.
25. **Gillespie, I. E., Clark, D. H., Kay, A. W., and Tankel, H. I.,** Effect of antrectomy, vagotomy with gastrojejunostomy and antrectomy and vagotomy on the spontaneous and maximal acid output in man, *Gastroenterology,* 38, 361, 1960.
26. **Peterson, J. and Grossman, M. I.,** Stimulation of gastric acid secretion by dimaprit in unanesthetized rats, *Agents Actions,* 8, 561, 1978.
27. **Nilsson, G., Simon, H., Yalow, R. S., and Berson, S. A.,** Plasma gastrin and gastric acid responses to sham feeding and feeding in dogs, *Gastroenterology,* 63, 51, 1972.
28. **Pavlov, I. P.,** *The Work of Digestive Glands,* 2nd ed., translated by W. H. Thompson, Griffin, London, 1910.
29. **Feldman, M., Richardson, C. T., and Fordtran, J. S.,** Effect of sham feeding on gastric acid secretion in healthy subjects and duodenal ulcer patients: evidence for increased basal vagal tone in some ulcer patients, *Gastroenterology,* 79, 796, 1980.
30. **Richardson, C. T., Walsh, J. H., Cooper, K. A., Feldman, M., and Fordtran, J. S.,** Studies on the role of cephalic-vagal stimulation in the acid secretory response to eating in normal human subjects, *J. Clin. Invest.,* 60, 435, 1977.
31. **Stenquist, B., Knutson, U., and Olbe, L.,** Gastric acid responses to adequate and modified sham feeding and to insulin hypoglycemia in duodenal ulcer patients, *Scand, J. Gastroenterol.,* 13, 357, 1978.
32. **Feldman, M.,** Gastric H^+ and HCO_3^- secretion in response to sham feeding in humans, *Am. J. Physiol.,* 248, G188, 1985.
33. **Tepperman, B. L., Walsh, J. H., and Preshaw, R. M.,** Effect of antral denervation on gastrin release by sham feeding and insulin hypoglycemia in dogs, *Gastroenterology,* 63, 973, 1973.
34. **Olbe, L. and Knutson, U.,** Gastric acid response to sham feeding in the dog and duodenal ulcer patients, *Acta Hepato-Gastroenterol.,* 23, 455, 1976.
35. **Stenquist, B., Rehfeld, J. F., and Olbe, L.,** The effect of proximal gastric vagotomy and anticholinergics on the acid and gastrin response to sham feeding in duodenal ulcer patients, *Gut,* 20, 1070, 1979.
36. **Feldman, M. and Richardson, C. T.,** Gastric acid secretion in humans, in *Physiology of the Gastrointestinal Tract,* Johnson, L. R., Ed., Raven Press, New York, 1981, 693.
37. **Stenquist, B., Nilsson, G., Rehfeld, J. F., and Olbe, L.,** Plasma gastrin concentration following sham feeding in duodenal ulcer patients, *Scand, J. Gastroenterol.,* 14, 305, 1979.
38. **Feldman, M., Richardson, C. T., Taylor, I. L., and Walsh, J. H.,** Effect of atropine on vagal release of gastrin and pancreatic polypeptide, *J. Clin. Invest.,* 63, 294, 1979.
39. **Debas, H. T. and Grossman, M. I.,** Chemicals bathing the oxyntic gland area stimulate acid secretion in the dog, *Gastroenterology,* 69, 651, 1975.
40. **Grotzinger, U., Bergegardh, S., and Olbe, L.,** Effect of fundic distension on gastric acid secretion in man, *Gut,* 18, 105, 1977.
41. **Strunz, U. T. and Grossman, M. I.,** Effect of intragastric pressure on gastric emptying and secretion, *Am. J. Physiol.,* 235, E552, 1978.
42. **Grotzinger, U., Bergegardh, S., and Olbe, L.,** The effect of atropine and proximal gastric vagotomy on the acid response to fundic distension in man, *Gut,* 18, 303, 1977.
43. **Pavlov, I. P. and Shumov-Simanovski, E. U.,** Innervation der magendruesen bein hunde, *Arch. Anat. Physiol.,* 53, 202, 1895.
44. **Delaney, J. P. and Grim, E.,** Experimentally induced variations in canine gastric blood flow and its distribution, *Am. J. Physiol.,* 208, 353, 1965.
45. **Guth, P. H. and Smith, E.,** Neural control of gastric mucosal blood flow in the rat, *Gastroenterology,* 69, 935, 1975.
46. **Grund, E. R., Reed, J. D., and Sanders, D. J.,** The effect of sympathetic nerve stimulation on acid secretion, regional blood flows, and oxygen usage by stomachs of anesthetized cats, *J. Physiol.,* 284, 639, 1975.
47. **Sanders, D. J.,** A review: the agents and actions of sympathetic nerve and catecholamine inhibition of gastric mucosal function, *Agents Actions,* 6, 385, 1976.
48. **Reed, J. D., Sanders, D. J., and Thorpe, V.,** The effects of splanchnic nerve stimulation on gastric secretion and mucosal blood flow in the anesthetized cat, *J. Physiol.,* 214, 1, 1971.

49. **Perry, M. A., Haedricke, G. J., Bulkley, G. B., Kvietys, P. R., and Granger, D. N.,** Relationship between acid secretion and blood flow in the canine stomach: role of oxygen consumption, *Gastroenterology,* 85, 529, 1983.
50. **Polansky, D. B., Shirazi, S. S., and Coon, D.,** Lack of correlation of gastric acid secretion and blood flow, *J. Surg. Res.,* 26, 320, 1979.
51. **Esplugues, J., Lloris, J. M., Marti-Bonmati, E., and Morcillo, E. J.,** Effects of β-adrenoreceptor drug stimulation on various models of gastric ulcer in rats, *Br. J. Pharmacol.,* 76, 587, 1982.
52. **Holton, P.,** Catecholamines and gastric secretion, in *The Pharmacology of Gastro-Intestinal Motility and Secretion, International Encyclopedia of Pharmacology and Therapeutics,* Holton, P., Section 39a, Vol.1, Pergamon Press, Oxford, 1973, A:287.
53. **Moraes, M. F., Nyhus, L. M., Kalahanis, N. G., Bombeck, C. T., and DasGupta, T. K.,** Role of sympathetic nervous system in peptic ulcer production in rats, *Surgery,* 83, 194, 1978.
54. **Oberhelman, H. A., Woodward, E. R., Smith, C. A., and Dragstedt, L. R.,** Effect of sympathectomy on gastric secretion in total pouch dogs, *Am. J. Physiol.,* 166, 679, 1951.
55. **Larson, G. M., Ahlman, B. H. J., Bombeck, C. T., and Nyhus, L. M.,** Gastric acid secretion after chemical sympathectomy, *Surgery,* 85, 534, 1979.
56. **Vizi, E. S.,** Interaction between adrenergic and cholinergic systems: presynaptic inhibitory effect of noradrenaline on acetylcholine release, *J. Neural Transmission,* Suppl. 11, 61, 1974.
57. **Baxter, S. G.,** Role of the sympathetic nervous system in gastric secretion, *Am. J. Dig. Dis.,* 1, 40, 1934.
58. **Brown, M. R.,** The effect of removal of the sympathetic chains and of the coeliac ganglia in gastric acidity, *Am. J. Physiol.,* 105, 399, 1933.
59. **Forrest, A. P. M. and Code, C. F.,** Effect of postganglionic sympathectomy on canine gastric secretion, *Am. J. Physiol.,* 177, 425, 1954.
60. **Hottenrot, C., Seufert, R. M., Kuhne, F. W., and Busing, M.,** Experimental gastric sympathectomy: an effective prophylaxis of gastric stress lesions, *Ann. Surg.,* 186, 762, 1977.
61. **Levine, B. A., Gaskill, H. V., and Sirinek, K. R.,** Gastric mucosal cytoprotection by splanchnicectomy is based on protection of gastric mucosal blood flow, *J. Trauma,* 23, 278, 1983.
62. **Rivilis, J. and Wlodek, G. K.,** Immunosympathectomy and gastric function in the rat, *Surg. Forum,* 21, 316, 1970.
63. **Heatley, N. G.,** Mucosubstance as a barrier to diffusion, *Gastroenterology,* 37, 313, 1959.
64. **Flemstrom, G. and Turnberg, L. A.,** Gastroduodenal defense mechanisms, *Clin. Gastroenterol.,* 13, 327, 1984.
65. **Allen, A. and Garner, A.,** Gastric mucus and bicarbonate secretion and their possible roles in mucosal protection, *Gut,* 21, 249, 1980.
66. **Allen, A., Holton, A., Pearson, J. P., and Sellers, L. A.,** Mucus glycoprotein structure, gel formation and gastrointestinal mucus function, in *Mucus and Mucosa,* CIBA Foundation Symposium, Pitman, London, 1984, 137.
67. **Gerard, A., Lev, R., and Glass, G. V. J.,** Histochemical study of the mucosubstances in the canine stomach. II. The effects of histamine, gastrin, urocholine, and food, *Lab. Invest.,* 19(1), 29, 1968.
68. **Zalewsky, C. A., Moody, F. G., Allen, M., and Davis, E. R.,** Stimulation of canine gastric mucus secretion with intraarterial acetylcholine chloride, *Gastroenterology,* 85, 1067, 1983.
69. **Florey, H. W.,** The secretion and function of intestinal mucus, *Gastroenterology,* 43, 326, 1962.
70. **Carne, S. J., Morrissey, S. M.,** and **Woods, R. J.,** A method for the quantitative estimation of gastric barrier mucus, *J. Physiol.,* 242, 116, 1974.
71. **Menguy, R. and Thompson, A. E.,** Regulation of secretion of mucus from the gastric antrum, *Ann. N. Y. Acad. Sci.,* 140, 797, 1967.
72. **Fandriks, L. and Delbro, D.,** Neural stimulation of gastric bicarbonate secretion in the cat: an involvement of vagal axon reflexes and substance P?, *Acta Physiol. Scand.,* 118, 301, 1983.
73. **McLeay, L. M. and Titchen, D. A.,** Gastric, antral and fundic pouch secretion in sheep, *J. Physiol. (London),* 248, 595, 1975.
74. **Feldman, M. and Schiller, L. S.,** Effect of bethanecol (urecholine) on gastric acid and non-parietal secretion in normal subjects and duodenal ulcer patients, *Gastroenterology,* 83, 262, 1982.
75. **Cheung, L. Y. and Newton, W. T.,** Cyclic guanosine monophosphate response to acetylcholine stimulation of gastric alkaline secretion, *Surgery,* 86, 156, 1979.
76. **Garner, A., Flemstrom, A. G., Allen, A., Heylings, J. R., and McQueen, S.,** Gastric mucosal protective mechanisms: roles of epithelial bicarbonate and mucus secretion, *Scand. J. Gastroenterology,* 19(Suppl. 101), 79, 1984.
77. **Fromm, D., Schwartz, J. H., Robertson, R., and Fuhro, R.,** Ion transport across isolated antral mucosa of the rabbit, *Am. J. Physiol.,* 231, 1783, 1976.
78. **Flemstrom, G.,** Effect of catecholamines, Ca^{++} and gastrin on gastric HCO_3^- secretion, in *Gastric Ion Transport,* Obrink, K. J. and Flemstrom, G., Eds., Almqvist & Wiksell, Uppsala, 1978, 81.

79. **Nylander, O. and Flemstrom, G.,** Effects of alpha-receptor agonists and antagonists on duodenal surface epithelial HCO_3^- secretion in the rat *in vivo, Acta Physiol. Scand.,* 126, 433, 1986.
80. **Bennett, A.,** Prostaglandins and the alimentary tract, in *Prostaglandins: Physiological, Pharmacological, and Pathological Aspects,* Karim, S. M. M., Ed., University Park Press, Baltimore, 1976, 247.
81. **Robert, A.,** Effects of prostaglandins on the stomach and the intestine, *Prostaglandins,* 6, 523, 1974.
82. **Robert, A.,** Prostaglandins and the digestive system, in *The Prostaglandins,* Ramwell, P. W., Ed., Plenum Press, New York, 1977, 225.
83. **Robert, A.,** Prostaglandins and the gastrointestinal tract, in *Physiology of the Gastrointestinal Tract,* Johnson, L. R., Ed., Raven Press, New York, 1981, 1407.
84. **Hawkey, C. J. and Rampton, D. S.,** Prostaglandins and the gastrointestinal mucosa: are they important in its function, disease, or treatment?, *Gastroenterology,* 89, 1162, 1985.
85. **Miller, T. A.,** Protective effects of prostaglandins against gastric mucosal damage: current knowledge and proposed mechanisms, *Am. J. Physiol.,* 245, G601, 1983.
86. **Helender, H. F., Johansson, C., Blom, H., and Uribe, A.,** Trophic actions of E_2 prostaglandins in the rat gastrointestinal mucosa, *Gastroenterology,* 89, 1393, 1985.
87. **Coceani, F., Pace-Asciak, C., Volta, F., and Wolfe, L. S.,** Effect of nerve stimulation on prostaglandin information and release from the rat stomach, *Am. J. Physiol.,* 213, 1056, 1967.
88. **Bennett, A., Friedman, C. A., and Vane, J. R.,** Release of prostaglandin E_1 from the rat stomach, *Nature,* 216, 873, 1967.
89. **Singh, J.,** Prostaglandin release from the rat stomach following vagal stimulation or administration of acetylcholine, *Eur. J. Pharmacol.,* 65, 39, 1980.
90. **Hall, A., Hickman, P., and Terblanche, J.,** Are acid and pepsin reduction the only effects of highly selective vagotomy? Evidence of changes in tissue levels of gastrin, prostaglandins, and lysosomal acid hydrolases in an experimental ulcer model, *Surg. Gastroenterol.,* 3, 34, 1984.
91. **Henagan, J. M., Smith, G. S., Seidel, E. R., and Miller, T. A.,** Influence of vagotomy on mucosal protection against alcohol-induced gastric damage in the rat, *Gastroenterology,* 87, 903, 1984.
92. **Miller, T. A., Henagan, J. M., Watkins, L. A., and Loy, T. M.,** Prostaglandin induced bicarbonate secretion in the canine stomach: characteristics and evidence for a cholinergic mechanism, *J. Surg. Res.,* 35, 106, 1983.
93. **Creaghe, S., Peskin, G., Greenburg, A. G., and Saik, R. P.,** Gastric tissue prostaglandin levels: effect of vagotomy, *Arch. Surg.,* 114, 331, 1979.
94. **Foschi, D., Ferrante, F., Varin, L., Del Soldeto, P., and Rovati, V.,** Protection of gastric mucosa in rats: differences between vagotomy, atropine, and PGE_2, *Dig. Dis. Sci.,* 31(3), 289, 1986.
95. **Pace-Asciak, C.,** Prostaglandin synthetase activity in the rat stomach fundus, *Biochim. Biophys. Acta,* 280, 161, 1972.
96. **Archibald, C. H., Moody, F. G., and Simons, M.,** Measurement of gastric blood flow with radioactive microspheres, *J. Appl. Physiol.,* 38(6), 1051, 1975.
97. **Delaney, J. P. and Grim, E.,** Canine gastric blood flow and its distribution, *Am. J. Physiol.* 207(6), 1195, 1964.
98. **Morishita, T. and Guth, P. H.,** Vagal nerve stimulation causes noncholinergic dilatation of gastric arterioles, *Am. J. Physiol.,* 250(13), G660, 1986.
99. **Mackie, D. B. and Turner, M. D.,** Vagotomy and submucosal blood flow, *Arch. Surg.,* 102, 626, 1971.
100. **Nakamura, K., Ishi, K., Kusano, M., and Hayashi, S.,** Acute and long term effects of vagotomy on gastric mucosal blood flow, in *Vagotomy: Latest Advances with Special Reference to Gastrin and Duodenal Ulcer,* Holle, F. and Anderson, S., Eds., Springer-Verlag, New York, 1974, 109.
101. **Delaney, J. P.,** Chronic alterations in gastrointestinal blood flow induced by vagotomy, *Surgery,* 62, 155, 1967.
102. **Guth, P. H. and Smith, E.,** Nervous regulation of the gastric microcirculation, in *Nerves and The Gut,* Brooks, F. P. and Evers, P. W., Eds., Charles B. Slack, New York, 1977, 365.
103. **Jansson, E. D., Kampp, M., Lundgren, O., and Martinson, J.,** Studies on the circulation of the stomach, *Acta Physiol. Scand.,* 68, (Suppl. 277), 91, 1966.
104. **Guth, P. H. and Smith, E.,** Escape from vasoconstriction in the gastric microcirculation, *Am. J. Physiol.,* 223, 1893, 1975.
105. **Arabehety, J. T., Dolcini, H. A., and Gray, S. J.,** Sympathetic influences on circulation of the gastric mucosa of the rat, *Am. J. Physiol.,* 197, 915, 1959.
106. **Zinner, M. J., Kerr, J. C., and Reynolds, D. J.,** Adrenergic mechanisms in canine gastric circulation, *Am. J. Physiol.,* 229, 977, 1975.
107. **Jacobson, E. D., Linford, R. H., and Grossman, M. I.,** Gastric secretion in relation to mucosal blood flow studied by clearance technic, *J. Clin. Invest.,* 45, 1, 1966.
108. **Jahnberg, T.,** Gastric adaptive relaxation: effects of vagal activation and vagotomy—an experimental study in dogs and in man, *Scand. J. Gastroenterol.,* 12, (Suppl. 46), 5, 1977.
109. **Staadas, J. O.,** Intragastric pressure/volume relationship before and after proximal truncal vagotomy, *Scand. J. Gastroenterol.,* 10, 129, 1975.

110. **Papasora, M. and Atanassova, E.,** Changes in bioelectric activity of the stomach after bilateral transthoracal vagotomy, *Bull. Inst. Physiol.,* 14, 121, 1972.
111. **Wilbur, B. G. and Kelly, K. A.,** Effects of proximal gastric, complete gastric, and truncal vagotomy on canine gastric electric activity, motility and emptying, *Ann. Surg.,* 178, 295, 1973.
112. **Roman, C. and Gonella, J.,** Extrinsic control of digestive tract motility, in *Physiology of the Gastrointestinal Tract,* 2nd ed., Johnson, L. R., Ed., Raven Press, New York, 1987, 507.
113. **Nakazato, Y., Saito, K., and Ohga, A.,** Gastric motor and inhibitor response to stimulation of the sympathetic nerve in the dog, *Jpn. J. Pharmacol.,* 20, 131, 1970.
114. **Creamer, B., Shorter, R. G., and Barnforth, J.,** The turnover and shedding of epithelial cells. I. The turnover in the gastrointestinal tract, *Gut,* 2, 110, 1961.
115. **McDonald, C., Trier, J. S., and Everett, B.,** Cell proliferation and migration in the stomach, duodenum and rectum of man, *Gastroenterology,* 46, 405, 1964.
116. **Johnson, L. R.,** New aspects of the trophic action of gastrointestinal hormones, *Gastroenterology,* 72, 788, 1977.
117. **Solomon, T. E.,** Trophic effects of pentagastrin on the gastrointestinal tract in fed and fasted rats, *Gastroenterology,* 91, 108, 1986.
118. **Johnson, L. R. and Guthrie, P. D.,** Stimulation of rat oxyntic gland mucosal growth by epidermal growth factor, *Am. J. Physiol.,* 238, G45, 1980.
119. **Schneyer, C. A. and Hall, H. D.,** Autonomic regulation of postnatal changes in cell number and size of rat parotid, *Am. J. Physiol.,* 219, 1268, 1970.
120. **Pearl, J. M., Ritchie, W. P., and Gilsdorf, R. B.,** Hypothalamic stimulation of feline gastric mucosal cellular populations, *JAMA,* 195, 141, 1966.
121. **Llavag, I. and Vaage, S.,** The effect of vagotomy and pyloroplasty on the gastrointestinal mucosa of the rat, *Scand. J. Gastroenterol.,* 7, 23, 1972.
122. **Crean, G. P., Gunn, A. A., and Rumsey, R. D. E.,** The effect of vagotomy on the gastric mucosa of the rat, *Scand. J. Gastroenterol.,* 4, 675, 1969.
123. **Ley, R., Willems, G., and Vansteenkiste, Y.,** Influence of vagotomy on parietal cell kinetics in the rat gastric mucosa, *Gastroenterology,* 65, 764, 1973.
124. **Hakanson, R., Vallgren, S., Ekelund, M., Rehfeld, J. F., and Sundler, F.,** The vagus exerts trophic control of the stomach in the rat, *Gastroenterology,* 86, 28, 1984.
125. **Eastwood, G. L.,** Effects of ulcerogens on gastroduodenal epithelial proliferation, in *Mechanisms of Mucosal Protection in the Upper Gastrointestinal Tract,* Allen, A., et al., Eds., Raven Press, New York, 1984, 27.
126. **Bullough, W. S. and Laurence, E. B.,** Mitotic control by internal secretion: the role of the chalone-adrenaline complex, *Exp. Cell Res.,* 33, 176, 1964.
127. **Epifanova, O. I. and Tchoumak, M. G.,** On the action of adrenalin upon the mitotic cycle of the intestinal epithelium in mice, *Cytologia,* 5, 455, 1963.
128. **Klein, R. M. and Torres, J., Jr.,** Analysis of intestinal cell proliferation after guanethidine-induced sympathectomy, *Cell. Tissue Res.,* 195, 239, 1978.
129. **Kuwayama, J., et al.,** Effects of vagotomy and of sympathectomy on gastric pH, serum gastrin, gastrin cell proliferation and epithelial proliferation in rat stomach, *Dig. Dis. Sci.,* 30(4), 1985.
130. **Legros, G. and Griffith, C. A.,** The anatomic basis for the variable adequacy of incomplete vagotomy. I. The various secretory and ulcerogenic potentials of various anatomic types of incomplete vagotomy in Shay rats, *Ann. Surg.,* 168, 1030, 1968.
131. **Brodie, D. A. and Chase, B. J.,** Role of gastric acid in aspirin-induced irritation in the rat, *Gastroenterology,* 63, 604, 1967.
132. **Davenport, H. W.,** Salicylate damage to the gastric mucosal barrier, *N. Engl. J. Med.,* 276, 1307, 1967.
133. **Brodie, D. A. and Chase, B. J.,** Evaluation of gastric acid as a factor in drug-induced gastric hemorrhage in the rat, *Gastroenterology,* 56, 206, 1969.
134. **Rovati, V., Foschi, D., Ferrante, F., Del Soldato, P., Daniotti, S., and Varin, L.,** Cytoprotection by PGE_2, atropine, pirenzipine, and vagotomy in rats, *Scand. J. Gastroenterol.,* 17(572), 261, 1982.
135. **Konturek, S. J., Brzozowski, T., Radecki, T., and Piastucki, I.,** Gastric cytoprotection by pirenzipine: role of endogenous prostaglandins, *Scand. J. Gastroenterol.,* 17(572), 255, 1982.
136. **Guth, P. H., Aures, D., and Paulson, G.,** Topical aspirin plus HCl gastric lesions in the rat: cytoprotective effects of prostaglandin, cimetidine, and probanthine, *Gastroenterology,* 76, 88, 1979.
137. **Mersereau, W. A. and Hinchey, E. J.,** Prevention of indomethacin-induced gastric hypercontractility: a mucosal protective mechanism of prostaglandin E_2, *Gastroenterology,* 78, 1221, 1980.
138. **Grijalva, C. V., Deregnaucourt, J., Code, C. F., and Novin, D.,** Gastric mucosal damage in rats induced by lateral hypothalamic lesions: protection by propantheline, cimetidine and vagotomy, *Proc. Soc. Exp. Biol. Med.,* 163, 528, 1980.

139. **Takeuchi, K., Ueki, S., and Okabe, S.,** Importance of gastric motility in the pathogenesis of indomethacin-induced gastric lesions in rats, *Dig. Dis. Sci.*, 31, 1114, 1986.
140. **Mersereau, W. A. and Hinchey, E. J.,** Prevention of phenylbutazone ulcer in the rat by glucose: role of a glycoprivic receptor system, *Am. J. Physiol.*, 242, G429, 1982.
141. **Qvist, G., Dormandy, J., Brown, C., Slome, D., and Scott, G. B. D.,** The experimental production of gastric ulcers by induced muscle spasm, *Br. J. Surg.*, 61, 259, 1974.
142. **Liebermann-Meffert, D., Muller, C., and Allgower, M.,** Gastric hypermotility and antro-pyloric dysfunction in gastric ulcer patients, *Br. J. Surg.*, 69, 11, 1982.
143. **Garrett, J. M., Summerskill, W. H. J., and Code, C. F.,** Antral motility in patients with gastric ulcer, *Am. J. Dig. Dis.*, 11, 780, 1966.
144. **Mozsik, G. Y., Moron, F., and Javor, T.,** Cellular mechanisms of the development of gastric mucosal damage and of gastrocytoprotection induced by prostacyclin in rats: a pharmacological study, *Prostaglandins Leukotrienes Med.*, 9, 71, 1982.
145. **Wallace, J. L., Morris, G. P., and Cohen, M. M.,** Gastric mucosal protection by chronic restraint: effects of vagotomy, *Am. J. Physiol.*, 248, G35, 1985.
146. **Foschi, D., Ferrante, F., Cavagna, G., Callioni, F., and Rovati, V.,** Role of the vagus nerve in gastric damage and protection: an experimental study in rats, *Dig. Surg.*, 1(Abstr.), 154, 1984.
147. **Miller, T. A.,** Gastroduodenal mucosal defense: factors responsible for the stomach and duodenum's ability to resist injury, *Surgery*, 103, 389, 1988.
148. **Holzer, P. and Sametz, W.,** Gastric mucosal protection against ulcerogenic factors in the rat mediated by capsaicin-sensitive afferent neurons, *Gastroenterology*, 91, 975, 1986.
149. **Szolcsanyi, J. and Bartho, L.,** Impaired defense mechanism to peptic ulcer in the capsaicin-desensitized rat, in *Gastrointestinal Defense Mechanisms*, Vol. 15, Mozsik, G. Y., Hanninen, O., and Javor, T., Eds., Pergamon Press and Akademiai Kiado, Oxford and Budapest, 1981, 39.
150. **Niijima, A.,** Electrophysiological study on nervous pathway from splanchnic nerve to vagus nerve in rat, *Am. J. Physiol.*, 244, R888, 1983.
151. **Westfall, T. C.,** Local regulation of adrenergic neurotransmission, *Physiol. Rev.*, 57, 659, 1977.
152. **Holmes, T. W., Jr.,** An evaluation of celiac ganglionectomy in the prevention of experimental peptic ulcer, *Ann. Surg.*, 138, 240, 1953.
153. **Hottenrott, C., Seufert, R. M., Kuhne, F. W., and Busing, M.,** Experimental gastric sympathectomy: an effective prophylaxis of stress lesions, *Arch. Surg.*, 186, 762, 1977.
154. **Menguy, R. and Masters, Y. F.,** Mechanism of stress ulcer: influence of alpha-adrenergic blockade on stress ulceration and gastric mucosal energy metabolism, *Am. J. Dig. Dis.*, 23, 493, 1978.
155. **Feifel, G.,** Experimentelle Untersuchungen zur Pathogenese Akuter Erosionen und Ulcera des Magens, Thesis University of Munich, 1971.
156. **Djahanguiri, B., Taubin, H. L., and Landsberg, L.,** Increased sympathetic activity in the pathogenesis of restraint ulcer in rats, *J. Pharm. Exp. Ther.*, 184, 163, 1973.
157. **Goldenberg, M. M.,** Stress-induced gastric lesions in spontaneously hypertensive rats, *Dig. Dis.*, 19, 353, 1974.
158. **Kamada, T., Sato, N., Kawano, S., et al.,** Gastric mucosal hemodynamics after thermal or head injury, *Gastroenterology*, 83, 535, 1982.
159. **Toth, T.,** The effect of chemiosympathectomy on the incidence of stress-induced gastric erosions, *Br. J. Exp. Pathol.*, 67, 349, 1986.
160. **Orlando, R. C., Hernandez, D. E., Prange, A. J., Jr., and Nemeroff, C. B.,** Role of the autonomic nervous system in the cytoprotective effect of neurotensin against gastric stress ulcers in rats, *Psychoneuroendocrinology*, 10, 149, 1985.
161. **Kivilaakso, E., Fromm, D., and Silen, W.,** The effect of the acid secretory state on intramural pH of rabbit gastric mucosa, *Gastroenterology*, 75, 641, 1978.
162. **Menguy, R., Desbaillets, L., and Masters, Y. F.,** Mechanism of stress ulcer: influence of hypovolemic shock on energy metabolism in the gastric mucosa, *Gastroenterology*, 66, 46, 1974.
163. **Kuwayama, H. and Eastwood, G. L.,** Effects of water immersion restraint stress and chronic indomethacin ingestion on gastric antral and fundic epithelial proliferation, *Gastroenterology*, 88, 362, 1985.
164. **Parks, D. A. and Granger, D. N.,** Ischemia-induced vascular changes: role of xanthine oxidase and hydroxyl radicals, *Am. J. Physiol.*, 245, G285, 1983.
165. **Granger, D. N., Rutili, G., and McCord, J. M.,** Superoxide radicals in feline intestinal ischemia, *Gastroenterology*, 81, 22, 1981.
166. **Lash, L. H., Hagen, T. M., and Jones, D. P.,** Exogenous glutathione protects intestinal epithelial cells from oxidative injury, *Proc. Natl. Acad. Sci. U. S. A.*, 83, 4641, 1986.

Chapter 5

GUT PEPTIDES IN PROTECTION AND DAMAGE OF THE GASTROINTESTINAL MUCOSA

Stanislaw J. Konturek

TABLE OF CONTENTS

I. INTRODUCTION

The gastrointestinal tract, particularly the stomach, is constantly exposed to various irritating and damaging factors, including its own acid-pepsin secretion, bile refluxed from the duodenum, foods at various temperatures and pH, microorganisms, and sometimes alcohol and drugs. In spite of the constant exposure to this hostile environment, the mucosa is usually able to maintain its integrity and withstand the presence of irritants and ulcerogens without being damaged. The protective mechanisms are not, however, unlimited and severe mucosal insults during reduced mucosal resistance may eventually lead to acute or chronic damage in the form of localized erosions, ulcerations, or gastritis.

The gastrointestinal mucosa has the capability to produce a variety of biologically active substances such as the metabolites of arachidonic acid, the hormonal peptides, biogenic amines, and others. These substances have been shown to affect different functions of the mucosa including secretion, blood flow, synthesis of biomolecules, permeability, growth, and integrity. The metabolites of arachidonic acid (eicosanoids), such as prostaglandins (PG), have been implicated in the protection of the cells (cytoprotection) of the gastrointestinal tract from damage induced by various irritants and ulcerogens. This phenomenon, studied most extensively in the stomach, has been divided into direct cytoprotection, in which the protective eicosanoid is administered exogenously, and adaptive cytoprotection, which is mediated by PG generated endogenously. Other products of arachidonate metabolism, such as thromboxanes (Tx) and leukotrienes (LT), appear to be mediators of tissue ischemia and damage.

The gastrointestinal tract is also the largest endocrine organ of the body containing a large number of biologically active peptides. Some of these peptides function as circulating hormones (e.g., gastrin, cholecystokinin, secretin), some are localized to nerve terminals and act as neurotransmitters (e.g., vasoactive intestinal peptide — VIP), some are active locally in the tissues having mainly paracrine effects (e.g., somatostatin), and others are released into the gut lumen (e.g., epidermal growth factor — EGF). The release of the hormonal peptides may be affected by feeding and remains, in part, under neural control.

This chapter reviews the involvement of the gut hormones in the maintenance of the integrity of the gastrointestinal mucosa and its protection against various ulcerogens. As mucosal integrity requires normal cell proliferation and growth and adequate blood supply to meet the metabolic needs, the hormonal peptides affecting mucosal growth and circulation have been implicated in the mucosal protection.

II. PROTECTION BY HORMONAL PEPTIDES AFFECTING MUCOSAL GROWTH AND REPAIR

The mucosa of the gastrointestinal tract is one of the most rapidly proliferating tissues in the body. Proliferation and growth are balanced by cell loss through exfoliation of the surface cells so that under normal conditions the cell population is maintained at a dynamic steady state.[1] Most newly produced cells migrate rapidly from the regenerative zone to the surface and differentiate into the mucous cells of the surface epithelium. The migration time required to replace the total surface epithelial cell layer is about 3 d in the rat[2] and 4 to 6 d in man.[3,4] Because of the rapid turnover of mucosal cell populations, any alteration in the processes regulating growth is likely to produce functional changes and may lead either to mucosal atrophy or ulcerations when the cell loss exceeds cell regeneration or to hyperplasia when the production of the cell is increased or their life is prolonged.

The growth of the mucosa is affected by a variety of factors, such as nongastrointestinal hormones (e.g., thyroxine, growth hormone) and gut hormonal peptides, particularly epidermal growth factor (EGF), gastrin, and somatostatin. Some of these are brought into play by ingestion and digestion of food and act by endocrine, paracrine, or exocrine (luminal) pathways.

Certain food products, as well as the exposure of the gastric mucosa to damaging agents such as aspirin,[4] ethanol,[5] bile salts,[6] hyperosmolar NaCl,[7] or stress,[8] may cause extensive injury of the surface epithelium with the loss of the continuity of this layer and denudation of the basal membrane. As described by Davenport,[9] such mucosal damage breaks the "mucosal barrier" which normally impedes diffusion of H^+ from the lumen to the mucosa and the movement of Na^+ from the interstitial space to the lumen. It also causes a profound decrease in the electrical potential difference (PD) across the mucosal membrane and this PD has been used as an index of the integrity of the mucosal barrier.[9] Hollander[11] suggested a two-component hypothesis for the gastric mucosal barrier, one being the surface mucus gel, and the other being the anatomical integrity of the surface epithelium. He was the first to recognize the extraordinary rapidity of the restoration of surface epithelium after injury, the phenomenon now called "restitution".[7,12] The restitution process occurs within minutes after mucosal damage and involves the migration of remaining viable cells from the area adjacent to or just beneath the injured surface cells to cover the denuded basal membrane. It does not depend upon cell differentiation and replication at the regeneration zone distinguishing it from the healing process, but does depend upon the inherent properties of the differentiated epithelial cells themselves to cover the superficial defect of the mucosa. It has been shown (e.g., in rat stomach exposed to luminal ethanol) that the early phase of restitution begins within 5 min of injury, and by 1 h after injury, greater than 90% of the mucosa is reepithelialized. Little is known about the nature of early reepithelialization after gastric mucosal damage, but recent reports indicate that the activation of ornithine decarboxylase (ODs), an enzyme responsible for polyamine synthesis, plays significant roles in protecting the mucosa from further damage and in mucosal restitution after damage.[13] Indeed, polyamines, which are absolutely required for the mucosal growth,[14] have been shown to protect the mucosa against the injury induced by ethanol.[15] The stimulation of ODs by hyperosmolar solutions of NaCl or by acidified aspirin has been suggested to account for the prevention of, or the recovery from, the damage caused by these irritants.[13] It remains to be determined what the influence of hormonal peptides protecting the mucosa is on the restitution process and polyamine synthesis.

III. EGF IN MUCOSAL PROTECTION AND INTEGRITY

EGF was originally isolated by Cohen[16] from the mouse submaxillary glands and shown by Savage et al.[17] to be a polypeptide containing 53 amino acids. It was found to resemble urogastrone, another peptide isolated from urine, composed of 37 amino acids which are identical to those of EGF.

Urogastrone was discovered following the observation that the extracts of urine from pregnant women had beneficial effects on healing of chronic ulcers in Mann-Williamson dogs.[18] Since urogastrone given parenterally caused a potent inhibition of gastric acid secretion, the question remained as to whether the observed ulcer healing could be attributed to its antisecretory effect or to another action. The fact that the increased ulcer healing occurred in a dose range that was incapable of inhibiting gastric secretion in normal or Mann-Williamson ulcer dogs was taken as evidence that some other factor than acid inhibition was the major factor in the antiulcer action of urogastrone.

EGF shares the gastric inhibitory effect or urogastrone that was demonstrated both *in vivo* in dogs with gastric fistulas and denervated fundic pouches[19] and in *in vitro* isolated gastric glands.[20] Moreover, urogastrone was found to compete with EGF for receptor sites on cultured human fibroblasts.[21]

Both EGF and urogastrone stimulated the growth of cultured fibroblasts[21] and increased the weight and the content of DNA and RNA in the gastric mucosa of rats,[22] indicating the potent growth-promoting action of these peptides on the gastroduodenal mucosa. Feldman et al.[23] demonstrated that EGF stimulates ODs activity in the stomach and duodenum of newborn mice.

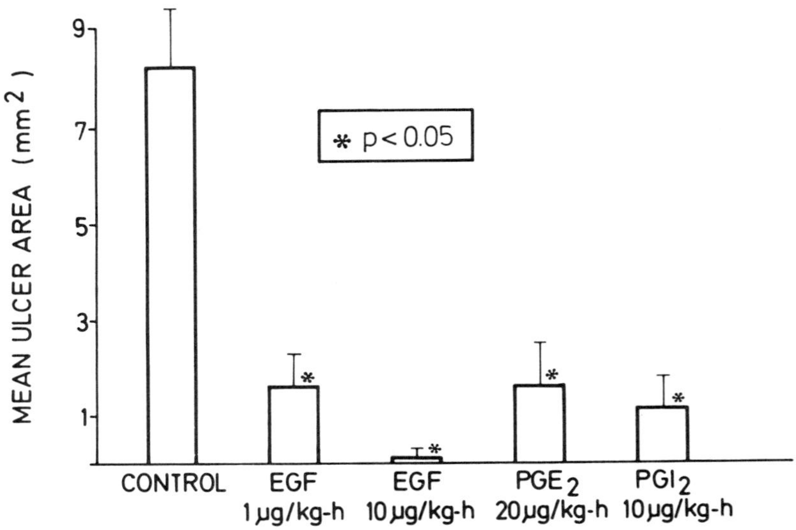

FIGURE 1. Effects of subcutaneous infusion of EGF at a dose of 1 or 10 µg/kg/h and of PGE_2 or PGI_2 at respective doses of 20 and 10 µg/kg/h given 30 min before and during 3 h intragastric administration of acidified ASA (100 mg/kg) on mean area of ASA-induced gastric ulcerations in rats. Each column represents mean ± SEM of 8 to 10 experiments. Asterisks indicate significant decreases below the control value obtained with ASA alone without EGF.

Since ODs is the rate-limiting enzyme in the synthesis of polyamines, which in turn are required for RNA synthesis[24] and for growth,[14] the induction of ODs activity by EGF may be used as an index of its trophic effect on the mucosa. Johnson and Guthrie,[25] who compared the trophic effects of EGF and gastrin, revealed that EGF was a potent stimulator of DNA synthesis with maximal effect similar to that of pentagastrin. Chronic administration of EGF (5 d) led to significant increases in gastric mucosal DNA, RNA, and protein content. These results confirmed and reinforced the finding that EGF is a trophic agent for the gastroduodenal mucosa and that EGF-induced mitogenesis is independent from its acid inhibitory effect.

Since it is unlikely that EGF is released into the bloodstream in physiologically important amounts, there is considerable interest in the peptide as a luminal growth factor. The major sources of luminal EGF are salivary and Brunner's glands.[26,27] EGF enters the gastrointestinal tract in large amounts with salivary and duodenal secretions,[28-31] and is quite resistant to both degradation by gastric proteases[16,17] and to absorption in the intestine.[32] It initiates its action by binding to specific receptors which have been found in the gastric and intestinal mucosa.[33,34] The trophic action of EGF was observed after its oral administration,[35,36] although oral EGF was without gastric inhibitory effects.[35] These findings indicate that luminal EGF may play an important physiological role in the stimulation of mucosal cell proliferation and maintenance of the integrity of the gastrointestinal mucosa.

The importance of the salivary glands in the protective mechanism and integrity of the gastrointestinal mucosa has been emphasized previously,[37,38] but the active component has not been identified. We[39] reported that EGF, given parenterally in nonantisecretory doses, dose-dependently prevented aspirin (acetylsalicylic acid — ASA)-induced ulcers and this effect was similar to that obtained with nonantisecretory doses of PGE_2 or PGI_2 (Figure 1). Since the formation of ASA-induced gastric ulcerations was accompanied by almost complete suppression of mucosal generation of PG and since EGF by itself did not affect the biosynthesis of PG in the intact mucosa nor was able to overcome the ASA-induced fall in PG formation (Figure 2), we concluded that the EGF-induced protection of the gastric mucosa against injury by ASA

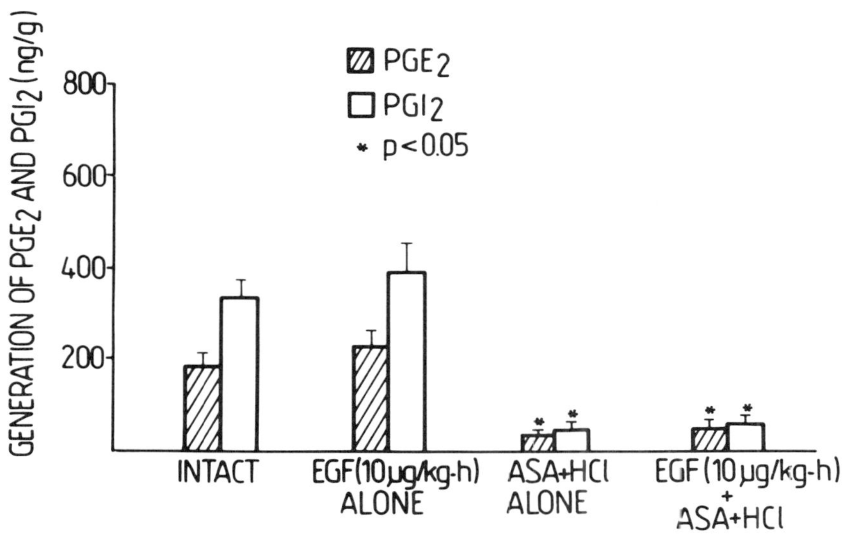

FIGURE 2. Mucosal generation of PGE_2 and PGI_2 determined by specific radioimmunoassay in the intact oxyntic mucosa and following pretreatment with s.c. EGF (10 µg/kg/h) alone for a 3-h period and after 3 h of exposure to acidified ASA alone or combined with s.c. EGF (10 µg/kg/h), as in the tests shown in Figure 1.

was unrelated to the generation of mucosal PG. Direct measurement of PG biosynthesizing capability of the gastric mucosa without and with exposure to ASA confirmed that EGF failed to influence the content of mucosal PG. Thus, the evidence was obtained that gastric cytoprotection is not the unique property of PG and that EGF could play a physiological role in mucosal protection. This has been supported by the finding[35] that intragastric administration of EGF in nonantisecretory doses also dose-dependently prevented the formation of ASA-induced gastric ulcers without affecting PG generation in the gastric mucosa (Figure 3).

The gastroprotective action of saliva and EGF has been confirmed by Olsen et al.,[41] who demonstrated that the removal of submandibular glands resulted in a dramatic fall (by about 90%) of the gastric content of EGF. Although the sialoadenectomized animals did not develop spontaneous gastric lesions, the administration of cysteamine prompted the formation of such ulcerations. Cysteamine by itself greatly suppressed the production of EGF by Brunner's glands (but not by salivary glands) and resulted in the formation of typical ulcerations only in the duodenum. Since intragastric administration of saliva containing EGF or EGF itself in a nonantisecretory dose prevented cysteamine-induced formation of gastric ulcers, it has been postulated that EGF in saliva is an active component responsible for the protection of the gastric mucosa.

It is of interest that EGF given intragastrically or parenterally only partly reduced the mucosal damage caused by necrotizing agents such as absolute ethanol or 25% NaCl, which are frequently used in studies of gastric cytoprotection[42] (Figure 4). This indicates that the spectrum of gastroprotective activity of EGF is limited to certain types of mucosal damage and is smaller than that of PG, which are highly effective against ethanol injury.

The mechanism by which EGF exerts its protective effects against acute gastric mucosal lesions and gastroduodenal ulcerations has not been explained. We[35,39] observed that damaging agents decreased DNA synthesis and that EGF given subcutaneously caused a dose-dependent increase in DNA synthesis, while preventing the formation of acute gastric damage induced by ASA or absolute ethanol (Figure 5). Similar increases in DNA synthesis were observed after intragastric administration of EGF at a dose which did not affect gastric acid secretion, but

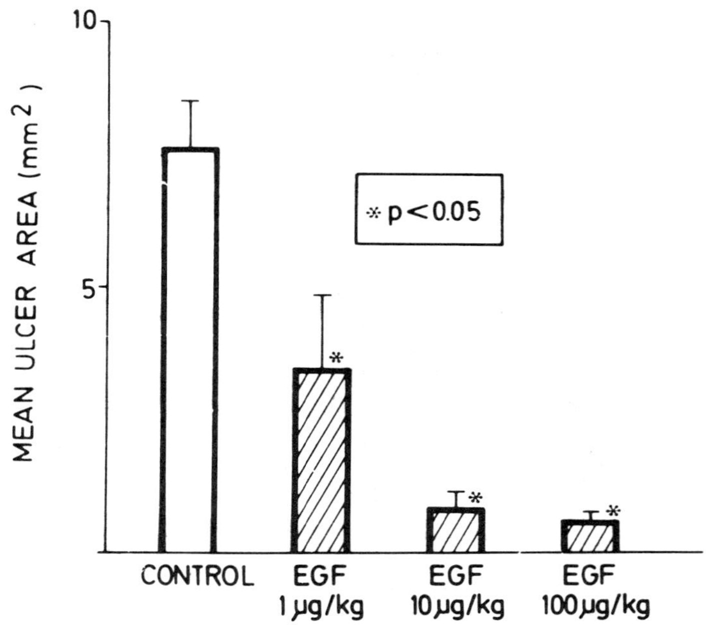

FIGURE 3. Effects of EGF at various doses (1 to 100 μg/kg) given intragastrically about 30 min before the start of administration of acidified ASA (100 mg/kg) on the area of gastric ulcerations caused by ASA. Each column represents mean ± SEM of 8 to 10 experiments on rats. Asterisk indicates significant decreases below the control value obtained with acidified ASA alone.

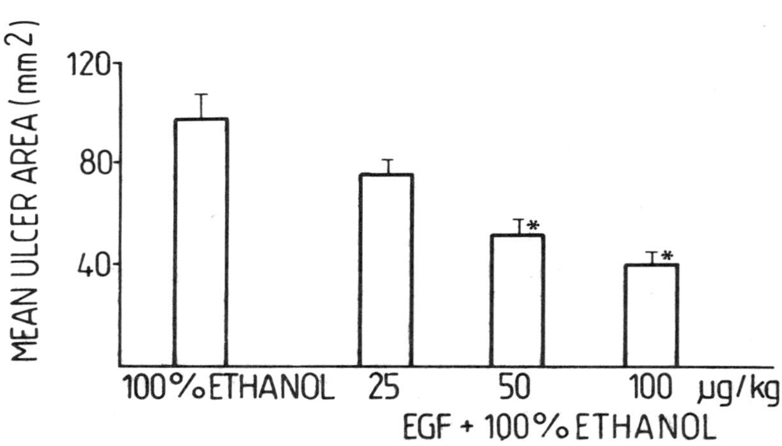

FIGURE 4. Effects of EGF at various doses (25 to 100 μg/kg) given subcutaneously 30 min before absolute ethanol on the area of gastric lesions measured 1 h after administration of ethanol. Each column represents the mean ± SEM of 10 to 12 experiments on rats. Asterisks indicate significant (p <0.05) decreases below the control value obtained with ethanol alone.

prevented ASA-induced ulceration (Figure 6). The reduction in mucosal DNA synthesis by various ulcerogens may simply be due to the destruction of large numbers of mucosal cells and subsequent decrease in the number of nuclei. It is not clear if the reduction in DNA synthesis could account for the formation of mucosal lesions, but it has been reported that similar

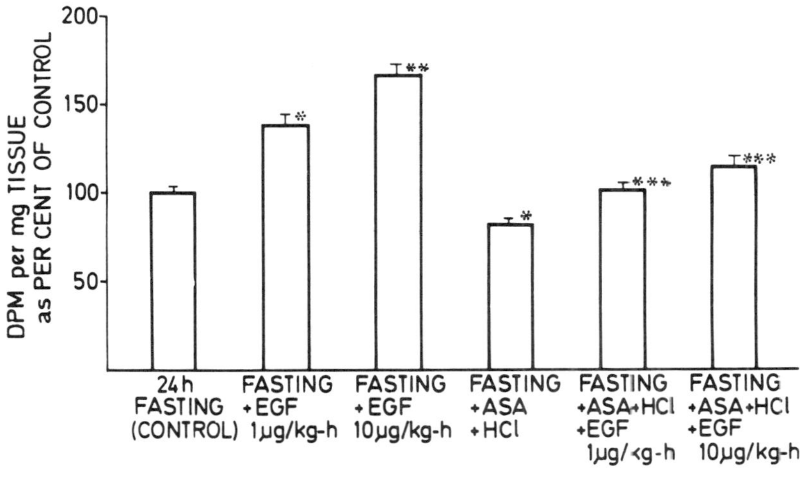

FIGURE 5. DNA synthesis as measured by *in vivo* incorporation of [^{3}H]-thymidine into DNA in the rat oxyntic mucosa after a 24-h fasting period without (control) and with s.c. administration of EGF (1 or 10 µg/kg/h) alone or combined with subsequent (30 min later) intragastric infusion of acidified ASA in tests as shown in Figure 1. Each column represents the mean ± SEM of 8 to 10 tests. A single asterisk indicates a significant (p <0.05) change from the control level observed in the intact mucosa. Double asterisks indicate significant increases above the value obtained from the mucosa pretreated with EGF. Triple asterisks indicate significant increases above the value obtained in ASA-treated mucosa.

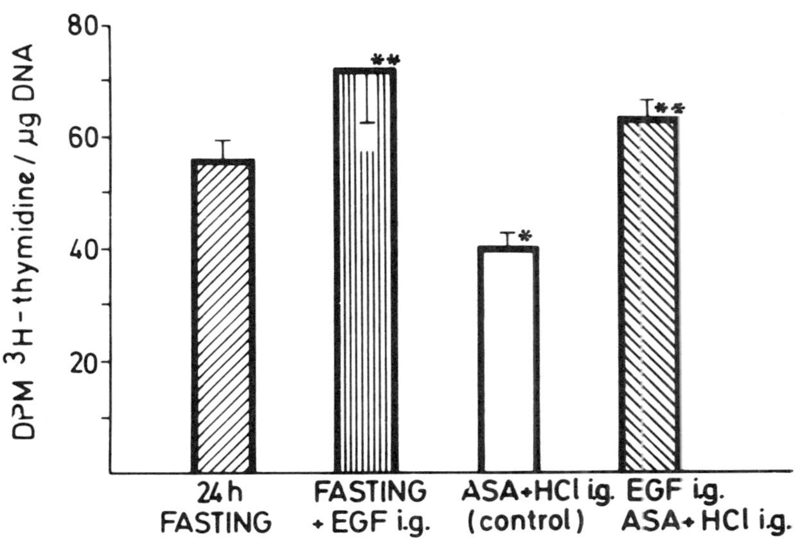

FIGURE 6. DNA synthesis as measured by *in vivo* incorporation of [^{3}H]-thymidine into the rat oxyntic mucosa after a 24-h fasting period without and with pretreatment with intragastric EGF (10 µg/kg) and after 3 h of adminstration of acidified ASA alone or combined with intragastric EGF (10 µg/kg), as in tests shown in Figure 3. Each column represents the mean ± SEM of 8 to 10 tests. A single asterisk indicates a significant decrease below the control value and double asterisks indicate significant increases above the control value obtained in the intact mucosa.

reductions in DNA synthesis by ASA[43] or by stress in fasting rats was accompanied by increased formation of gastric ulcerations.[44] ASA-induced gastric ulcerations were found to be accompanied by a dose-dependent increase in cell loss and by a reduction in DNA synthesis, such that a highly significant positive correlation between ulcer index and the ratio of DNA loss to DNA synthesis was observed.[43]

Both ASA- and stress-induced ulcerations were prevented by the administration of trophic hormones such as growth hormone[45] or pentagastrin[43,44] and this prevention was closely correlated with an increase in DNA synthesis. The major argument against the contribution of DNA synthesis to the gastroprotective or antiulcer action of EGF is that such stimulation of DNA synthesis and the subsequent increase in mitotic activity induced by EGF requires a long latency period. The observed changes in DNA synthesis, namely the return of DNA synthesis to normal level in the EGF pretreated stomach, could be interpreted as the result rather than the cause of protective action of EGF. It is likely that the gastroprotective effect of EGF may be associated with the early steps of DNA synthesis, such as polyamine formation, as a result of increased activity of ODs.[13] Alternatively, the gastroprotective effects of EGF may be due to the physical properties or the secretory rate of the protective mucus layer. This is supported by the finding that EGF stimulates mucosal cells to uptake and incorporate glucosamine into glycoproteins,[46,47] the main constituents of the protective mucus gel adherent to the surface of the stomach and duodenum.

IV. EGF AND ULCER HEALING

As mentioned previously, the beneficial action of urogastrone in the healing of chronic peptic ulcers was described long ago[18] and was clearly dissociated from the gastric antisecretory action of this substance. More recently, it has been confirmed that oral administration of synthetic human EGF does enhance the healing of chronic duodenal ulcers induced by cysteamine.[48] This enhancement of healing was comparable to that induced by cimetidine, but since oral EGF did not affect gastric secretion (whereas cimetidine did), it has been postulated that EGF acts directly on the duodenal mucosa, possibly via the promotion of mucosal growth and the stimulation of the reepithelialization. The same group of investigators[49] reported that the removal of submandibulary glands delayed the healing chronic gastric ulcers induced by serosal application of acetic acid. Orally administered human EGF stimulated ulcer healing and augmented the healing effect of cimetidine in this model. It has thus been suggested that submandibular glands play an important role in ulcer healing.

The mode of antiulcer action of EGF has not been established. Again, mucosal cell regeneration[22,50] and increased synthesis of hialuronic acid and protein in surface epithelial cells,[46,47] as well as an increase of fibroblasts[26] and collagen,[51] have been implicated.

We[52] attempted to correlate EGF-induced healing of chronic acetic acid gastroduodenal ulcers with biochemical indices of mucosal growth in rats with intact and resected submandibular glands. It was confirmed that the extirpation of salivary glands delayed ulcer healing, although neither gastric acid secretion nor serum gastrin were affected by this procedure (Figures 7 and 8). The delay in healing was accompanied by a marked decrease in mucosal growth parameters such as DNA and RNA content. Repeated administration of EGF either subcutaneously or orally (30 μg/kg/d) reversed the delay in ulcer healing, demonstrating that EGF plays a crucial role in ulcer healing by stimulation of the growth of the gastroduodenal mucosa.

Recent studies in humans and animals with chronic gastroduodenal ulcerations have emphasized an important role of endogenous EGF in the promotion of ulcer healing. It was found that EGF accumulates in the area of ulcerations, partly by direct binding to the cells at the edge of the ulcer (Figure 9), and partly by complexing with gastroprotective drugs such as sucralfate[53] or De-Nol.[54] Following intragastric administration of these drugs, most of the endogenous EGF

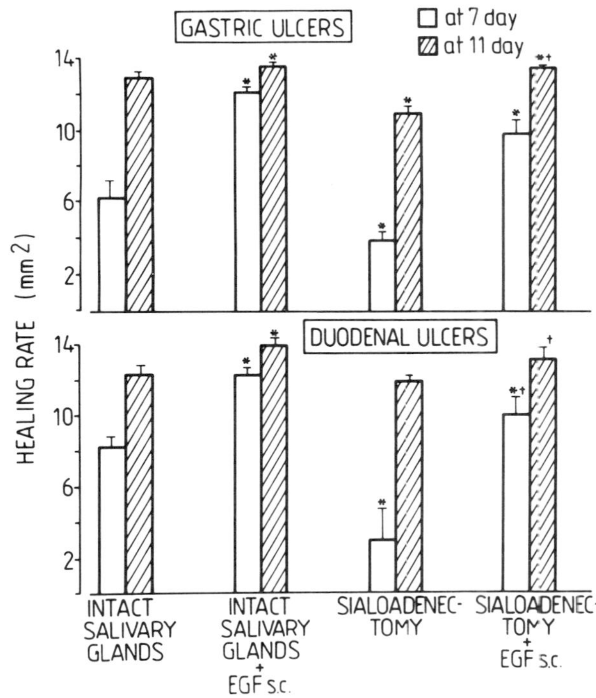

FIGURE 7. Healing rates of chronic gastric and duodenal ulcerations induced by serosal application of acetic acid on an area of 13.8 mm^2 at 7 and 11 d after ulcer induction in rats with intact salivary glands without and with s.c. injection of EGF (30 μg/kg/d), and in rats following the resection of submandibulary glands without or with s.c. injection of EGF (30 μg/kg/d). Each column represents the mean ± SEM of 10 to 12 tests. Asterisks indicate significant (p <0.05) changes as compared to control values obtained in rats with intact salivary glands, while crosses indicate significant increases above the values obtained in sialoadenectomized rats without treatment with EGF.

becomes bound to the drug, particularly at lower intragastric pH, and this prolongs EGF availability in the ulcer area for a longer period of time than when EGF is given alone. The accumulation of EGF in larger concentrations in the ulcer area by sucralfate or De-Nol may explain their well-known beneficial effects on ulcer healing. On the other hand, the deficiency of EGF in saliva observed in patients with active ulcer[30] may contribute to the formation of ulcers and/or to the resistance to antiulcer therapy.

V. GASTRIN AND SECRETIN FAMILIES OF PEPTIDES IN MUCOSAL PROTECTION AND ULCER HEALING

As discussed above, a normal mucosa is the manifestation of a balance between forces acting to destroy the lining of the gastrointestinal tract and those acting to maintain or rebuild it. Destructive forces, such as ethanol, aspirin, bile acids or stress, are known to decrease the rate of cell proliferation and DNA synthesis, as well as to destroy the lining by direct necrotizing actions on the mucosal cells.

Previous studies demonstrated that out of numerous factors, the most important in the control of mucosal proliferation was growth hormone (GH), as general promoter of body and tissue growth, and gastrin, as a specific stimulant of growth of the gut mucosa.[55] Enoch and Johnson[56,57]

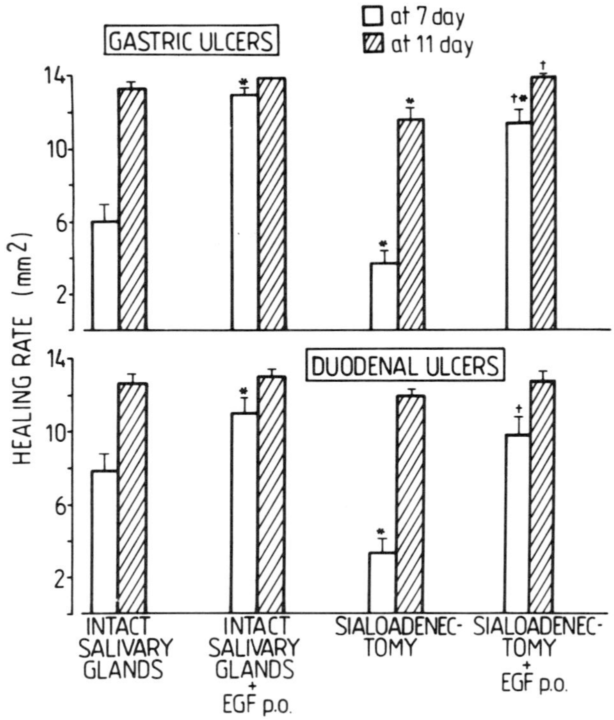

FIGURE 8. Healing rates of chronic gastric and duodenal ulcerations induced by serosal application of acetic acid on an area of 13.8 mm^2 at 7 and 11 d after ulcer induction in rats with intact salivary glands without and with p.o. administration of EGF (30 μg/kg/d) and in rats following the resection of submandibular glands without and with p.o. administration of EGF (30 μg/kg/d). Each column represents the mean ± SEM of 10 to 12 tests. Asterisks indicate significant (p <0.05) changes as compared to control values obtained in rats with intact salivary glands, while crosses indicate significant increases above the values obtained in sialoadenectomized rats without treatment with EGF.

who studied the interdependence of GH and gastrin with respect to mucosal growth, suggested that adequate levels of circulating GH is permissive for the release and synthesis of gastrin. On the other hand, GH-release-inhibiting hormone, somatostatin, which is present in large quantities in the stomach,[59-61] has been shown to inhibit gastrin release.[62,63]

The trophic effect of GH on the gastric mucosa has been implicated as a possible mechanism for the protective effect of this hormone against stress- or steroid-induced gastric ulcers.[44,45] In view of the permissive influence of GH on the synthesis and release of gastrin, the possibility that gastrin is the major factor mediating the protective action of GH on the gastric mucosa cannot be excluded. It is doubtful that the gastroprotective effects of GH could be attributed to its direct trophic action on the mucosa, particularly since the stimulation of DNA synthesis[57] and cell division[65] requires on the order of 16 to 20 h, while the protection by GH occurs within 4 to 7 h.

The possible role of gastrin in gastroprotection against stress ulceration has been documented by Takeuchi and Johnson[44] and by Sakamoto et al.[66] Using rats depleted of gastrin by feeding a liquid diet, they found a marked decrease in DNA synthesis in the oyxntic mucosa, which by itself did not lead to ulcer formation, but greatly increased the ulcerogenicity of restraint-stress. Thus, rats with low endogenous gastrin release and reduced DNA synthesis were found to be

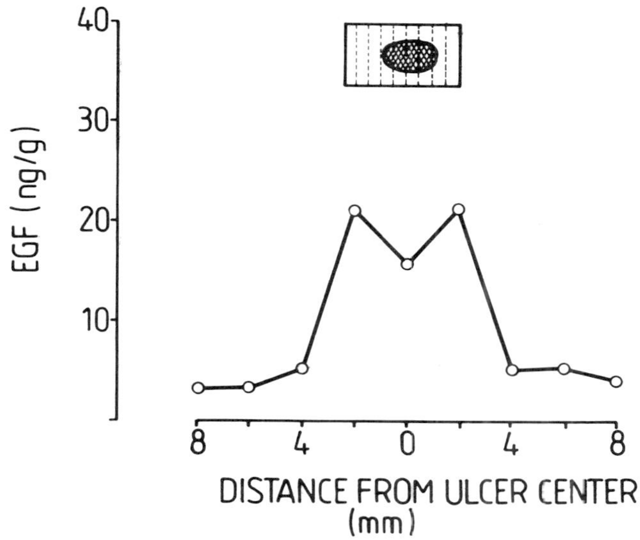

FIGURE 9. Distribution of EGF in the area of chronic ulcerations as measured by radioimmunoassay in the biopsy samples taken at each 1 to 2 mm distance from the ulcer center. Ulcers were induced by serosal application of acetic acid on an area of 13.8 mm^2 for a period of 20 s. The biopsy samples for the EGF distribution were taken 2 d after ulcer induction.

more susceptible to stress ulceration. Injection of pentagastrin, which reversed the effects of the liquid diet on DNA synthesis, significantly protected against stress ulcerations, suggesting that the strengthening of regenerative factors for the gastric mucosa may be an important protective mechanism. Sakamoto et al.[66] confirmed that pentagastrin prevented stress ulcer formation, but this was attributed to increased release of endogenous somatostatin in the stomach and to the involvement of this peptide in mucosal protection.

It is of interest that stress ulcerations induced by water immersion and restraint were observed only in animals with depleted gastrin and reduced DNA synthesis.[44] Pentagastrin given to such animals increased DNA synthesis while protecting the mucosa from ulcer formation.[44]

Pentagastrin was also found to reduce ASA-induced gastric ulceration, particularly in gastrin-depleted animals.[43] Although no direct correlation was observed between ulcer index and either cell (DNA) loss or DNA synthesis, there was a highly significant, positive correlation between ulcer index and the ratio of DNA loss to DNA synthesis. It was concluded that the decreased proliferative capacity of the mucosa by gastrin depletion increased ASA-induced mucosal damage and this was reversed in part by increasing cell proliferation with exogenous gastrin.[43]

We were unable to confirm these findings. According to our experience, gastric lesions induced by acidified ASA were unaffected by pentagastrin[42] (Figure 10); however, we only used rats with normal plasma gastrin kept on chow diet, so it is possible that in animals with reduced gastrin release and decreased proliferative capacity the protective effects of gastrin may have been demonstrated. The major difference between ethanol- and ASA-induced lesions is that the former are accompanied by increased mucosal generation of protective PG, while the latter are associated with suppression of PG formation and only moderate decreases in DNA synthesis. Although pentagastrin by itself, or when combined with ethanol, did not affect PG generation in the oxyntic mucosa, it is likely that the presence of endogenous PG is a prerequisite of the gastroprotective action of pentagastrin against ethanol-induced damage. Since ASA blocked the

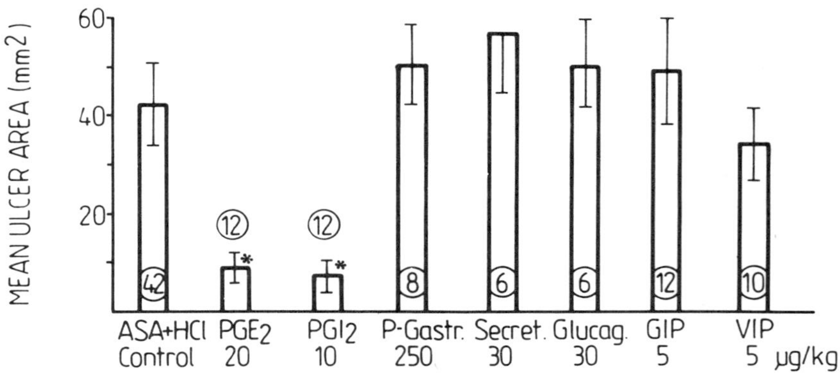

FIGURE 10. Means (± SEM) area of gastric ulceration induced by acidified ASA (100 mg/kg given for a 3-h period) in rats without (control) and with s.c. administration of PGE_2, PGI_2, pentagastrin, secretin, glucagon, GIP, or VIP, given 30 min before the start of infusion of ASA. Numbers in circles indicate the number of animals used in each series of experiments. Asterisks indicate significant ($p < 0.05$) decreases below the control value obtained with acidified ASA alone.

formation of mucosal PG while causing only a moderate decrease in DNA synthesis, the major mechanisms of the protective action of pentagastrin were eliminated. Moreover, injected pentagastrin stimulated HCl secretion by the oxyntic mucosa exposed to ASA and the increased luminal H^+ in the stomach may have increased the ulcerogenicity of ASA. In the case of absolute ethanol, this could not play any role because the exposure of mucosa to this irritant leads to complete achlorhydria.

It is not clear if gastrin can protect against acute mucosal damage caused by necrotizing substances such as absolute ethanol. According to our experience,[42] pentagastrin at a dose of 25 µg/kg/h did not affect gastric secretion and was ineffective against ethanol-induced damage, but a larger dose (250 µg/kg/h) of the peptide, which significantly stimulated acid secretion, was protective in ethanol model (Figure 11). It is of interest that pentagastrin at the protective dose prevented a marked suppression of DNA synthesis caused by ethanol. The mechanism of pentagastrin-induced protection against ethanol is unknown, but again, the strengthening of mucosal integrity by promoting the early phase of cell proliferation and sulfhydryl biosynthesis may be involved.

The mucosal growth-promoting effect of pentagastrin may contribute not only to the prevention of acute gastric lesions, such as those induced by ethanol or restraint stress, but also appear to be involved in the healing of chronic ulcerations. Takeuchi and Johnson[67] recently demonstrated that in gastrin-depleted rats kept on a liquid diet, the healing of chronic gastric and duodenal ulcers produced by acetic acid was remarkably reduced and this reduction could be reversed by injection of pentagastrin. The delay of ulcer healing in gastrin-depleted animals was accompanied by a reduction in DNA synthesis and total DNA and RNA content. All these biochemical indices of mucosa growth were returned to normal values by the pretreatment with pentagastrin. This study reinforces the concept that cell proliferation accomplished by growth-promoting factors such as gastrin is an important factor in healing of gastroduodenal ulceration. Furthermore, feeding appropriate diets, which cause adequate release of endogenous gastrin may exert a beneficial influence on this healing.

Previous studies demonstrated that the peptides of the secretin family, particularly secretin and glucagon,[58] inhibited the production of experimental duodenal ulcers in various species. This antiulcer action has been attributed to inhibition of gastric acid secretion and to increased duodenal secretion; however, the tested peptides of the secretin family of hormones, such as secretin, glucagon, and gastrin-inhibiting peptide (GIP), did not exhibit any protective action

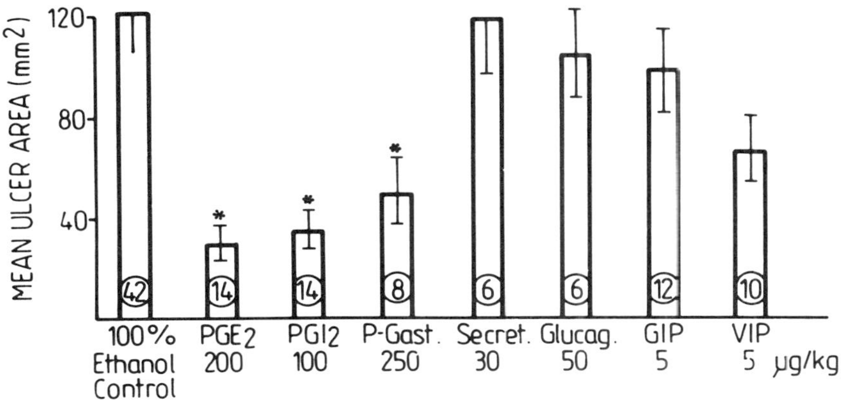

FIGURE 11. Mean (± SEM) of area of gastric lesions induced by intragastric administration of absolute ethanol (for a 1-h period) in rats without (control) and with s.c. administration of PGE_2, PGI_2, pentagastrin, secretin, glucagon, GIP, or VIP, given 30 min before application of ethanol. Numbers in circles indicate the number of animals used in each series of experiments. Asterisks indicate significant ($p < 0.05$) decreases below the control value obtained with absolute ethanol alone.

against ethanol- or ASA-induced gastric lesions, even when used in large gastric inhibitory doses (Figures 10 and 11). Since none of these peptides has any influence on the growth parameters of the gastric mucosa,[55] it is possible that this might explain their failure to protect the gastric mucosa. The only exception was VIP, which caused a small but significant decrease in ethanol-induced gastric damage, possibly attributable to the increase in the mucosal blood flow[68] or to prevention of the mucosal vasocongestion and hemorrhage caused by ethanol.

VI. PROTECTIVE AND ANTIULCER PROPERTIES OF SOMATOSTATIN

Somatostatin (SS), originally isolated from the hypothalamus and identified by its inhibitory action on the release of growth hormone (GH), has been detected in large amounts in the gastrointestinal tract and pancreas, both in the neurons of the autonomic nervous system and endocrine-paracrine cells.[59-61] Both small (SS-14) and larger (SS-28) molecular forms of the peptide have been extracted and identified in the mucosa[69] and in the plasma.[70]

The spectrum of biological actions of somatostatin is quite impressive.[71] In addition to its major inhibitory action on the release of pituitary hormones such as GH, it suppresses both exo- and endocrine functions of the gastroenteropancreatic system, reduces splanchnic blood flow, inhibits motor activity of the gut, and decreases the growth of the mucosa and the pancreas, partly by suppressing the release and action of trophic peptides such as gastrin[62,63] and/or by acting directly on the progenitor cells.[72] It may act by endocrine (via circulation), neurocrine (via SS-containing nerves), or exocrine (via luminal release) pathways, but the physiological action of somatostatin on the digestive system seems to mainly involve the paracrine route.[70]

The antiulcer effects of somatostatin were described[73] long before the cytoprotection phenomenon was recognized.[74] Somatostatin was found to reduce the formation of gastric and duodenal ulcerations produced by potent secretagogues such as pentagastrin or histamine, but this effect was entirely attributable to the inhibition of gastric acid secretion.[73]

More recently, it was demonstrated that somatostatin displays a potent protective activity against stress-[75] and cysteamine-induced gastroduodenal ulceration[76,77] and against ethanol-induced gastric damage.[78,79] The common feature of stress and cysteamine ulcerations is an important role of increased acid-pepsin secretion and gastrin release in the pathogenesis of the formation of these mucosal defects. The protection by somatostatin against these ulcerations could simply be attributed to the inhibition of gastric secretion by direct action on the oxyntic glands and indirectly by suppressing gastrin release and gastric acid secretion. Cysteamine also causes the depletion of somatostatin from the gastroduodenal mucosa, as well as from other organs including the pancreas and the hypothalamus.[77] The protective effect of somatostatin against cysteamine-ulcerations may be due to the replacement in the gastroduodenal mucosa of the peptide required to inhibit gastric secretion and to reduce duodenal hypermotility. It is of interest that the well-recognized antitrophic effect of somatostatin on the gastric or duodenal mucosa[73] apparently does not interfere with the protective action of the peptide. The same is true with regard to the reduction of the mucosal blood flow caused by somatostatin.[80] It is likely that the gastric antisecretory action is so potent that the antitrophic and vasoconstrictive effects do not interfere with gastroprotection by somatostatin.

Somatostatin and its potent analogs, particularly of cyclic forms, are also effective against ethanol-induced gastric damage.[81] Since gastric acid plays little role in the formation of ethanol-induced gastric erosions, it is obvious that somatostatin protection of such lesions should involve other mechanisms than inhibition of gastric secretion. Diel and Szabo[79] observed that the extent of protection by cyclic somatostatin correlated with the number of mast cells in the gastric mucosa. By showing the release of histamine-containing granules and by prevention of mast cell degranulation, somatostatin could reduce tissue content of histamine to prevent the vasocongestion and mucosal hemorrhage, which are the main features of mucosal damage by ethanol.

According to our experience,[42] somatostatin was protective against both ethanol- and aspirin-induced gastric lesions (Figures 12 and 13), confirming that this peptide does display a gastroprotective activity. Since the mucosal generation of PG was not affected by this dose of somatostatin (Figure 14), we excluded the possibility of mediation by endogenous PG, which were once believed to be released by the peptide[82] but has since been disproved.[83] Intragastric administration of somatostatin was without any influence on ethanol or ASA-induced damage or on mucosal generation of PG (Figures 12 and 13).

Long-acting somatostatin analogs have been successively used in the therapy of acute bleeding due to peptic ulceration[84] and the beneficial effects have been attributed to the reduction in the splanchnic blood flow and the suppression of gastric acid-pepsin secretion. This indicates that somatostatin or its potent analogs might be useful in the prevention or treatment of certain forms of ulcerations.

ACKNOWLEDGMENT

The studies described in this chapter were supported in part by a Polish Academy of Sciences Research Grant (CPBP-06.03.3.6).

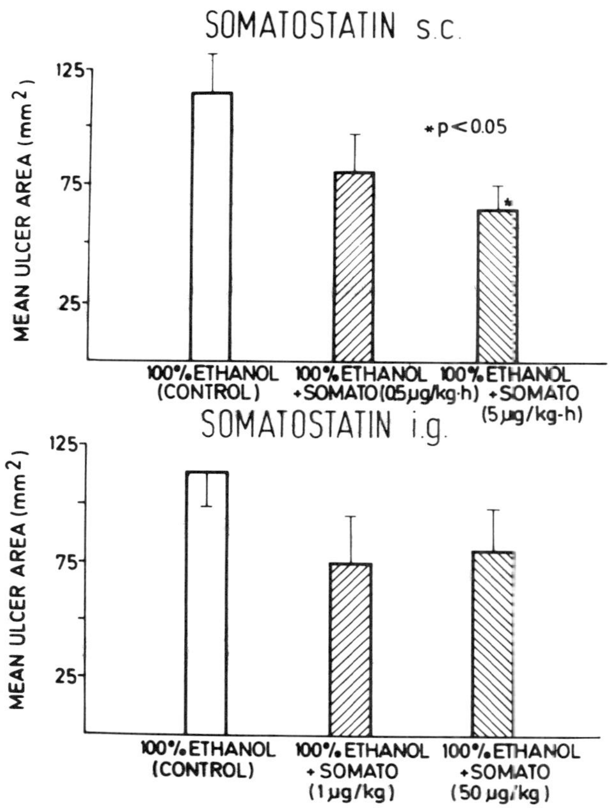

FIGURE 12. Effects of somatostatin (somato) administered subcutaneously or intragastrically on mean area of gastric ulcerations produced by absolute ethanol. Each column represents the mean (± SEM) of 8 to 12 experiments on rats. Asterisks indicate significant ($p < 0.05$) decreases below the control value obtained with 100% ethanol alone. The doses of somatostatin used (1 and 5 µg/kg/h) did not affect gastric acid secretion in rats with chronic gastric fistula.

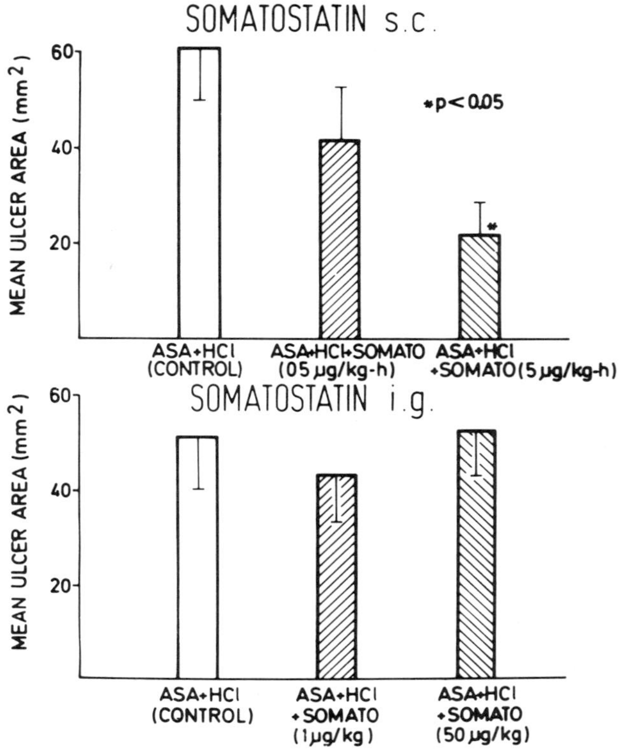

FIGURE 13. Effects of somatostatin (somato) administered subcutaneously or intragastrically on mean area of gastric ulcerations produced by acidified ASA (100 mg/kg/h) during 3 h. Each column represents the mean (± SEM) decreases below the control value obtained with acidified ASA (p <0.05). The doses of somatostatin used (1 and 5 µg/kg/h) did not affect gastric acid secretion in rats with chronic gastric fistula.

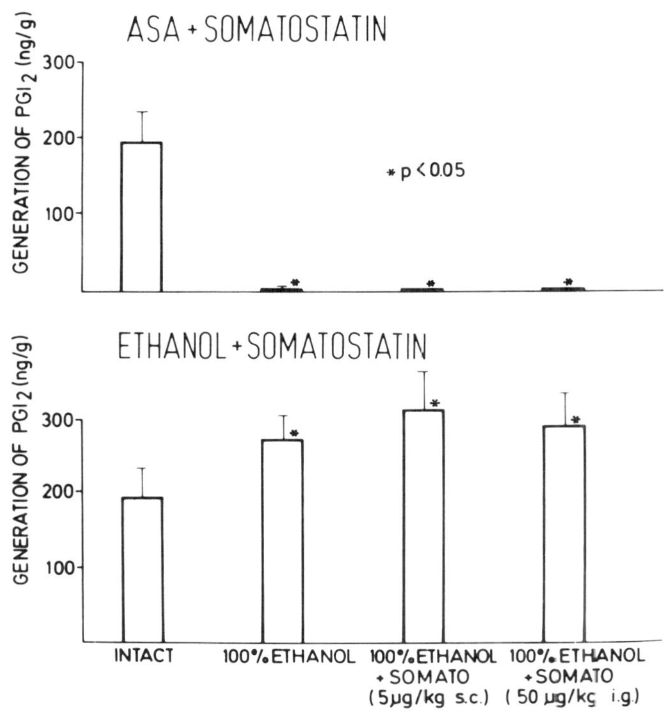

FIGURE 14. Generation of PGE_2 and PGI_2 in the oxyntic mucosa of intact rats and following exposure to acidified ASA (for 3 h) or absolute ethanol (for 1 h) with or without the pretreatment with somatostatin given subcutaneously (5 µg/kg) or intragastrically (50 µg/kg) 30 min before the start of administration of ASA or ethanol.

REFERENCES

1. **Creamer, B., Shorter, R. G., and Barnforth, J.,** Turnover of shedding of epithelial cells. I. Turnover in the gastrointestinal tract, *Gut,* 2, 110, 1961.
2. **Grant, R., Grossman, M. I., and Ivy, A. C.,** Histological changes in gastric mucosa growth, *Gastroenterology,* 25, 218, 1953.
3. **McDonald, C., Trier, J. S., and Everett, B.,** Cell proliferation and migration in the stomach, duodenum and rectum of man, *Gastroenterology,* 46, 405, 1964.
4. **Hingson, D. J. and Ito, S.,** Effect of aspirin and related compounds on the fine structure of mouse gastric mucosa, *Gastroenterology,* 61, 156, 1971.
5. **Eastwood, G. L. and Kirchner, J. P.,** Changes in the fine structure of mouse gastric epithelium produced by ethanol and area, *Gastroenterology,* 67, 71, 1974.
6. **Forte, T. M., Silen, W., and Forte, J. G.,** Ultrastructural lesions in gastric mucosa exposed to deoxycholate. Implications toward the barrier concept, in *Gastric Hydrogen Ion Secretion,* Kasbekar, D. K., Sachs, G., and Rehm, W. S., Eds., Marcel Dekker, New York, 1976, 1.
7. **Svanes, K., Ito, S., Takeuchi, K., and Silen, W.,** Restitution of the surface epithelium of the *in vitro* gastric mucosa after damage with hyperosmolar sodium chloride. Morphological and physiological characteristics, *Gastroenterology,* 82, 1409, 1982.
8. **Morris, G. P., Harding, P. K., and Wallace, J. L.,** A functional model for extracellular gastric mucus in the rat, *Virchows Arch. (Cell Pathol.),* 46, 239, 1984.

9. **Davenport, H. W.,** The gastric mucosal barrier, *Digestion,* 5, 162, 1972.
10. **Ivey, K. J.,** Gastric mucosal barrier, *Gastroenterology,* 61, 247, 1971.
11. **Hollander, F.,** The two component mucus barrier. Its activity in protecting the gastroduodenal mucosa against peptic ulceration, *Arch. Intern. Med.,* 93, 107, 1948.
12. **Rutten, M. J. and Ito, S.,** Morphology and electrophysiology of guinea pig gastric mucosal repair *in vitro, Am. J. Physiol.,* 244, G171, 1983.
13. **Thirumalai, C. H., Tseng, C.-C., Tabata, K., Fitzpatrick, L. R., and Johnson, L. R.,** Relationship between ornithine decarboxylase activity and gastric damage, *Am. J. Physiol.,* 253, G1, 1987.
14. **Tabor, C. W. and Tabor, H.,** Polyamines, *Ann. Rev. Biochem.,* 53, 749, 1984.
15. **Mizui, T. and Doteuchi, M.,** Effect of polyamines on acidified ethanol-induced gastric lesions in rats., *Jpn. J. Pharmacol.,* 33, 939, 1983.
16. **Cohen, S.,** Isolation of a mouse submaxillary gland protein accelerating incisor eruption and eyelid opening of newborn animal, *J. Biol. Chem.,* 237, 1155, 1962.
17. **Savage, C. R., Jr., Inagami, T., and Cohen, S.,** The primary structure of epidermal growth factor, *J. Biol. Chem.,* 247, 7612, 1972.
18. **Sandweiss, D. J. and Friedman, M. H. F.,** Is the beneficial effect of urine extract on M-W ulcers due to gastric secretory depressant in urine?, *Am. J. Dig. Dis.,* 9, 166, 1942.
19. **Konturek, S. J., Cieszkowski, M., Jaworek, J., Brzozowski, T., and Gregory, H.,** Effects of epidermal growth factor on gastrointestinal secretion, *Am. J. Physiol.,* 246, G580, 1984.
20. **Dembinski, A., Drozdowicz, D., Gregory, H., Konturek, S. J., and Warzecha, Z.,** Inhibition of acid formation by epidermal growth factor in the isolated rabbit gastric glands, *J. Physiol. (London),* 378, 347, 1986.
21. **Carpenter, G. and Cohen, S.,** Human epidermal growth factor and the proliferation of human fibroblasts, *J. Cell. Physiol.,* 88, 227, 1976.
22. **Dembinski, A., Gregory, H., Konturek, S. J., and Polanski, M.,** Trophic action of epidermal growth factor on the pancreas and gastrointestinal mucosa in rats, *J. Physiol. (London),* 325, 35, 1982.
23. **Feldman, E. J., Aures, D., and Grossman, M. I.,** Epidermal growth factor stimulates ornithine decarboxylase activity in the digestive tract of the mouse, *Proc. Soc. Exp. Biol. Med.,* 159, 400, 1978.
24. **Russel, D. H., Byrus, C. V., and Manen, C. A.,** Proposed model of major sequential biochemical events of a trophic response, *Life Sci.,* 19, 1927, 1976.
25. **Johnson, L. R. and Guthrie, P. D.,** Stimulation of rat oxyntic gland mucosal growth by epidermal growth factor, *Am. J. Physiol.,* 238, G45, 1978.
26. **Heitz, Ph. V., Kasper, M., Noordenn, S. V., Polak, J. M., Gregory, H., and Pearse, A. G. E.,** Immunohistochemical localization of urogastrone to human submandibulary glands, *Gut,* 19, 408, 1978.
27. **Gresik, E. W., Noen, H., and Barka, H.,** Epidermal growth-like material in rat submandibular gland, *Am. J. Anat.,* 156, 83, 1979.
28. **Gregory, H., Walsh, S., and Hopking, C. R.,** The identification of urogastrone in serum saliva and gastric juice, *Gastroenterology,* 77, 313, 1979.
29. **Nexo, E., Olsen, P. S., and Poulson, K.,** Exocrine and endocrine secretion of renin and epidermal growth factor from the mouse submandibular glands, *Regul. Peptides,* 8, 327, 1984.
30. **Ohmura, E., Emoto, N., Tsushima, T., Watanabe, S., Takeuchi, T., Kawamura, M., Shigemoto, M., and Shizume, K.,** Salivary immunoreactive human epidermal growth factor (IR-EGF) in patients with peptic ulcer disease, *Hepato-Gastroenterol.,* 34, 160, 1987.
31. **Olsen, P. S., Poulsen, S. S., and Kirkegaard, P.,** Adrenergic effects on secretion of epidermal growth factor from Brunner's glands, *Gut,* 26, 920, 1985.
32. **Gregory, H.,** Isolation and structure of urogastrone and its relationship to epidermal growth factor, *Nature,* 257, 325, 1975.
33. **Das, M.,** Epidermal growth factor: mechanisms of action, *Int. Rev. Cytol.,* 78, 233, 1982.
34. **Forgue-Lafitte, M.-E., Kobari, L., Gespach, C., Chamblier, M.-C., and Rosselin, G.,** Characterization of epidermal growth factor — urogastrone receptors in gastric glands isolated from young and adult guinea pigs, *Biochem. Biophys. Acta,* 798, 192, 1984.
35. **Konturek, S. J., Brzozowski, T., Piastucki, I., Dembinski, A., Radecki, T., Dembinska-Kiec, A., Zmuda, A., and Gregory, H.,** Role of mucosal prostaglandins and DNA synthesis in gastric protection by luminal epidermal growth factor, *Gut,* 22, 927, 1981.
36. **Ulshen, M. H., Lyn-Cook, L. E., and Raasch, R. H.,** Effects of luminal epidermal growth factor on mucosal proliferation in the small intestine of adult rats, *Gastroenterology,* 91, 1134, 1986.
37. **Barker, J. H., Lund, J. P., and Delow, P. G.,** Desalivation and the incidence of experimental gastric ulcerations, *Proc. Soc. Fed. Biol.,* 12, 62, 1969.
38. **Skinner, K. A. and Tepperman, B. L.,** Influence of desalivation on acid secretory output and gastric mucosal integrity in the rat, *Gastroenterology,* 81, 335, 1981.

39. **Konturek, S. J., Radecki, T., Brzozowki, T., Piastucki, I., Dembinski, A., Dembinska-Kiec, A., Zmuda, A., Gryglewski, R., and Gregory, H.**, Gastric cytoprotection by epidermal growth factor. Role of endogenous prostaglandins and DNA synthesis, *Gastroenterology,* 81, 438, 1981.
40. **Kirkegaard, P., Olsen, P. S., Poulsen, S. S., and Nexo, E.**, Epidermal growth factor inhibits cysteamine-induced duodenal ulcers, *Gastroenterology,* 85, 1283, 1983.
41. **Olsen, P. S., Poulsen, S. S., Kirkegaard, P., and Nexo, E.**, Role of submandibular saliva and epidermal growth factor in gastric cytoprotection, *Gastroenterology,* 87, 103, 1984.
42. **Konturek, S. J., Brzozowski, T., Radecki, T., Piastucki, I., and Dembinski, A.**, Cytoprotective effects of gastrointestinal hormones, in *Gut Peptides and Hormones,* Miyoshi, A., Ed., Biomedical Research Foundation, Tokyo, 1982, 411.
43. **Takeuchi, K. and Johnson, L. R.**, Effect of cell proliferation and loss on aspirin-induced gastric damage in the rat, *Am. J. Physiol.,* 243, G463, 1982.
44. **Takeuchi, K. and Johnson, L. R.**, Pentagastrin protects against stress ulcerations in rats, *Gastroenterology,* 76, 327, 1979.
45. **Vanemee, P., Winawer, S. J., and Sherlock, R.**, Decreased incidence of restraint stress induced gastric erosions in rats treated with bovine growth hormone, *Proc. Soc. Exp. Biol. Med.,* 135, 259, 1970.
46. **Lembach, K. J.**, Enhanced synthesis and extracellular accumulation of hyaluronic acid during stimulation of quiescent human fibroblasts by mouse epidermal growth factor, *J. Cell. Physiol.,* 89, 277, 1976.
47. **Chen, L. B., Gudor, R. C., Sun, T.-T., Chen, A. B., and Mosesson, M. W.**, Control of a cell surface major glycoprotein by epidermal growth factor, *Science,* 197, 776, 1977.
48. **Olsen, P. S., Poulsen, S. S., Therkelsen, K., and Nexo, E.**, Oral administration of synthetic human urogastrone promotes healing of chronic duodenal ulcers in rats, *Gastroenterology,* 90, 911, 1986.
49. **Olsen, P. S., Poulsen, S. S., Therkelsen, K., and Nexo, E.**, Effects of sialoadenectomy and synthetic human urogastrone on healing of chronic gastric ulcers in rats, *Gut,* 27, 1443, 1986.
50. **Al-Nafussi, A. L. and Wright, N. A.**, The effect of epidermal growth factor (EGF) on cell proliferation of the gastrointestinal mucosa in rodents, *Virchows. Arch.,* 40, 63, 1982.
51. **Kumegawa, M., Hiramatsu, M., Yajima, T., Hatakeyema, K., and Hoseda, M.**, Effect of epidermal growth factor on collagen formation in liver- deprived epithelial clonic cells, *Endocrinology,* 110, 607, 1982.
52. **Konturek, S. J., Dembinski, A., Warzecha, Z., and Gregory, H.**, Role of epidermal growth factor in healing of chronic gastroduodenal ulcers in rats, *Gastroenterology,* 94, 1300, 1988.
53. **Nexo, E., and Poulsen, S. S.**, Does epidermal growth factor play a role in the action of sucralfate?, *Scand. J. Gastroenterol.,* 22(Suppl.), 127, 45, 1987.
54. **Konturek, S. J., Dembinski, A., Warzecha, Z., and Bielanski, W.**, Epidermal growth factor (EGF) in the gastroprotective and ulcer healing action of colloidal bismuth subcitrate, *Gut,* 29, 894, 1988.
55. **Johnson, L. R.**, Regulation of gastrointestinal growth, in *Physiology of the Gastrointestinal Tract,* Johnson, L. R., Ed., Raven Press, New York, 1987, 301.
56. **Enoch, M. R. and Johnson, L. R.**, Effect of hypophysectomy and growth hormone on serum and antral gatrin levels in the rat, *Gastroenterology,* 70, 727, 1976.
57. **Enoch, M. R. and Johnson, L. R.**, Changes in protein and nucleic acid synthesis in rat gastric mucosa after pentagastrin, *Am. J. Physiol.,* 233, E223, 1977.
58. **Konturek, S. J., Radecki, T., Thor, P., and Kwiecien, N.**, Effect of intestinal hormones on pentagastrin- and histamine-evoked gastric acid secretion and duodenal ulcerations in cats, *Dig. Dis.,* 18, 135, 1973.
59. **Vinik, G., Gaginella, T., O'Dorisio, T., Shapiro, B., and Wagner, L.**, The distribution and characterization of somatostatin-like immunoreactivity in epithelial cells, submucosa, and muscle of the rat stomach and intestine, *Endocrinology,* 109, 1921, 1981.
60. **Chaywialle, J. A., Miyata, M., Rayford, P. L., and Thompson, J. C.**, Immunoreactive somatostatin and vasoactive intestinal peptide in the digestive tract of cat, *Gastroenterology,* 79, 837, 1980.
61. **Penman, E., Wass, J., Butler, M., Penny, E., Price, J., Wu, P., and Ress, L.**, Distribution and characterization of immunoreactive somatostatin in human gastrointestinal tract, *Regul. Peptides,* 7, 53, 1983.
62. **Konturek, S. J., Tasler, J., Cieszkowski, M., Coy, D. H., and Schally, A. V.**, Effect of growth hormone release-inhibiting hormone on gastrin secretion, mucosal blood flow and serum gastrin, *Gastroenterology,* 70, 737, 1976.
63. **Creutzfeldt, W. and Arnold, R.**, Somatostatin and the stomach: exocrine and endocrine aspects, *Metabolism,* 27, 1309, 1975.
64. **Robert, A., Phillips, J. P., and Nezamis, J. E.**, Gastric secretion and ulcer formation after hypophysectomy and administration of somatotrophic hormone, *Am. J. Dig. Dis.,* 11, 546, 1966.
65. **Willems, G., Vansteenkiste, Y., and Limbosch, J. M.**, Stimulation of effect of gastrin on cell proliferation kinetics in canine fundic mucosa, *Gastroenterology,* 62, 385, 1972.

66. **Sakamoto, T., Swierczek, J. S., Ogden, D., and Thompson, J. C.,** Cytoprotective effect of pentagastrin and epidermal growth factor on stress ulcer formation, *Ann. Surg.*, 201, 290, 1985.
67. **Takeuchi, K. and Johnson, L. R.,** Effect of proliferation of healing of gastric and duodenal ulcers in rats, *Digestion,* 33, 92, 1986.
68. **Said, S. I.,** Vasoactive intestinal peptide (VIP): isolation, distribution, biological actions, structure-function relations, and possible functions, in *Gastrointestinal Hormones,* Glass, J. G. B., Ed., Raven Press, New York, 1987, 245.
69. **Baskin, D. and Ensinck, J.,** Somatostatin in epithelial cells of intestinal mucosa is present primarily as somatostatin 28, *Peptides,* 5, 615, 1984.
70. **Polansky, K., Shoelson, S., and Docherty, H.,** Plasma somatostatin 28 increases in response to feeding in man, *J. Clin. Invest.,* 71, 1514, 1983.
71. **Walsh, J. H.,** Gastrointestinal hormones, in *Physiology of the Gastrointestinal Tract,* Johnson, L. R., Ed., Raven Press, New York, 1987, 181.
72. **Lehy, T., Dubrasquet, M., and Bonfils, S.,** Effect of somatostatin on normal and gastrin-stimulated cell proliferation in the gastric and intestinal mucosae of the rat, *Digestion,* 19, 99, 1979.
73. **Konturek, S. J., Radecki, T., Pucher, A., Coy, D. H., and Schally, A. V.,** Effect of somatostatin on gastrointestinal secretion and peptic ulcer production in cats, *Scand. J. Gastroenterol.,* 12, 379, 1977.
74. **Robert, A.,** Cytoprotection by prostaglandins, *Gastroenterology,* 77, 761, 1979.
75. **Zierden, E., Hengst, K., Wagner, H., and Gerlach, V.,** Inhibition of stress ulcer formation with somatostatin in rats, *Exp. Med.,* 168, 199, 1976.
76. **Schwedes, V., Vsadel, K., and Szabo, S.,** Somatostatin prevents cysteamine- induced duodenal ulcer, *Eur. J. Pharmacol.,* 44, 195, 1977.
77. **Szabo, S. and Reichlin, S.,** Somatostatin depletion by cysteamine: mechanism and implication for duodenal ulcer, *Fed. Proc.,* 44, 2540, 1985.
78. **Szabo, S., Usadel and K. -K.,** Cytoprotection-organoprotection: gastric and hepatic lesions, *Experientia,* 38, 254, 1982.
79. **Diel, F. and Szabo, S.,** Dose-dependent effects of linear and cyclic somatostatin on ethanol-induced gastric erosions. The role of mast cells and increased vascular permeability, *Regul. Peptides,* 13, 235, 1986.
80. **Moreau, J. P. and De-Fendis, F. V.,** Pharmacological studies of somatostatin and somatostatin analogues; therapeutic advances and perspectives, *Life Sci.,* 40, 419, 1987.
81. **Kusterer, K., Rohr, G., Schwedes, V., Usadel, K. H., and Szabo, S.,** Gastric mucosal protection by somatostatins, *Klin. Wochenshr.,* 64(Suppl. VII), 97, 1986.
82. **Ligumsky, M., Goto, Y., Debas, H., and Yamada, T.,** Prostaglandins mediate inhibition of gastric acid secretion by somatostatin in the rat, *Science,* 219, 301, 1982.
83. **Moragd, M. H., Kauffman, G. L., Phelevanian, M., Golanska, E., Elashoff, J. D., and Walsh, J. H.,** Prostaglandins may not mediate inhibition of gastric acid secretion by somatostatin in the rat, *Regul. Peptides,* 10, 213, 1985.
84. **Christiansen, J. and Yotis, A.,** The role of somatostatin and long-acting analogue, SMS, 201-995 in acute bleeding due to peptic ulceration, *Scand. J. Gastroenterol.,* 21(Suppl., 119), 109, 1986.

Chapter 6

ROLE OF THROMBOXANE A_2 AND OTHER CYCLOOXYGENASE PRODUCTS IN GASTRIC DAMAGE

Brendan J. R. Whittle

TABLE OF CONTENTS

I. INTRODUCTION

Eicosanoids are the products of the endogenous fatty acid, arachidonic acid, that are formed through action of the cyclooxygenase and lipoxygenase enzymes. Following its liberation from membrane-bound phospholipids by the action of phospholipases, predominantly phospholipase A_2, arachidonic acid is converted into prostanoids by the action of an enzyme complex, now termed cyclooxygenase.[1] This enzyme converts arachidonic acid into unstable intermediate endoperoxides, and it is at this biosynthetic step that aspirin, indomethacin, and similar drugs act to inhibit the formation of prostanoids.[2] These labile endoperoxides, prostaglandin G_2 (PGG_2) and PGH_2 (Figure 1), can be readily converted to PGE_2 via the action of an endoperoxide isomerase enzyme, while activity of a reductase enzyme may be involved with $PGF_{2\alpha}$ formation; however, both PGE_2 and $PGF_{2\alpha}$ can also arise nonenzymatically, since the endoperoxides can spontaneously decompose in aqueous solution to form PGE_2, $PGF_{2\alpha}$, and PGD_2.

Although the endoperoxides are unstable in aqueous solution and can be readily converted to other products, these intermediates may have intrinsic biological activity acting at specific receptors, including thromboxane receptor sites. Both PGG_2 and PGH_2 can contract vascular tissue and gastrointestinal smooth muscle *in vitro,* whereas in vascular beds *in vivo,* the vasodilatation that is usually observed is due to its conversion to prostacyclin (PGI_2) in the vessel wall.[1]

PGE_2 and PGI_2 are formed by a wide variety of tissues and cells, including gastric mucosal tissue.[3] These prostanoids can inhibit gastric acid secretion, stimulate gastric bicarbonate and mucus secretion, affect mucosal sodium and chloride ionic flux, and can induce vasodilation in the mucosal microcirculation and prevent the vascular stasis induced by damaging agents.[3-5] These prostanoids and their synthetic analogs protect the gastric mucosa from damage, an action which may be brought about by their effects on several of the above parameters;[3-5] however, the other arachidonate metabolites may be involved in the pathogenesis of gastric damage. Thus, the cyclooxygenase product, thromboxane A_2(TXA_2) (Figure 1), has been demonstrated to exert potent pro-ulcerogenic actions.[6]

TXA_2 is a highly active but unstable metabolite, enzymatically formed from the endoperoxides.[1] The chemical half-life in aqueous solution at 37°C is 30 s and it decomposes to TXB_2 which has insignificant biological activity. TXA_2, which is synthesized in substantial quantities by platelets, is a powerful stimulant of platelet aggregation and constricts vascular smooth muscle *in vitro* while it is also a potent vasoconstrictor agent in most vascular beds *in vivo.*[7] The enzyme involved in the biosynthesis of these thromboxanes has been characterized and can be selectively inhibited by several experimental compounds, notably derivatives of imidazole.

Thromboxanes have been demonstrated to be biosynthesized in gastric mucosal tissue from several species. Thus, a radiolabeled metabolite with the same chromatographic mobility as TXB_2 is formed in microsomal preparations from both bovine and dog mucosa.[8-10] The biosynthesis of TXB_2 by gastric mucosal tissue homogenates of rat, rabbit, dog, pig, guinea pig, and man has been demonstrated following incubation with radiolabeled PGH_2 or arachidonic acid, or following extraction for the determination of endogenous formation by specific radioimmunoassay.[11-16] Using short-term culture of biopsy specimens of human gastric mucosa, the release of TXB_2, as well as the prostaglandins, 6-oxo-$PGF_{1\alpha}$ and PGE_2, have likewise been determined by radioimmunoassay.[17] Whether cells within the mucosa contain the thromboxane synthetase enzyme has yet to be defined clearly since platelets entrapped in the gastric microcirculation would be an active source of thromboxanes; however, the synthesis of TXB_2 by primary cultures of mucus-producing epithelial cells from the rat gastric mucosa has been observed.[18]

In this chapter, the adverse actions of TXA_2 and its mimetics and the effects of prostaglandin depletion on gastric mucosal function and integrity are discussed, along with the involvement of prostanoids in the regulation of gastric mucosal hemostasis.

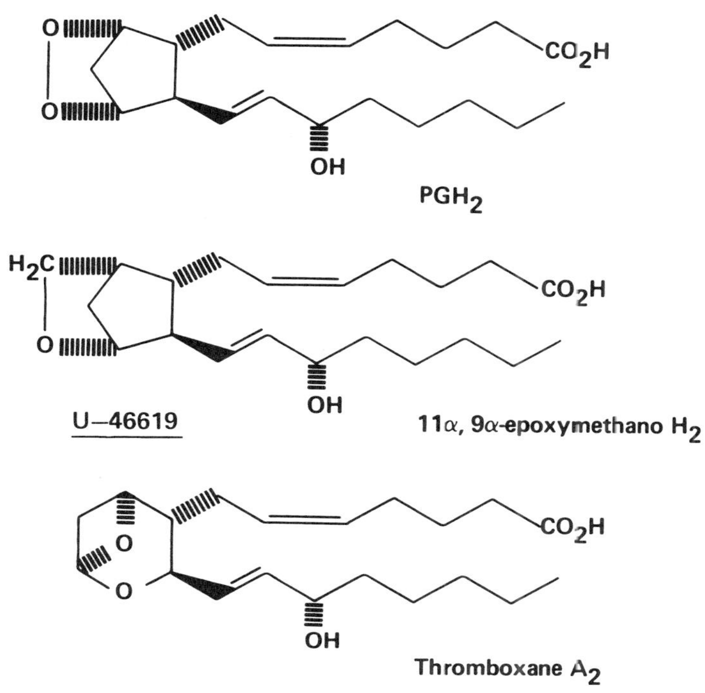

FIGURE 1. Structure of the endogenous endoperoxide prostaglandin H_2, thromboxane A_2, and the chemically stable synthetic endoperoxide analog (U-46619) which acts as a thromboxane mimetic.

II. GASTRIC ACTIONS OF PROSTAGLANDIN $F_{2\alpha}$

$PGF_{2\alpha}$ had no demonstrable gastric antisecretory activity in the chronic fistula dog[4] and had variable actions in the cat following parenteral administration.[19] An inconsistent antisecretory effect of high concentrations of $PGF_{2\alpha}$ was observed on canine isolated parietal cells,[20] while studies in man with $PGF_{2\alpha}$ demonstrated a transient antisecretory action after intravenous administration.[21] The 15-methyl analog of $PGF_{2\alpha}$ weakly inhibited pentagastrin-stimulated acid output in the rat following intravenous infusion.[22] This analog likewise inhibited acid output while enhancing gastric emptying in the rhesus monkey.[23]

Local intraarterial administration of $PGF_{2\alpha}$ into the blood-perfused exteriorized segment of dog stomach *in situ* increased vascular resistance[24] as shown in Figure 2. Likewise, in the rabbit-isolated gastric circulation, bolus administration of $PGF_{2\alpha}$ induced vasoconstriction, as indicated by an increase in perfusion pressure.[25] Direct visualization of the rat gastric microcirculation indicated a preferential vasoconstriction in the submucosal venules after topical application of $PGF_{2\alpha}$ to the submucosa.[26] As discussed later, such actions could reduce the integrity of the mucosa and predispose it to damage.

III. GASTRIC ACTIONS OF THROMBOXANE A_2

The prostanoid precusor, arachidonic acid, inhibited gastric acid secretion when incubated *in vitro* in the isolated rat gastric mucosa[27] and in canine isolated parietal cells.[20] Since this action was abolished by indomethacin, these actions resulted from the biotransformation of arachidonic acid to an antisecretory prostanoid by these gastric preparations. In studies *in vivo,* intravenous infusion of arachidonic acid inhibited gastric acid secretion in the rat and dog *in vivo,* while elevating the ratio of mucosal blood flow to acid output.[27,28] In studies where blood flow

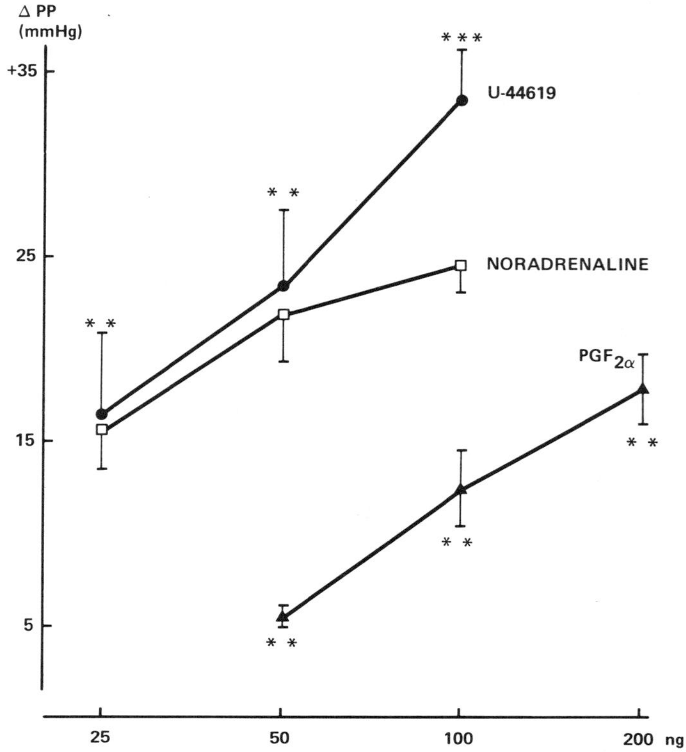

FIGURE 2. Gastric vasoconstriction in the blood-perfused chambered segment of the canine stomach *in situ* induced by close arterial injection of $PGF_{2\alpha}$, noradrenaline, and the stable thromboxane mimetic, 11α,9α-epoxymethano-PGH_2 (U-46619). Results, shown as the increase in perfusion pressure (ΔPP, mmHg), are the mean ± s.e. mean of 4 to 6 experiments, where statistical significant changes from resting values are shown as $^{**}p < 0.01$, $^{***}p < 0.001$. Data are adapted from Kauffman and Whittle.[26]

in the dog stomach was measured via a flow probe, direct infusion of low doses of arachidonic acid into the gastric artery produced vasodilatation.[29,30] In contrast, however, when high doses of arachidonic acid were infused close intraarterially into an exteriorized chambered segment of the gastric mucosa, acid inhibition was accompanied by a fall in the ratio of blood flow to acid output, suggesting a vasoconstrictor action.[31,32] Thus, the profile of vascular responses to arachidonic acid are closely dependent on the experimental conditions, on the dose of arachidonic acid, and the time in which it can incubate with blood *in vivo*.

When administered by close intraarterial injection to the canine stomach in low doses, arachidonic acid produced gastric vasodilatation (Figure 3), which could be abolished by indomethacin. This is likely to reflect the biosynthesis of a vasodilator prostaglandin, either PGE_2 or PGI_2 in the gastric microvasculature.[24] Indeed, elevated levels of the PGI_2 breakdown product 6-oxo-$PGF_{1\alpha}$ have been detected in the venous effluent draining the gastric segment following arachidonic acid administration;[33] however, when arachidonic acid was injected into a delay coil to allow its incubation with the flowing arterial blood for 30 s before reaching the stomach, vasoconstriction was observed[6] as shown in Figure 3. This response was abolished by indomethacin and reflects the biotransformation of arachidonic acid by the blood-borne platelets to TXA_2,[33] which was detected by RIA as the breakdown product, TXB_2. This was further confirmed by use of the specific thromboxane synthetase inhibitor, 1-benzyl imidazole (BZI), which abolished this vasoconstriction, reversing it to a vasodilator response.[6] Thus, under these

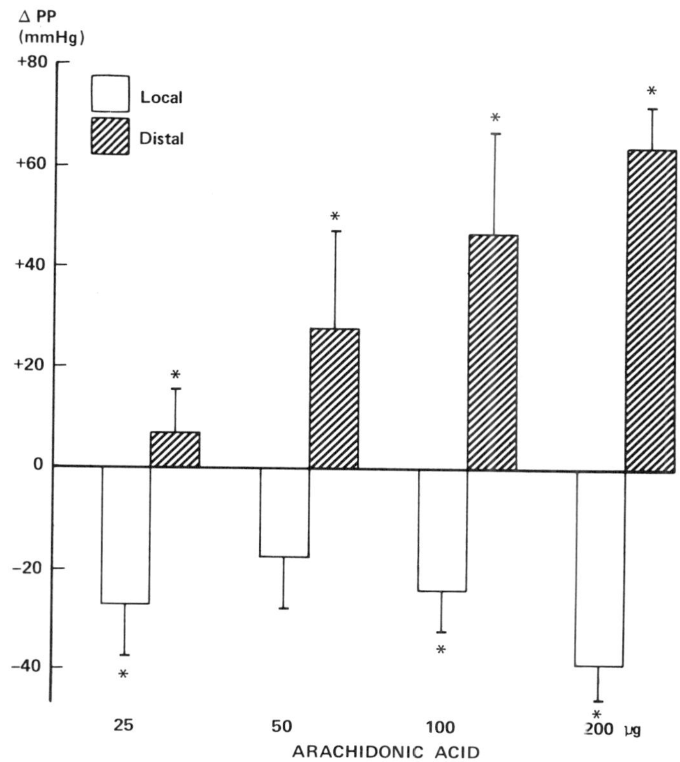

FIGURE 3. Vascular effects of local intraarterial administration of arachidonic acid on the blood-perfused chambered segment of the canine stomach *in situ*. Arachidonic acid (25 to 200 μg) was injected either into local port (so as to reach the stomach within 3 s), shown by open columns, or into a distal port (so as to reach the stomach after 30 s incubation in blood), shown by hatched columns. Results shown as changes in gastric perfusion pressure (ΔPP), are the mean ± s.e. mean of 3 to 8 experiments where $^{*}p < 0.05$. Data are adapted from Kauffman and Whittle.[26]

conditions, since arachidonic acid was no longer converted to TXA_2 by the platelets, it was presumably available for bioconversion into vasodilator prostanoids in the gastric vasculature. Indeed, such vasodilation by arachidonic acid was subsequently abolished by administration of indomethacin, indicating the involvement of a cyclooxygenase metabolite.[6]

IV. GASTRIC ACTIONS OF THE THROMBOXANE MIMETIC

The instability of TXA_2 limits the extent and nature of the pharmacological investigations that can be carried out, and such studies necessitate the de novo synthesis of TXA_2 when required. Thus, to extend these observations further, studies have been conducted using the chemically stable endoperoxide analog, 11α-9α epoxy-methano-PGH_2 (U-46619; Figure 1) which has been pharmacologically characterized as a thromboxane mimetic acting at thromboxane-sensitive sites.[34] Intravenous infusion of this thromboxane mimetic inhibited acid secretion in the monkey[36] and the dog,[37] an effect attributed to a primary reduction in gastric mucosal blood flow. Oral administration of U-46619 did not inhibit gastric acid secretion in the rat, yet stimulated the secretion of mucus and fluid.[38]

To study the actions of the thromboxane mimetic on the gastric vasculature and subsequently on mucosal integrity, a segment of acid-secreting fundic mucosa of the stomach of the

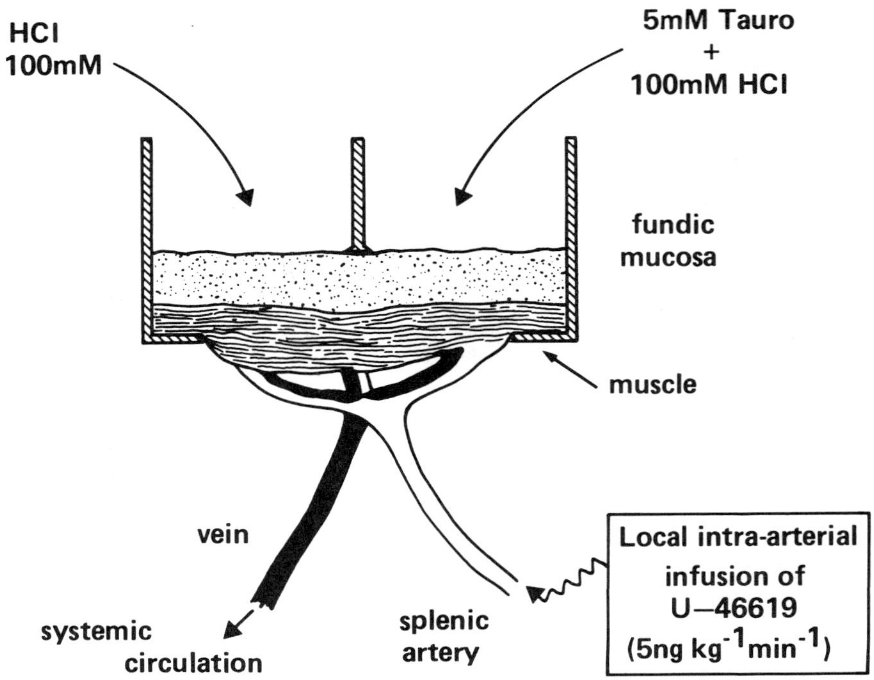

FIGURE 4. Technique for the investigation of the effects of local intraarterial infusion of the thromboxane mimetic, U-46619, on the chambered segment of the canine stomach *in situ*. The surface of the gastric mucosa was bathed with either acid (100 m*M* HCl) or acidified-taurocholate (5 m*M* sodium taurocholate, 100 m*M* HCl), utilizing a two-compartment perspex chamber.

pentobarbital-anesthetized dog was encased *in situ* in a lucite chamber consisting of two compartments.[24] The vasculature was pump-perfused with blood (10 ml min^{-1}) from a cannulated femoral artery, as shown in Figure 4, and the thromboxane mimetic was administered locally into the arterial bloodline, close to the stomach. Intraarterial injection of U-46619 induced dose-related increases in gastric vascular perfusion pressure, indicating marked vasoconstriction in the gastric circulation (Figure 2). Likewise, in the isolated gastric circulation of the rat and rabbit, perfused *in vitro* with Krebs' solution, U-46619 induced rises in perfusion pressure, again showing direct vasoconstrictor effects.[25]

To investigate further this vascular action of the thromboxane mimetic, its actions on the rat gastric microcirculation *in vivo* was studied. The *in vivo* microscopy technique described by Guth and colleagues[39,40] was used to determine gastric submucosal arteriolar and venular responses in the pentobarbital-anesthetized rat. A fiberoptic light carrier rod was inserted into the gastric lumen via an incision in the forestomach to transilluminate the stomach wall. After removal of the serosal and muscle layers, a shallow disk with a 5-mm orifice was sealed over the exposed submucosa for the local application of Krebs' solution and the compounds under investigation. This system allowed direct microscopical visualization and measurement of the submucosal vascular networks, which were video recorded via a television camera. Arterioles and venules of resting diameter 20 and 50 μm, respectively, were selected for study. Changes in the diameter of the microvessels were subsequently determined by an image-splitting monitor.

Topical application of U-46619 to the exposed submucosal vascular bed reduced vessel diameter in both arterioles and venules (Figure 5) reaching plateau responses within 2 min of application.[26] At the highest concentration studied, the reduction in vessel diameter was

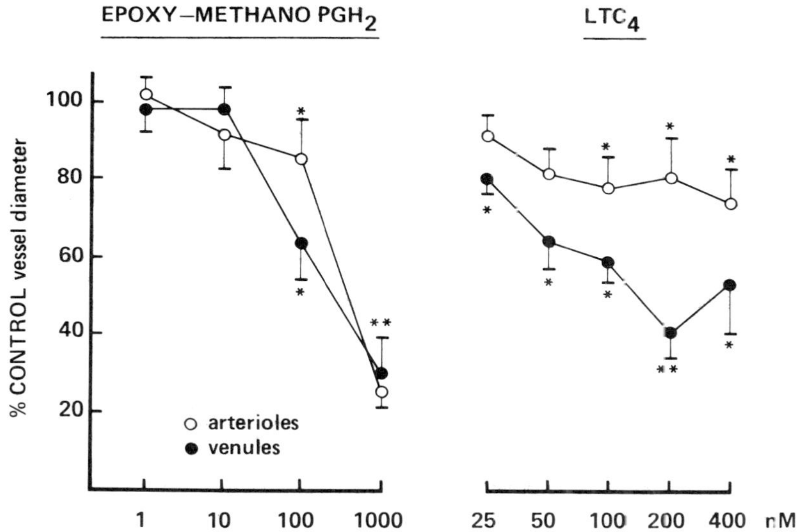

FIGURE 5. Vasoconstriction in the rat gastric submucosal arterioles (o—o) and venules (•—•) following a 5-min local application of the thromboxane mimetic, U-46619 (11α-9α epoxy-methano PGH_2) and LTC_4. The results, expressed as the change in vessel diameter percent of the control, are the mean ± s.e. mean of 6 and 10 studies respectively, where significant changes are shown as $*p < 0.05$, $**p < 0.01$. Data are adapted from Whittle et al.[26]

comparable for both arterioles and venules (Figure 5). Also shown are the effects of local application of the lipoxygenase product, leukotriene C_4 (LTC_4), which induced vasoconstriction in the venules, which was more pronounced than in the arterioles, reaching peak responses within 1.5 min. With both LTC_4 and the thromboxane mimetic, intense focal vasoconstriction in the venules was clearly demonstrated, leading to sluggish blood flow and stasis within the vessels.[26] Preliminary studies using a laser doppler technique to determine blood flow in the rat gastric mucosa have likewise demonstrated a reduction in vascular perfusion following intravenous administration of U-46619, which was inhibited by a thromboxane-receptor antagonist.[40]

V. THROMBOXANE A_2 IN GASTRIC PATHOLOGY

A. GASTRIC DAMAGE INDUCED BY TXA_2 AND ITS MIMETIC

To investigate the pro-ulcerogenic actions of TXA_2 and its mimetic, the chambered exteriorized segment of the canine stomach was utilized (Figure 4), and the mucosa exposed to either an acid solution or a solution containing an acidified bile salt.

Topical instillation into the gastric chamber of acid (100 m*M* HCl) or an acid-taurocholate mixture (5 m*M* in 100 m*M* HCl) caused only a low incidence of macroscopically visible gastric mucosal damage during the 30 min observation period.[6] Intraarterial infusion of arachidonic acid during exposure to the acid solution alone also failed to substantially damage the mucosa (Figure 6). Likewise, intraarterial infusion of U-46619 (5 ng kg^{-1} min^{-1}) in a dose that increased gastric perfusion pressure of Δ 66 ± 5 mmHg (n = 6; $p < 0.001$), indicating marked vasoconstriction in the gastric circulation, did not induce macroscopic damage;[41] however, when the mucosa was exposed to acid-taurocholate, extensive mucosal damage developed during the 30 min infusion of arachidonic acid or the thromboxane mimetic (Figure 6). Thus, with TXA_2 generated *in situ* from arachidonic acid or the thromboxane mimetic, localized areas of blanching, followed by engorgement and stasis could clearly be observed during their administration.

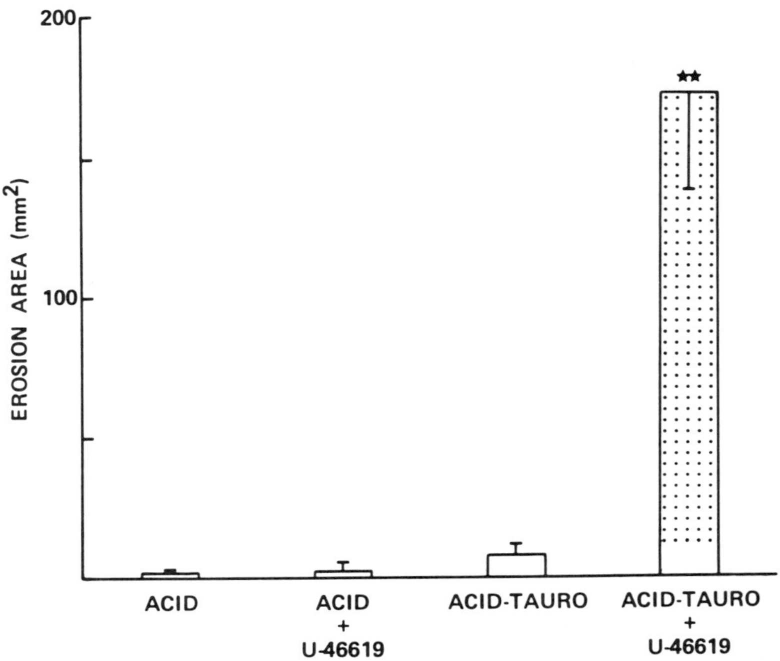

FIGURE 6. Gastric mucosal damage in the canine chambered stomach *in situ* following local intraarterial infusion of the thromboxane mimetic (U-46619; 5 ng kg^{-1} min^{-1}) during a 30-min period of topical application of acid (100 m*M* HCl) or acidified bile salt (5 m*M* sodium taurocholate in 10 m*M* HCl). Results, shown as the area of macroscopically apparent damage (mm^2), are expressed as mean ± s.e. mean of 5 experiments, where significant difference from acid alone is shown as $**p < 0.01$.

These areas often were the initial or predominant sites for necrosis and punctate bleeding, which became apparent within 10 to 15 min of the infusion. Sloughing of the mucosal epithelial tissue led to extensive bleeding from the exposed underlying tissue following termination of the infusion.

In other studies, this thromboxane mimetic (1.5 mg/kg) administered orally to rats, was found to stimulate fluid and mucus secretion and cause some attenuation of macroscopically assessed ethanol-induced gastric damage.[37] More recently, high oral doses of U-46619 likewise have been shown to reduce ethanol-induced gastric lesions in the rat, with an ID_{50} (dose reducing gastric damage by 50% of 100 μg/kg, while stimulating nonparietal gastric secretion at doses up to 1 mg/kg;[42] however, the latter authors concluded that such protective actions of U-46619 administered orally did not necessarily reflect the effects of endogenous TXA_2, and that these actions were probably not related to activity at the thromboxane receptor. Indeed, pretreatment with indomethacin reduced this nonparietal secretory response and protective effects of U-46619.[42] Furthermore, the gastric antisecretory actions of this compound *in vitro* on the rat isolated gastric mucosa was substantially attenuated by concurrent incubation with indomethacin.[43] These results, therefore, suggest a nonspecific protective action of high oral doses of U-46619 involving endogenous prostaglandin stimulation, perhaps as a result of local mild irritation of the superficial mucosa.

In more recent studies in our laboratories using U-46619 in the rat, a novel technique for the close arterial administration of substances via a cannula inserted into the left gastric artery has been utilized.[44] Intraarterial infusion of U-46619 (100 to 500 ng kg^{-1} min^{-1} for 10 min), in doses having no effect on systemic arterial blood pressure, induced extensive damage in both the antral and corpus regions of the gastric mucosa, as assessed macroscopically and histologically. The antral damage was apparent macroscopically as deep penetrating ulcers.[44] In the presence of a dilute concentration of intraluminal ethanol (10%), intraarterial infusion of lower doses of U-46619 (25 to 100 ng kg^{-1} min^{-1}) induced hemorrhagic and necrotic mucosal damage. These pro-ulcerogenic actions of U-46619 were abolished by pretreatment with the selective thromboxane antagonist, BM 13,177.

These findings indicate that the damage induced by U-46619 was not a nonspecific action, but was the result of interaction with thromboxane receptor sites in the mucosa. Such receptor sites may be located in the microvasculature since local application of U-46619 to the exposed submucosa induced profound focal vasoconstriction in both the arterioles and venules, leading to stasis of blood flow.[26] The resultant mucosal ischemia would account for the damage observed and would also predispose the mucosa to injury by weak irritants such as dilute ethanol; however, this thromboxane mimetic may, in addition, activate or aggregate platelets or other blood cells in the microcirculation leading to the occlusion of the microvessels as well as to the release of further tissue-destructive mediators including TXA_2 itself, lipoxygenase products, lysosomal enzymes, and free radicals. Furthermore, TXA_2 and its mimetic could exert direct cytolytic actions on the gastric microvasculature or mucosal cells, as suggested from previous studies in the liver,[45] endothelium,[46] and erythrocytes.[47]

B. PROTECTIVE ACTIONS OF A THROMBOXANE SYNTHASE INHIBITOR

To investigate the role of locally generated TXA_2 in the pathogenesis of gastric mucosal damage, the protective actions of the thromboxane synthase inhibitor, BZI, against ethanol-induced lesions in the rat was studied.[48] Gastric mucosal lesions were induced by the oral administration of 1 ml of an acidified-ethanol mixture (40% ethanol in 100 m*M* HCl) via a rubber intragastric tube. The degree of gastric damage was assessed 2 h after treatment, with each mucosa being coded to avoid observer bias and assigned a lesion score based on the incidence and severity of the lesions macroscopically visible as discrete hemorrhagic erosions.

Oral pretreatment with BZI as the fumerate salt 30 min prior to challenge reduced the incidence and severity of the gastric erosions seen 2 h after acid-ethanol treatment, as shown in Figure 7. The ID_{50} (dose inhibiting gastric lesions by 50%) was calculated to be 3.2 mg kg^{-1}. BZI was also effective following subcutaneous injection, administered 1 h prior to challenge, the ID_{50} being 3.8 mg kg^{-1}.[48] This indicates that the protective action was not the result of a local buffering action of BZI in the gastric lumen or from a local weak irritant action, which has been shown to confer some protection to the gastric mucosa.

Other studies with selective thromboxane synthase inhibitors in experimental models also give support to the concept that TXA_2 is involved in the pathogenesis of gastric damage. Thus, OKY-1581 reduced bile-salt induced gastric necrosis in the rat, although it failed to inhibit that induced by ethanol.[49] Furthermore, oral administration of dazmegrel, in doses reducing TXB_2 synthesis by the rat gastric mucosa, likewise reduced macroscopically assessed mucosal damage induced by acidified taurocholate.[50] In preliminary studies, the thromboxane synthase inhibitor, dazoxiben, as well as thromboxane antagonists reduced enthanol-induced gastric lesions;[51] however, in our studies, while BZI substantially inhibited gastric damage induced by acid-ethanol, it also inhibited indomethacin-induced erosions.[48] Since the dose of indomethacin used would inhibit cyclooxygenase, and therefore itself would reduce TXA_2 formation, the mechanisms of its protective action under these conditions are not fully clear. However, the involvement of TXA_2 in gastric damage resulting from local ischemia and other microcirculatory disordered thus requires further consideration.

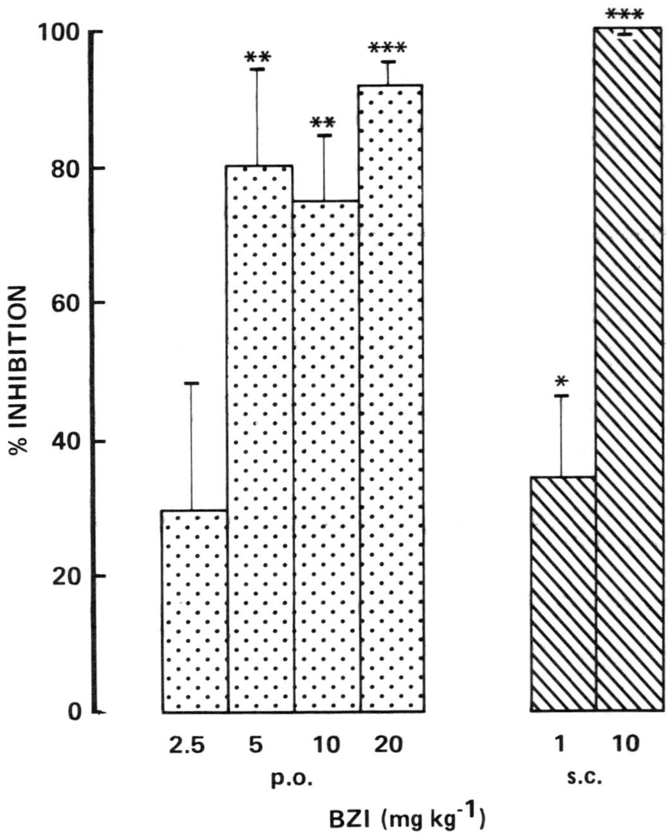

FIGURE 7. Inhibition by the thromboxane synthase inhibitor, BZI, of macroscopically assessed gastric mucosal damage in the rat. Rats were pretreated with BZI either by the oral or subcutaneous route 30 min prior to challenge with 1 ml acidified ethanol (40% in 100 m*M* HCl) via an intragastric tube. Results, shown as percent inhibition of the control damage, are the mean ± s.e. mean of 6 to 12 rats in each group, where $*p < 0.05$, $**p < 0.01$, $***p < 0.001$.

VI. ENDOGENOUS PROTECTIVE PROSTANOIDS IN MUCOSAL INTEGRITY

Since prostanoids of the E and I series exert such potent actions on gastric function and integrity,[3-5] it is not surprising that alterations in local prostaglandin formation have been implicated as a mechanism underlying gastric damage and disease.[52] The depletion of endogenous prostanoids by nonsteroidal anti-inflammatory agents, which directly inhibit the cyclooxygenase enzyme, is a likely mechanism contributing to the gastric mucosal damage induced by these drugs, both in experimental models and in their clinical use. Local alterations in prostanoid turnover have also been implicated in the pathogenesis peptic ulcer disease.[3-5]

Nonsteroidal anti-inflammatory drugs (NSAID) are recognized to cause local irritant actions on the gastric mucosa, allowing acid to diffuse back into the tissue. This "barrier-breaking" activity does not appear to be related to the inhibition of endogenous prostaglandin biosynthesis[53,54] and results from a direct action initially exerted on the surface epithelial cells. Indeed, agents such as isobutyric acid and hyperosmotic glucose that are not regarded as cyclooxygenase inhibitors likewise affect gastric "barrier" integrity.[55] Both local irritancy and the inhibition of prostaglandin biosynthesis are of importance, however, when considering the gastric toxicity of nonsteroidal anti-inflammatory agents, especially since both processes interact synergistically to produce more extensive gastric injury than either activity alone.

The gastric damage that follows challenge with low concentrations of topical irritants such as acidified bile salts or ethanol is greatly augmented by concurrent administration of cyclooxygenase inhibitors.[53] Intravenous or subcutaneous administration of such agents in doses inhibiting mucosal cyclooxygenase by greater than 60% significantly potentiated mucosal damage by topical irritants such as acidified taurocholate or ethanol in the rat or dog.[41,56,57] Such potentiation of injury may reflect changes in the mucosal microcirculation brought about by a reduction in endogenous prostanoid biosynthesis. These findings give support for a role of endogenous prostanoids in the maintenance of mucosal integrity. Thus, although cyclooxygenase products do not appear to regulate mucosal barrier function, their actions on the mucosal microcirculation and other potentially protective processes appear to be of physiological importance. Significant suppression of endogenous prostanoid biosynthesis thus greatly augments the susceptibility of the mucosal tissue to damage by normally weak irritants.

VII. THROMBOXANE A_2 AND HEMOSTASIS IN THE GASTRIC MUCOSA

Platelet adhesion, aggregation, and subsequent plug formation play a major role in the control of cutaneous and vascular hemostasis.[58] Since TXA_2 is a potent inducer of platelet aggregation, it has been implicated as a mediator in the process of hemostasis. Thus, inhibition of thromboxane synthesis can reduce platelet aggregation[1,7] and prolong cutaneous bleeding time in man.[59,60] Although bleeding of the gastric mucosa from ulcer sites and following damage by aspirin-like drugs and topical irritants is common, little is known about the hemostatic process and the role of TXA_2 in this microcirculation. Bleeding from a standard incision in the rat gastric mucosa has therefore been investigated.[61] The actions of PGI_2, which directly prevents platelet aggregation[1,7] and of the thromboxane synthase inhibitor, BZI, as well as those of low doses of heparin which interfere with blood coagulation, have been compared on bleeding time in the gastric mucosa and in the mesenteric artery.

Rats were anesthetised with pentobarbitone, the stomach was opened along the greater curvature and mounted in a plexiglass chamber with its vascular supply intact. Ileal mesentery was placed over a similar chamber. Gastric mucosal bleeding was produced by a 2-mm blade cut through a rugal fold, while mesenteric bleeding was induced by puncturing a mesenteric artery close to the ileal wall with a 25-gauge needle. Warmed isotonic saline was superfused over the surface, collected at timed intervals, and the hemoglobin output determined using spectrophotometric techniques.

Gastric bleeding time was not significantly prolonged by intravenous infusion of prostacyclin (0.5 $\mu g\ kg^{-1}\ min^{-1}$) in a dose which inhibits platelet aggregation *ex vivo*. Likewise, administration of BZI (50 mg kg^{-1} i.v.), 10 min prior to the incision, in a dose reducing TXB_2 formation in clotting blood by 90 ± 2% (n = 5), did not significantly prolong bleeding time (Figure 8). Intravenous injection of heparin (100 U kg^{-1}), however, prolonged the bleeding time beyond 15 min. In contrast, in the mesenteric artery, the bleeding time, which was comparable to gastric bleeding time, was significantly prolonged by administration of PGI_2 or BZI, but not by heparin (Figure 8). Similar findings were obtained in studies on the gastric mucosa of rabbit and dog, where heparin, but not PGI_2 or BZI, prolonged gastric bleeding from the standard incision.[61]

These findings confirm the importance of platelet aggregation and TXA_2 in the hemostatic processes that terminate primary bleeding from arterial vasculature. In contrast in the gastric mucosa, neither PGI_2 nor BZI had any significant action on bleeding, yet heparin substantially prolonged the bleeding time. These findings therefore suggest that hemostasis in the gastric mucosal microcirculation is more dependent on the coagulation system than on platelet

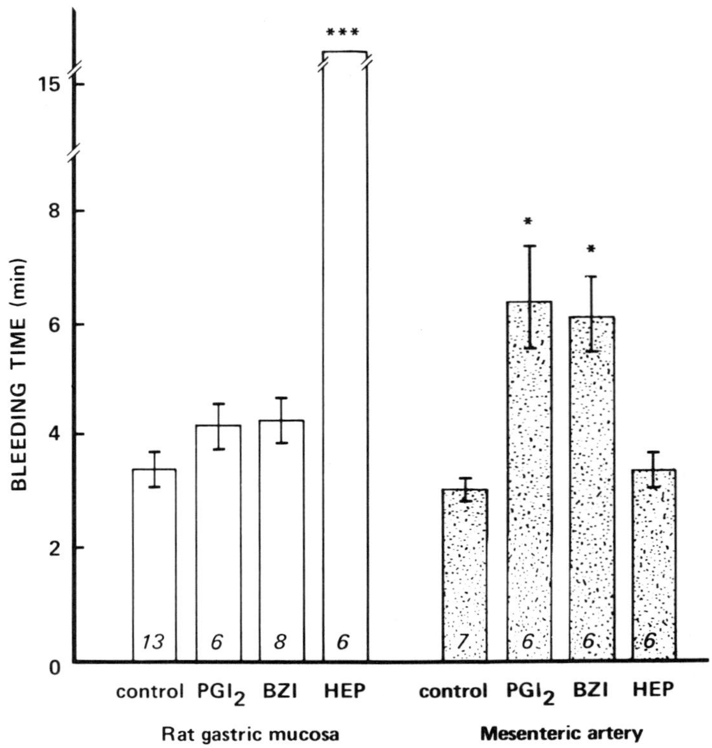

FIGURE 8. Effect of platelet antiaggregatory doses of PGI_2 (0.5 µg kg^{-1} min^{-1}, i.v.), doses of BZI (50 mg kg^{-1}, i.v.) sufficient to reduce platelet thromboxane formation by 90%, and the anticoagulant heparin (100 U kg^{-1}, i.v.) on the duration of bleeding from the rat gastric mucosa and mesenteric artery. Results are shown as the bleeding time (the time taken for hemoglobin output from the standard incision to decline to <0.1 mg min^{-1}) and expressed as mean ± s.e. mean of (n) rats, where statistical difference from the control value is $*p < 0.05$, $***p < 0.001$.

aggregation or local TXA_2 formation. Furthermore, local or systemic administration of NSAID in doses sufficient to inhibit cyclooxygenase, did not prolong such gastric bleeding.[61] Indeed, these results now explain the findings of an earlier clinical study in which acute or chronic aspirin administration failed to enhance mucosal bleeding from gastric biopsy sites in human volunteers in doses sufficient to prolong the skin bleeding time.[60] Thus, interference with TXA_2 formation or platelet aggregation appears to play little part in the bleeding associated with the gastric irritancy associated with these anti-inflammatory agents.

VIII. CONCLUSIONS

Although the cyclooxygenase product, TXA_2, does not appear to be involved with the primary hemostatic events that terminate bleeding in the gastric mucosa, TXA_2 generated by platelets in arterial blood from arachidonic acid and the thromboxane mimetic are potent vasoconstrictors in the gastric microcirculation. Local intraarterial administration of U-46619 can induce mucosal disruption in the rat, while both U-46619 and TXA_2 cause extensive gastric mucosal hemorrhage and necrosis in the dog in the presence of weak irritants such as topically applied acidified bile salts. Thus, these thromboxanes reduce the ability of the mucosa to withstand challenge from normally mild irritants, an action which may be related to their vasoconstrictor properties. Direct cytolytic actions of these thromboxanes on the mucosal cells cannot yet, however, be entirely excluded.

These potent actions of the thromboxanes point to the possibility that endogenous TXA_2 may be involved in the pathogenesis of gastric ulceration. Thus, following platelet activation in the microcirculation as a result of local trauma, or in stress or shocked states resulting from hemorrhage or during bacterial infection and resultant disseminated intravascular coagulation, local generation of TXA_2 may contribute to the associated gastrointestinal injury.

REFERENCES

1. **Moncada, S. and Vane, J. R.,** Pharmacology and endogenous roles of prostaglandin endoperoxides, thromboxane A_2, and prostacyclin, *Pharmacol Rev.,* 30, 293, 1979.
2. **Vane, J. R.,** Inhibition of prostaglandin synthesis as a mechanism of action of aspirin-like drugs, *Nature (London) New Biol.,* 231, 232, 1971.
3. **Whittle, B. J. R. and Vane, J. R.,** Prostanoids are regulators of gastrointestinal function, in *Physiology of the Gastrointestinal Tract,* 2nd ed., Vol. 1, Johnson, L. R., Ed., Raven Press, New York, 1987, 601.
4. **Robert, A.,** Prostaglandins and the gastrointestinal tract, in *Physiology of the Gastrointestinal Tract,* Johnson, L. R., Ed., Raven Press, New York, 1981, 1407.
5. **Hawkey, C. J. and Rampton, D. S.,** Prostaglandins in the gastrointestinal mucosa: are they important in its function, disease or treatment?, *Gastroenterology,* 89, 1162, 1985.
6. **Whittle, B. J. R., Kauffman, G. L.,** and **Moncada, S.,** Vasoconstriction with thromboxane A_2 induces ulceration of the gastric mucosa, *Nature,* 292, 472, 1981.
7. **Whittle, B. J. R. and Moncada, S.,** The pharmacological interactions between prostacyclin and thromboxanes, *Br. Med. Bull.,* 39, 232, 1983.
8. **Zemecnik, A. M., Cerskus, J., Stoessl, A. L., Barnett, A. J., and McDonald, J. W. D.,** Synthesis of thromboxane B_2 and prostaglandins by bovine gastric mucosal microsomes, *Prostaglandins,* 14, 819, 1977.
9. **LeDuc, L. E. and Needleman, P.,** Regional localization of prostacyclin and thromboxane synthesis in dog stomach and intestinal tract, *J. Pharm. Exp. Ther.,* 211, 181, 1979.
10. **Ali, M. and McDonald, J. W. D.,** Synthesis of thromboxane B_2 and 6-keto-prostaglandin $F_{1\alpha}$ in bovine gastric mucosal and muscle microsomes, *Prostaglandins,* 20, 245, 1980.
11. **Ahlquist, D. A., Duenes, J. A., Madson, T. H., Romero, J. C., Dozois, R. R., and Malagelada, J. R.,** Prostaglandin generation from gastroduodenal mucosa: regional and species differences, *Prostaglandins,* 24, 115, 1982.
12. **Ahlquist, D. A., Madson, T. H., Romero, J. C., Dozois, R. R., and Malagelada, J. R.,** Factors influencing metabolism of arachidonic acid in guinea-pig gastric mucosa, *Am. J. Physiol.,* 244, G131, 1983.
13. **Aly, A., Johansson, C., Slezak, P., and Green, K.,** Bioconversion of arachidonic acid in the human gastrointestinal tract, *Biochem. Med.,* 31, 319, 1984.
14. **Whittle, B. J. R. and Boughton-Smith, N. K.,** Biosynthesis of endogenous arachidonate products involved in gastric damage and protection, in *Proceedings of IUPHAR 9th International Congress of Pharmacology,* Vol. 3, Paton, W., Mitchell, J., and Turner, P., Eds., Macmillan, London, 1984, 345.
15. **Wallace, J. L. and Whittle, B. J. R.,** Role of prostanoids in the protective actions of BW755C on the gastric mucosa, *Eur. J. Pharmacol.,* 115, 45, 1985.
16. **Hawkey, C. J.,** Synthesis of prostaglandin E_2 and thromboxane B_2 and prostaglandin catabolism in gastritis and gastric ulcer, *Gut,* 12, 1484, 1986.
17. **Rachmilewitz, D., Branski, D., Sharon, P., and Karmeli, F.,** Possible role of endogenous prostanoids in the pathogenesis of peptic ulcer, in *Mechanisms of Mucosal Protection in the Upper Gastrointestinal Tract,* Allen, A., Flemstrom, G., Garner, A., Silen, W., and Turnberg, L. A., Eds., Raven Press, New York, 1984, 329.
18. **Hiraishi, H., Terano, A., Ota, S., Shiga, J., Kobayashi, T., Harada, H., Ishii, M., Ivey, K. J., and Sugimoto, T.,** Prostaglandin production in cultured gastric mucosal cells: role of cAMP on its modulation, *Prostaglandins,* 32, 259, 1986.
19. **Gascoigne, A. D. and Hirst, B. H.,** Prostaglandins alter the relationship between gastric hydrogen ion concentration and flow: evidence for the stimulation of non-parietal secretion in the cat, *J. Physiol.,* 316, 427, 1981.
20. **Skoglund, M. L., Nies, A. S., and Gerber, J. G.,** Inhibition of acid secretion in isolated canine parietal cells by prostaglandins, *J. Pharm. Exp. Ther.,* 229, 371, 1982.

21. **Newman, A., Prado, J., de Moraes-Fiho, P., Philippakos, P., and Misiewicz, J. J.,** The effect of intravenous infusions of prostaglandins E_2 and $F_{2\alpha}$ on human gastric function, *Gut,* 16, 272, 1975.
22. **Whittle, B. J. R.,** Relationship between the prevention of rat gastric erosions and the inhibition of acid secretion by prostaglandins, *Eur. J. Pharmacol.,* 40, 233, 1976.
23. **Shea-Donohue, T., Nompleggi, D., Myers, L., and Dubois, A.,** A comparison of the effects of prostacyclin and the 15(S),15-methyl analogs of PGE_2 and $PGF_{2\alpha}$ on gastric parietal and non-parietal secretion, *Dig. Dis. Sci.,* 27, 17, 1982.
24. **Kauffman, G. L. and Whittle, B. J. R.,** Gastric vascular actions of prostanoids and the dual effect of arachidonic acid, *Am. J. Physiol.,* 242, G582, 1982.
25. **Salvati, P. and Whittle, B. J. R.,** Investigation of the vascular actions of arachidonate lipoxygenase and cyclo-oxygenase products on the isolated perfused stomach of rat and rabbit, *Prostaglandins,* 22, 141, 1981.
26. **Whittle, B. J. R., Oren-Wolman, N., and Guth, P. H.,** Gastric vasoconstrictor actions of leukotriene C_4, $PGF_{2\alpha}$, and thromboxane mimetic U-46619 on rat submucosal microcirculation *in vivo, Am. J. Physiol.,* 248, G580, 1985.
27. **Frame, M. H. and Main, I. H. M.,** Effects of arachidonic acid on rat gastric secretion in response to different secretagogues; inhibition of these effects by indomethacin, *Br. J. Pharmacol.,* 69, 171, 1980.
28. **Connolly, M. E., Bieck, P. R., Payne, N. A., Adkins, B., and Oates, J. A.,** Effect of the prostaglandin precursor, arachidonic acid, on histamine stimulated gastric secretion in the conscious dog, and the observations on the effect of inhibiting endogenous prostaglandin synthesis, *Gut,* 18, 429, 1977.
29. **Gerber, J. G.** and **Hies, A. S.,** Canine gastric mucosal vasodilation with prostaglandins and histamine analogs, *Dig. Dis. Sci.,* 27, 870, 1982.
30. **Gerkens, J. F., Shand, D. G., Flexner, C., Hies, A. S., Oates, J. A., and Data, J. L.,** Effect of indomethacin and aspirin on gastric blood flow and acid secretion, *J. Pharmacol. Exp. Ther.,* 203, 646, 1977.
31. **Konturek, S. J., Mikos, E., Pawlik, W., and Walus, K.,** Direct inhibition of gastric acid secretion and mucosal blood flow by arachidonic acid, *J. Physiol. (London),* 286, 15, 1979.
32. **Walus, K. M., Gustaw, P., and Konturek, S. J.,** Differential effects of prostaglandins and arachidonic acid on gastric circulation and oxygen consumption, *Prostaglandins,* 20, 1080, 1980.
33. **Kauffman, G. L., Whittle, B. J. R., and Salmon, J. A.,** Gastric venous prostaglandin concentrations during basal and stimulated acid secretion in the dog, *Proc. Soc. Exp. Med.,* 169, 233, 1982.
34. **Coleman, R. A., Humphrey, P. P. A., Kennedy, I., Levy, G. P.,** and **Lumley, P.,** Comparison of the actions of U-46619, a prostaglandin H_2-analogue, with those of prostaglandin H_2 and thromboxane A_2 on some isolated smooth muscle preparations, *Br. J. Pharmacol.,* 73, 773, 1981.
35. **Shea-Donohue, P. T., Nompleggi, D., Myers, L.,** and **Dubois, A.,** A prostaglandin endoperoxide analog increases gastric emptying and suppresses gastric secretion in rhesus monkeys, *J. Pharm. Exp. Ther.,* 222, 379, 1982.
36. **Tao, P., Scruggs, W.,** and **Wilson, D. E.,** The effects of an endoperoxide analogue on canine gastric acid and mucus secretion, *Dig. Dis. Sci.,* 24, 449, 1979.
37. **Tao, P. and Wilson, D. E.,** Effects of prostaglandin E_2, 16,16-dimethyl prostaglandin E_2 and a prostaglandin endoperoxide analogue (U-46619) on gastric secretory volume, (H^+) and mucus synthesis and secretion in the rat, *Prostaglandins,* 28, 353, 1984.
38. **Guth, P. H. and Moler, T. L.,** The role of endogenous prostanoids in the response of the rat gastric microcirculation to vasoactive agents, *Microvasc. Res.,* 23, 336, 1982.
39. **Guth, P. H., Paulsen, G., and Nagata, H.,** Histologic and microcirculatory changes in alcohol-induced gastric lesions in the rat. Effect of prostaglandin cytoprotection, *Gastroenterology,* 87, 1083, 1984.
40. **Currington, A., Pipkin, G., Price, C. A., and Swayne, G. T.,** The effect of U-46619 on rat gastric blood flow using laser doppler velocimetry, *Br. J. Pharmacol.,* 90, 233P, 1987.
41. **Whittle, B. J. R. and Moncada, S.,** Ulceration induced by an endoperoxide analogue and by indomethacin in the canine stomach, in *Advances in Prostaglandin, Thromboxane and Leukotriene Research,* Vol. 12, Samuelsson, B., Paoletti, R., and Ramwell, P., Eds., Raven Press, New York, 1983, 373.
42. **Bunce, K. T. and Clayton, N. M.,** The effects of the stable thromboxane A_2-mimetic, U-46619, on gastric mucosal damage and gastric non-parietal secretion in the rat, *Br. J. Pharmacol.,* 91, 23, 1987.
43. **Reeves, J. J. and Stables, R.,** Effects of indomethacin, piroxicam and selected prostanoids on gastric acid secretion by the rat isolated gastric mucosa, *Br. J. Pharmacol.,* 86, 677, 1985.
44. **Esplugues, J. V. and Whittle, B. J. R.,** Gastric mucosal damage induced by local intra-arterial administration of a thromboxane mimetic and PAF in the rat, *Gastroenterology,* 92, 1385, 1987.
45. **Lefer, A. M., Smith, E. F., III, Araki, H., Smith, J. B., Aharony, D., Claremon, D. A., Magolda, R. L., and Nicolaou, K. C.,** Dissociation of vasoconstrictor and platelet aggregatory activities of thromboxane by carbocyclic thromboxane A_2, a stable analog of thromboxane A_2, *Proc. Natl. Acad. Sci. U.S.A.,* 77, 1706, 1980.
46. **DeClerck, F., Loots, W., Somers, Y., Van Gorp, L., Verheyen, A., and Wouters, L.,** Thromboxane A_2-induced vascular endothelial cell damage and respiratory smooth muscle cell contraction: inhibition by flunarizine, a Ca^{2+}-overload blocker, *Arch. Int. Pharmacodyn, Ther.,* 274, 4, 1985.

47. **Brezinski, M. E., Lefer, D. J., Bowker, B., and Lefer, A. M.,** Thromboxane induced red blood cell lysis, *Prostaglandins,* 83, 75, 1987.
48. **Whittle, B. J. R.,** Cellular mediators in gastric damage: actions of thromboxane A_2 and its inhibitors, in *Mechanisms of Mucosal Protection in the Upper Gastrointestinal Track,* Allen, A., Garner, A., Flemstrom, G., Silen, W., and Turnberg, L. A., Eds., Raven Press, New York, 1984, 295.
49. **Konturek, S. J., Brzozowski, T., Piastucki, I., Radecki, T., and Dembinska-Kiec, A.,** Role of prostaglandin and thromboxane biosynthesis in gastric necrosis produced by taurocholate and ethanol, *Dig. Dis. Sci.,* 28, 154, 1983.
50. **Walt, R. P., Kemp, R. T., Filipowicz, B., Davies, J. G., Bhaskar, N. K., and Hawkey, C. J.,** Gastric mucosal protection with selective inhibition of thromboxane synthesis, *Gut,* 28, 541 1987.
51. **Price, C. A., Pipkin, G., Currington, A., Davies, L., Darling, L., and Parsons, M. E.,** Thromboxanes and gastric mucosal damage, *Gut,* 26, A1145, 1985.
52. **Whittle, B. J. R.,** Mechanisms of damage by non-steroid anti-inflammatory drugs, in *Biological Protection with Prostaglandins,* Vol. 2, Cohen, M. M., Ed., CRC Press, Boca Raton, FL, 1985, 1.
53. **Whittle, B. J. R.,** Mechanisms underlying gastric mucosal damage induced by indomethacin and bile salts, and the actions of prostaglandins, *Br. J. Pharmacol.,* 60, 455, 1977.
54. **Ligumsky, M., Grossman, M. I., and Kauffman, G. L., Jr.,** Endogenous gastric mucosal prostaglandins: their role in mucosal integrity, *Am. J. Physiol.,* 242, G337, 1982.
55. **Morris, G. P., Wallace, J. L., Harding, P. L., Krausse, E. J., and Lolle, S. J.,** Correlations between changes in indicators of gastric mucosal barrier integrity at time of exposure to "barrier breakers" and extent of hemorrhagic erosions one hour later, *Dig. Dis. Sci.,* 29, 6, 1984.
56. **Lewi, H. J. and Carter, D. C.,** Intravenous prostaglandin synthetase inhibitors potentiate the effect of topical taurocholate on transmucosal ion flux, in *Gastrointestinal Mucosal Blood Flow,* Fielding, L. P., Ed., Churchill Livingstone, London, 1980, 192.
57. **Whittle, B. J. R.,** The potentiation of taurocholate-induced rat gastric erosions following parenteral administration of cyclo-oxygenase inhibitors, *Br. J. Pharmacol.,* 80, 545, 1983.
58. **Sixma, J. J. and Wester, J.,** The hemostatic plug, *Sem. Hematol.,* 14, 165, 1977.
59. **Fitzgerald, G. A., Brash, A. R., Oates, J. A., and Pedersen, A. K.,** Endogenous prostacyclin biosynthesis and platelet function during selective inhibition of thromboxane synthase in man, *J. Clin. Invest.,* 71, 1336, 1983.
60. **O'Laughlin, J. C., Hoftiezer, J. W., Mahoney, J. P., and Ivey, K. J.,** Does aspirin prolong bleeding from gastric biopsies in man?, *Gastro. Endosc.,* 27, 1, 1981.
61. **Whittle, B. J. R., Kauffman, G. L., and Moncada, S.,** Hemostatic mechanisms, independent of platelet aggregation arrest gastric mucosal bleeding, *Proc. Natl. Acad. Sci. U.S.A.,* 83, 5683, 1986.

Chapter 7

LIPOXYGENASE PRODUCTS OF ARACHIDONIC ACID AS MEDIATORS OF GASTROINTESTINAL DAMAGE

Brigitta M. Peskar

TABLE OF CONTENTS

I. INTRODUCTION

Arachidonic acid, a 20-carbon polyunsaturated fatty acid, is the most common fatty acid incorporated in mammalian cellular phospholipids, and is the precursor of a number of mediators with important biologic activities. Arachidonic acid is liberated from phospholipid stores by the action of phospholipases. Metabolism of the free fatty acid can occur via several different pathways. Via the cyclooxygenase pathway arachidonic acid is transformed to the unstable endoperoxide intermediates prostaglandin (PG) G_2 and PGH_2, which are subsequently metabolized to the prostaglandins PGE_2, $PGF_{2\alpha}$, PGD_2, and thromboxane (TX) A_2. While PGE_2, $PGF_{2\alpha}$, and PGD_2 are chemically stable, PGI_2 and TXA_2 are rapidly converted nonenzymatically to the stable but biologically inactive compounds 6-keto-$PGF_{1\alpha}$ and TXB_2. Prostaglandins have been shown to possess a wide spectrum of gastrointestinal effects such as contraction or relaxation of gastrointestinal smooth muscle, stimulation of mucus and alkaline secretion, vasoconstriction or vasodilatation, inhibition of acid secretion, and modulation of ion transport processes (see also References 1 and 2 and Chapter 6).

Among the most remarkable properties of prostaglandins, described by Robert[3] in 1976, is their ability to protect the gastrointestinal mucosa against the damaging effect of a great number of noxious agents. Although the mechanism underlying this protective activity is still a matter of debate and its relevance for the beneficial effect of prostaglandins in the treatment of ulcer disease in man has recently been questioned,[4,5] the concept of mucosal protection as a phenomenon independent of inhibition of acid secretion has contributed considerably to our understanding of the events involved in mucosal integrity and damage. Contrary to the protective actions of prostaglandins, TXA_2, which is also formed via the cyclooxygenase pathway of arachidonate metabolism, was found to produce severe mucosal damage in the canine stomach in the presence of intraluminal bile salts, probably due to its potent vasoconstrictor actions.[6]

In 1974, an alternative pathway of arachidonate oxygenation was described. In platelets, arachidonic acid was found to be metabolized by a lipoxygenase enzyme to form 12-L-hydroperoxy-5,8,10,14-eicosatetraenoic acid (12-HPETE) which is then reduced by glutathione peroxydase to 12-L-hydroxy-5,8,10,14-eicosatetraenoic acid (12-HETE).[7] Arachidonate metabolism by other lipoxygenase enzymes may result in formation of other open-chain hydroxy acids such as 5-, 11-, and 15-HPETE and 15-HETE, respectively. Oxygenation of arachidonic acid at C-5 is also the initial step in formation of a family of biologically highly active compounds named the leukotrienes (LT).[8]

While formation and biologic actions of cyclooxygenase-derived products of arachidonate metabolism in the gastrointestinal tract have been studied extensively during recent years, only limited information on a possible physiological and/or pathophysiological role of lipoxygenase-derived arachidonate metabolites in this organ system is available. Gastrointestinal tissues of various species, including man, synthesize lipoxygenase products from endogenous substrate and recent studies indicate that increased formation of these arachidonate metabolites occurs in intestinal inflammation and certain types of mucosal injury. This chapter reviews the evidence suggesting a mediator role of lipoxygenase products in mucosal damage of the upper gastrointestinal tract.

II. BIOSYSNTHESIS AND METABOLISM OF LIPOXYGENASE PRODUCTS OF ARACHIDONATE

A. BIOSYNTHESIS OF LIPOXYGENASE PRODUCTS

After liberation from phospholipids arachidonic acid may undergo peroxidation which is or is not followed by cyclization. The first pathway is catalyzed by the enzyme complex cyclooxygenase and results in formation of the various prostaglandins and thromboxanes. The second pathway is mediated by various lipoxygenase enzymes and leads to the production of noncyclized monohydroxy and hydroperoxy acids (HETEs and HPETEs) and the leukotrienes.

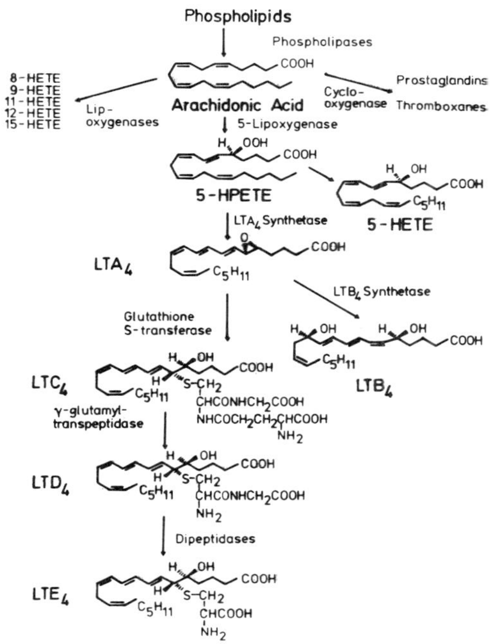

FIGURE 1. Metabolism of arachidonic acid via the 5-lipoxygenase pathway.

Plant lipoxygenases, such as soybean lipoxygenases, have been known for a long time and have been studied extensively. Hamberg and Samuelsson[7] in 1974 and Nugteren[9] in 1975 were the first to demonstrate the existence of such enzymes in mammalian cells. Lipoxygenation occurs following abstraction of hydrogen ions at position 7 (yielding either 5- or 9-HETE), position 10 (yielding either 8- or 12-HETE) or position 13 (yielding either 11- or 15-HETE), with subsequent peroxidation with molecular oxygen at the appropriate position. In these reactions there is a high preference for the 5-, 12-, and 15- products. Oxygenation of 11-products can occur either by the activity of a specific lipoxygenase or by incomplete operation of cyclooxygenation.[10]

5-HPETE, which is formed from arachidonic acid by the activity of 5-lipoxygenase, is either enzymatically or nonenzymatically processed to 5-HETE or acts as precursor in the biosynthesis of the leukotrienes. Leukotrienes are a group of compounds with a wide spectrum of biologic activities and a chemical structure containing a conjugated triene configuration. Further conversion of 5-HPETE by the enzyme 5-lipoxygenase yields the instable intermediary 5,6-epoxide LTA_4. LTA_4 can be spontaneously nonenzymatically hydrolyzed to several stereochemically distinct 5,12-dihydroxyeicosatetraenoic acids (5,12-diHETE). Alternatively, LTA_4 can be enzymatically hydrated to form LTB_4, a specific 5,12-diHETE (5S,12R-dihydroxy-6,14-*cis*-8,10-*trans*-eicosatetraenoic acid).[11-13] Contrary to the enzymatically formed LTB_4, the chemical hydrolysis products have only minor biologic activity.[14,15]

An alternative pathway of metabolism of LTA_4 is mediated by addition of glutathione by the enzyme glutathione-*S*-transferase leading to the formation of LTC_4 (5S-hydroxy-6R-gluthathionyl-7,9-*trans*-11,14-*cis*-eicosatetraenoic acid).[16,17] Successive shortening of the peptide side chain results in conversion of LTC_4 to LTD_4 and further to LTE_4. With respect to the related chemical structure and similarity in biological activities these compounds as a group are named the cysteinyl or sulfidopeptide leukotrienes.

The metabolic pathway of arachidonic acid via 5-lipoxygenase is shown in Figure 1. A number of excellent reviews provide more detailed information on these topics.[10,18-23]

B. METABOLISM AND INACTIVATION OF LIPOXYGENASE PRODUCTS

Metabolism of LTB_4 occurs by ω-hydroxylation resulting in formation of 20-hydroxy-LTB_4 and subsequently 20-carboxy LTB_4[24] via a cytochrome P-450 enzyme.[25] High activities of this enzyme have been found in human polymorphonuclear leukocytes, but not in human monocytes, lymphocytes and platelets, and polymorphonuclear leukocytes from other species. Formation of 19-hydroxy LTB_4[26] and various trihydroxy derivatives of eicosatetraenoic acid has been described as additional pathways of LTB_4 metabolism.[26,27]

The initial step in the metabolism of LTC_4 involves removal of the γ-glutamyl group leading to formation of LTD_4.[28,29] This reaction is catalyzed by the membrane-bound emzyme γ-glutamyl transferase. Removal of the glycine residue of LTD_4 by the activity of dipeptidases results in formation of LTE_4.[30,31] LTE_4 can be further metabolized to LTF_4[32] by addition of glutamic acid to the cysteine residue by the activity of γ-glutamyl transferase. Alternatively, acetylation to *N*-acetyl LTE_4 has been observed in certain tissues.[33] The route of excretion and the structure of metabolites *in vivo* is species specific. Thus, in rodents cysteinyl leukotrienes are excreted mainly in the bile in the form of *N*-acetyl LTE_4, while metabolites of LTC_4 in man are predominantly excreted in the urine in the form of LTE_4.[34]

Although LTC_4, LTD_4, and LTE_4 may exhibit certain differences in their biological activities, metabolism of LTC_4 by peptide cleavage is usually not an inactivation process, but represents bioconversion from one active mediator to another. Rapid biological inactivation of cysteinyl leukotrienes by the peroxydase-hydrogen/peroxide-halide system, however, has been observed in certain cells such as human polymorphonuclear leukocytes resulting from conversion to the biologically inactive 6-*trans*-LTB_4 and 6-*trans*-12-epi-LTB_4 and to the *S*-diastereoisomeric sulfoxides.[35] For details of leukotriene metabolism, see reviews by Hammarström et al.[34] and Drazen and Austen.[36]

The numerical subscript in the leukotriene nomenclature refers to the number of double bonds in the precursor fatty acid. Leukotrienes of the series 4 are products of arachidonic acid. Leukotrienes derived from 5,8,11-eicosatetraenoic acid are given the subscript 3 (LTB_3, LTC_3, etc.) and products of 5,8,11,14,17-eicosapentaenoic acid are given the subscript 5 (LTB_5, LTC_5, etc.) Although formation of the leukotrienes of series 3 and series 5 from the corresponding precursor fatty acids has been described under certain circumstances, leukotrienes of series 4 are the most important, because under normal conditions only arachidonic acid is present in significant amounts in human phospholipids.

III. CELLULAR SOURCES OF LIPOXYGENASE PRODUCTS

While cyclooxygenase, the enzyme initiating formation of prostaglandins and thromboxanes from arachidonic acid, is found in almost every mammalian cell, lipoxygenase enzymes are not as widely distributed. Furthermore, the type of lipoxygenase found differs in various cell types leading to the introduction of hydroperoxy groups at specific locations in the fatty acid molecule. Platelet lipoxygenase adds the hydroperoxy group to arachidonate at the 12-carbon position, while in neutrophils the 5-lipoxygenase is the predominant enzyme. Several lipoxygenases may be present in one cell type. Thus, in addition to products of the 5-lipoxygenase pathway of arachidonate neutrophils may also generate 15- , 11- , 8- and 9-HETE.[22]

The range of cell types to metabolize arachidonate via lipoxygenase pathways is limited. Cells of bone marrow origin are an important source of lipoxygenase-derived products. Formation of 5-lipoxygenase products (5-HETE and leukotrienes) has been found in basophilic leukemia cells, mouse mastocytoma cells, peritoneal, alveolar and blood monocytes, neutrophils, eosinophils, human blood basophils, rat peritoneal and human lung mast cells, human leukemic basophils, and various sensitized lung systems,[22] however, not all lipoxygenase metabolites of arachidonate produced by various tissues or organ systems may originate from bone marrow-derived cells. Recently, formation of LTB_4 and cysteinyl leukotrienes from LTA_4, but not from arachidonic acid, has been demonstrated in human endothelial cells.[37] Furthermore, rat pancreatic islet cells were found to metabolize arachidonate to 12-HETE in addition to several cyclooxygenase products.[38]

IV. BIOLOGICAL ACTIONS OF LIPOXYGENASE PRODUCTS

A. GENERAL ASPECTS

While the primary actions of the cysteinyl leukotrienes LTC_4, LTD_4, and LTE_4 are directed to smooth muscle, blood vessels, and secretory cells, those of LTB_4 relate to functions of different types of leukocytes. In 1980, Ford-Hutchinson at al.[39] reported that LTB_4 is a potent chemokinetic and aggregating agent on human and rat polymorphonuclear cells, respectively. Extensive studies in this field have clearly demonstrated that LTB_4 is a highly potent chemotactic factor for polymorphonuclear leukocytes such as neutrophils and eosinophils, as well as for monocytes such as macrophages and fibroblasts.[40] In addition, LTB_4 is a potent chemokinetic agent which increases the random movement of polymorphonuclear leukocytes and monocytes from experimental animals and man.[40] Superfusion of the hamster cheek pouch with LTB_4 caused adherence of leukocytes to the vascular endothelium followed by diapedesis.[41] Intradermal injection or topical application of LTB_4 resulted in a marked accumulation of polymorphonuclear cells in several species, including man.[42,43] In addition to effects on cell movement, LTB_4 stimulates human and animal leukocyte lysosomal enzyme secretion. This activity is, however, considerably less pronounced than that of agents such as C5a and FMLP.[44-46] LTB_4, and to a lesser extent 5-, 12-, or 15-HPETE, caused plasma exudation in various experimental models by a leukocyte-dependent mechanism and enhanced the increase in vascular permeability elicited by vasodilating agents such as bradykinin and PGE_2.[47,48] Finally, LTB_4 has been shown to modulate a variety of other lymphocyte functions primarily related to an enhancement of T-suppressor cell activity and modulation of interleukin-I formation.[49,50] Several reviews on the role of lipoxygenase products as mediators of inflammatory reactions have recently been published.[40,51-53]

The spasmogenic activity of cysteinyl leukotrienes was described as early as 1938 when Feldberg and Kellaway[54] observed the release of a smooth muscle-contracting principle from rat and guinea pig lung during perfusion with cobra venom. Anaphylactic stimulation of the perfused sensitized guinea pig lung caused release of a substance with similar properties which was named slow-reacting substance of anaphylaxis (SRS-A).[55] The smooth muscle-contracting activity of SRS-A is now attributed to the release of cysteinyl leukotrienes by the anaphylactic reaction.[16,56] LTC_4, LTD_4, and LTE_4 contract smooth muscle cells of blood vessels, pulmonary airways, the gastrointestinal tract, and myocardial, endothelial, and glandular epithelial cells. These contractions are characterized by a slow onset and prolonged time course.[19,22] LTC_4, LTD_4, and LTE_4 contract isolated airways and arouse bronchoconstriction in experimental animals and man.[57] The bronchoconstricting effect of leukotrienes is partially mediated by stimulation of TXA_2 formation depending on species and route of administration.[58] Various HETEs, particularly 12- and 15-HETE, and/or LTC_4 and LTD_4 stimulate mucus secretion from human bronchi *in vitro*[58,59] and increase mucus secretion after systemic or topical administration in experimental animals *in vivo*.[58] LTC_4 and LTD_4 cause arteriolar constriction in most vascular beds such as in the hamster cheek pouch, canine renal arteries, and rat and cat coronary arteries,[53,58] but increase microvascular flow in human skin.[60] Vascular actions of cysteinyl leukotrienes include a marked increase in permeability with exudation of fluid, electrolytes, and plasma proteins.[41,53,58] Leukotrienes have complex effects on blood pressure and heart rate. Generally, intravenous injection of LTC_4 or LTD_4 causes an initial transient increase in systemic blood pressure followed by a sustained systemic hypotension probably resulting from both cardiodepressive effects and hemoconcentration as a result of increased plasma exudation.[58]

B. GASTROINTESTINAL EFFECTS OF LIPOXYGENASE PRODUCTS

1. Effects on Gastrointestinal Smooth Muscle

Cysteinyl leukotrienes induce contractions of isolated gastrointestinal smooth muscle preparations *in vitro* and affect gastrointestinal motility *in vivo*. Large species and regional differences have been found in the response of gastrointestinal tissues. The isolated guinea pig ileum is contracted by all cysteinyl leukotrienes, LTD_4 being more active than LTC_4 and LTE_4, while LTF_4 has only minor spasmogenic activity.[19] In contrast, muscular tissue of human stomach, jejunum, ileum, and colon does not respond to SRS-A released from guinea pig lung.[61] Regional differences in the reactivity to the leukotrienes were described in the rat gastrointestinal tract. Thus, both LTC_4 and LTD_4 elicited concentration-dependent contractions of the isolated rat stomach and colon which were inhibited by the cysteinyl leukotriene antagonist FPL 55712. In contrast, rat duodenum and ileum failed to respond to either LTC_4 or LTD_4,[62] possibly indicating regional differences in the distribution of leukotriene receptors. LTC_4, LTD_4, and LTE_4 were also found to produce contractions of the guinea pig gall bladder.[63]

LTD_4-induced contractions of the isolated guinea pig ileum are partially inhibited by tetrodotoxin, suggesting that part of the spasmogenic activity of the leukotriene is mediated by release of a neurotransmitter.[64] Partial inhibition of the LTD_4-induced contractions by substance P desensitization and by a substance P antagonist may indicate that increased release of substance P is involved in the spasmogenic activity of LTD_4.[64]

In contrast to the smooth muscle contracting activity of cysteinyl leukotrienes observed *in vitro*, in the anesthetized dog, intraarterial LTD_4 caused a prolonged suppression of smooth muscle responsiveness to neural stimuli in the gastric antrum, jejunum, and ileum, but not colon, resulting in delayed emptying.[65] Furthermore, in conscious rhesus monkeys administration of the lipoxygenase inhibitor nordihydroguaiaretic acid was found to stimulate gastric emptying.[66]

2. Effects on Gastrointestinal Blood Flow

Effects of leukotrienes on gastric blood flow were studied in the rat. Using direct microscopy Whittle et al.[67] demonstrated a potent vasoconstricting action of LTC_4 on gastric submucosal vessels. The vasoconstricting response was more pronounced in the venules than the arterioles and was characterized by a segmental and focal nature. This segmental vasoconstriction resulted in extensive stasis and sluggish blood flow. LTD_4 and LTB_4 had no significant vasoactive actions on the rat submucosal microcirculation. The vasoconstrictor action of LTC_4 was not due to the release of arachidonate cyclooxygenase products such as TXA_2, since the action was insensitive to pretreatment with indomethacin.[67] The stasis of mucosal blood flow and vasocongestion caused by LTC_4 resembled the microcirculatory disturbances observed in certain models of experimental gastric mucosal damage[68] including those caused by topical irritants such as ethanol. Dose-dependent reduction in gastric mucosal blood flow (as measured by H_2 gas clearance) in rats *in vivo* was also observed after subcutaneous infusion of LTC_4.[69] In addition, LTC_4 elicited potent vasoconstrictor actions on the rat mesenteric vascular bed *in vivo* and *in vitro*[70] and in the isolated perfused mesenteric artery of the guinea pig *in vitro*.[71] In contrast to the vasoconstrictor effect of LTC_4, various hydroperoxy acid derivatives of arachidonate were found to be vasodilators in the isolated vascularly perfused whole stomach of rat and rabbit. To both species the rank order of potency was 12-HPETE > 11-HPETE > 5-HPETE > 15-HPETE.[72]

3. Effects on Gastrointestinal Secretory Functions

The information available regarding the effects of leukotrienes on gastric secretory functions is conflicting and may be species specific. Magous et al.[73] reported stimulation of acid secretion in isolated rabbit gastric cells by LTC_4, LTD_4, and LTE_4. This effect was not influenced by histamine, carbachol, or isobutyl methylxanthine, suggesting specific actions of the leukotrienes on parietal cells. Using isolated rabbit gastric glands Pendleton et al.[74] found no effect of LTD_4 on acid secretion but a significant increase in pepsin secretion. In the cat *in vivo* treatment with LTC_4, LTD_4, and LTE_4 likewise did not affect acid secretion but increased pepsin secretion and caused significant decreases in transgastric electrical potential difference.[74] LTB_4 had no effect upon any of these parameters. L-649,923, a selective LTD_4 antagonist, completely blocked the stimulatory action of LTD_4 on pepsin secretion, while the potential difference response was unaffected, suggesting the existence of functionally different leukotriene receptor subtypes in the gastric mucosa.[75] In gastric fistula rats subcutaneous infusion of LTC_4 caused little changes in gastric acid or pepsin secretion,[69] while LTC_4 was found to be a potent inhibitor of gastric acid secretion induced in vagally innervated and denervated portions of the stomach of conscious dogs by a variety of stimulants such as histamine, pentagastrin, and meat feeding *in vivo*.[76] In contrast to the report by Magous et al.,[73] in the latter study LTC_4 was also an effective inhibitor of acid formation in isolated rabbit gastric glands stimulated by histamine or dibutyryl cyclic adenosine monophosphate (cAMP).[76] This effect was not mediated by increased formation of prostaglandins. In addition, LTC_4 stimulated gastric alkaline secretion. This action was accompanied by increased luminal PGE_2 release and was prevented by pretreatment with indomethacin.[76] LTC_4 inhibited pancreatic secretion of bicarbonate and protein and reduced plasma insulin and pancreatic polypeptide levels in dogs *in vivo*.[77] LTC_4, however, failed to affect enzyme release from dispersed pancreatic acini cells *in vitro*, suggesting that contrary to the effects on acid secretion, the inhibitory action of LTC_4 on pancreatic secretion is a consequence of reduction of blood supply.

Lipoxygenase products of arachidonate metabolism have also been reported to modulate intestinal secretion of fluid and electrolytes. Musch et al.[78] were the first to report stimulation of secretion in the rabbit colon by various hydroxy fatty acids. Recently, Montzka et al.[79] reported a stimulatory action of LTC_4 and LTD_4 on rat small intestinal fluid secretion and ion transport processes. Whether lipoxygenase-derived arachidonate metabolites which are generated in increased amounts by intestinal mucosa of patients with inflammatory bowel diseases contribute to the diarrhea in these patients remains to be elucidated. In one study LTB_4 was reported to stimulate gastric mucus synthesis by rabbit antral mucosa.[80] Changes in gastric mucus production, however, could not be observed after treatment of rhesus monkeys with a lipoxygenase inhibitor.[66]

V. BIOSYNTHESIS OF ARACHIDONATE LIPOXYGENASE PRODUCTS BY GASTROINTESTINAL TISSUES

A. EXPERIMENTAL ANIMALS

Numerous studies have shown that gastrointestinal tissues of various species including man have a high capacity to generate cyclooxygenase products of arachidonate metabolism.[4] Recently, it has been demonstrated that tissues of the gastrointestinal system also synthesize lipoxygenase products from exogenous as well as endogenous arachidonic acid. In the tissues studied so far formation of cyclooxygenase products exceeded formation of arachidonate metabolites generated via lipoxygenase pathways. Thus, gastric and colonic mucosa of ovalbumin-sensitized guinea pigs incubated *in vitro* in the absence of antigen release large amounts of prostaglandins and thromboxanes, but only small amounts of cysteinyl leukotrienes.[81,82] Leukotriene release is, however, increased up to 20-fold when the antigen is added to the incubation medium[81-83] and Figure 2. Furthermore, antigen challenge causes release of material from the tissues that elicits contractions of the isolated guinea pig ileum (SRS-A), which are prevented by the cysteinyl leukotriene antagonist FPL 55712.[81,83] Antigen challenge does not increase release of cysteinyl leukotrienes or SRS-A-like material from gastric or colonic mucosa of nonsensitized guinea pigs. In contrast to the marked response in leukotriene

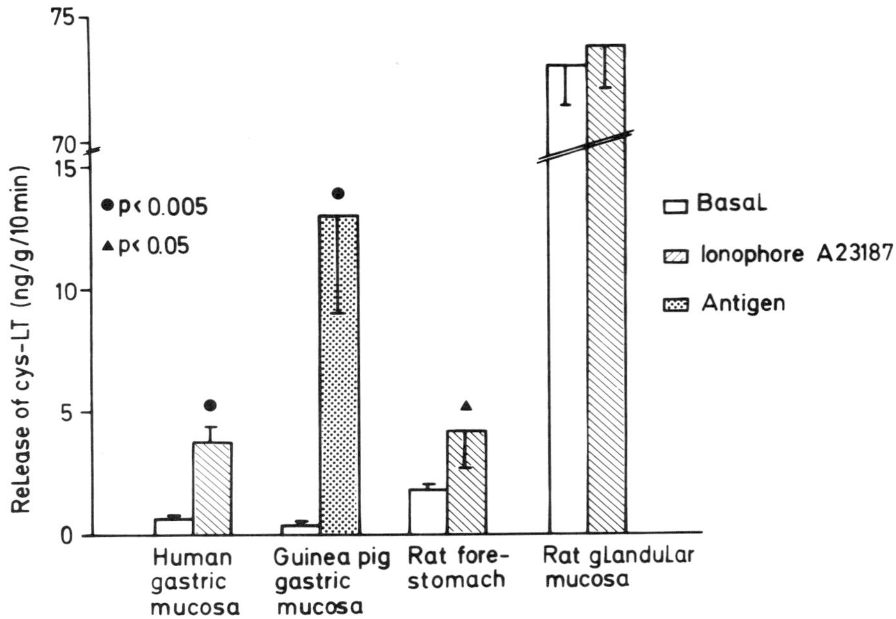

FIGURE 2. Release of cysteinyl leukotrienes by gastric tissues of man, guinea pig, and rat. Tissues were incubated in Tyrode solution for 10 min (basal incubations) and thereafter in the presence of antigen or ionophore A23187. For details of methods used, see References 81, 83, 85, and 89.

release, antigen challenge of gastric or colonic mucosa of sensitized guinea pigs does not affect release of cyclooxygenase-derived products of arachidonate metabolism.[81-83] These findings indicate that a certain stimulus can selectively activate one pathway of arachidonate conversion without affecting other routes of metabolism. This specificity could either be due to a stimulus-selective effect on the various enzymes of arachidonate metabolism or result from activation of certain cell types which exhibit a preferential pathway of arachidonate metabolism.

The profile of cyclooxygenase and lipoxygenase products formed differs in the various layers of the gastrointestinal tract (Figure 3). In the ovalbumin-sensitized guinea pig colon antigen challenge *in vitro* caused the most pronounced release of cysteinyl leukotrienes in the mucosal layer, while leukotriene formation by the smooth muscle and subserosal layer was negligible. Formation of cyclooxygenase products, on the other hand, was most marked in the subserosa and considerably lower in the mucosal and muscular tissues.[81,84]

Mucosa of the glandular part of the rat stomach has a particularly high biosynthetic capacity for leukotrienes. In this tissue LTC_4 is released spontaneously during incubation *in vitro* in amounts exceeding those generated by guinea pig or human gastric mucosa by a factor of up to 100.[85] Release of LTC_4 from rat gastric mucosal fragments is not stimulated by the divalent cation ionophore A23187, indicating that phospholipase and 5-lipoxygenase are not further activated by influx of calcium ions. Fragments obtained from the rat forestomach which also contain smooth muscle tissue release more 6-keto-$PGF_{1\alpha}$, but considerably less LTC_4 than fragments of mucosal tissues of the glandular gastric region.

Interestingly, in the forestomach leukotriene formation is stimulated by ionophore A23187, indicating again selective responses of different gastrointestinal tissues to a given stimulus. The species-specific release of cysteinyl leukotrienes from gastric tissues upon various stimuli is shown in Figure 2. In addition to LTC_4, rat gastric mucosa also synthesizes LTB_4, the amounts are, however, low compared to the amounts of LTC_4 generated.[86]

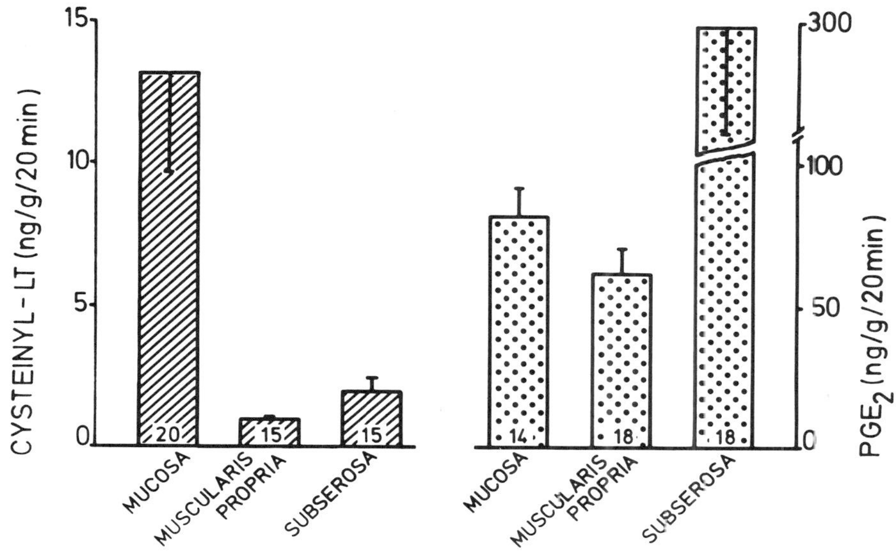

FIGURE 3. Profile of formation of cysteinyl leukotrienes (hatched bars) and PGE_2 (dotted bars) by the mucosal smooth muscle and subserosal layer of the guinea pig colon.[84]

B. HUMAN GASTROINTESTINAL TISSUES

Formation of lipoxygenase products of arachidonate metabolism by human gastrointestinal tissues was first reported by Bennett et al.[87] These authors could detect 12-HETE in extracts of human colonic, ileal, and gastric mucosa and smooth muscle. Homogenates of human colonic mucosa metabolized (^{14}C) arachidonic acid to 11-, 12-, and 15-HETE. in addition to various cyclooxygenase products.[88] Human gastrointestinal tissues also synthesize leukotrienes from endogenous substrate. Thus, fragments prepared from gastric, small intestinal, and colonic mucosa or smooth muscle generate cysteinyl leukotrienes and LTB_4 during incubation *in vitro*.[89] Release of lipoxygenase-derived products by human gastrointestinal tissues is small compared to the formation of cyclooxygenase metabolites of arachidonic acid. Ionophore A23187 stimulates mucosal and muscular release of LTB_4 and cysteinyl leukotrienes, but not of cyclooxygenase products. Similar to the guinea pig gastrointestinal tract, human mucosal tissues generate more leukotrienes, but less prostaglandins than the corresponding muscular tissues.[89]

C. METABOLISM OF LEUKOTRIENE C_4 BY GASTROINTESTINAL TISSUES

High pressure liquid chromatography (HPLC) analysis revealed that the cysteinyl leukotrienes released by fragments of guinea pig or human gastrointestinal mucosal and muscular tissues under basal conditions as well as during stimulation by antigen or ionophore A23187, respectively, consist of a mixture of LTC_4, LTD_4, and LTE_4[84,89] (Figure 4). Furthermore, during incubation *in vitro* human gastrointestinal tissues release enzymes into the incubation media that rapidly convert exogenous LTC_4 to LTD_4 and LTE_4.[89] The reaction is blocked by addition of glutathione to the incubation media. These findings show that gastrointestinal tissues of guinea pig and man possess the enzymatic machinery to process LTC_4 to LTD_4 and LTE_4. In contrast, fragments of rat gastric mucosa incubated *in vitro* generate practically exclusively LTC_4 and only trace amounts of LTD_4 and LTE_4[85] (Figure 4). The specific profile of cysteinyl leukotrienes released by rat gastric mucosa during incubation *in vitro* may either be due to a lack of γ-glutamyl-transpeptidase in this tissue or could result from the high concentrations of glutathione present in the gastric mucosa of rodents[90] which may prevent metabolism of LTC_4 in chopped tissue preparations.

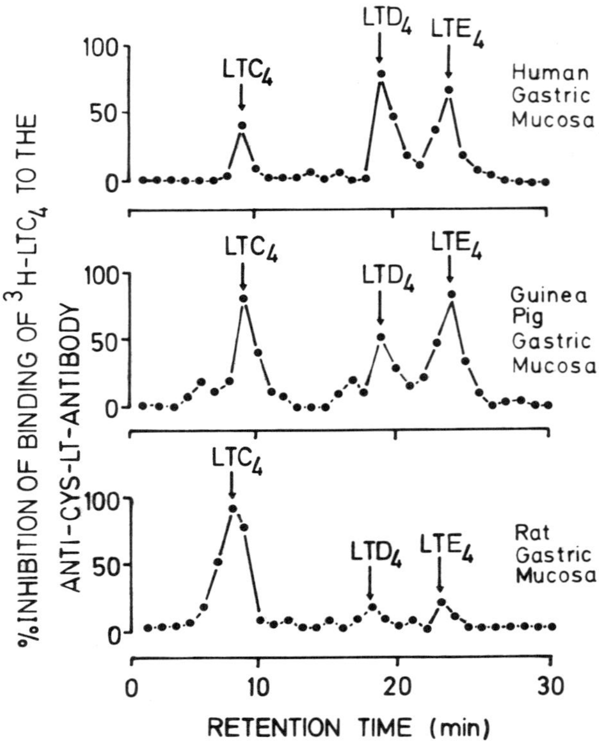

FIGURE 4. Profile of cysteinyl leukotrienes released by human, guinea pig, and rat gastric mucosa *in vitro*. Leukotriene formation was stimulated by ionophore A2187 (human and guinea pig gastric mucosa) or *in vivo* exposure to ethanol (rat gastric mucosa). Leukotrienes were separated by reversed phase HPLC and were determined radioimmunologically in 1 min elution fractions using an antibody that recognizes LTC_4, LTD_4, and LTE_4.

D. SOURCE OF GASTROINTESTINAL LEUKOTRIENES

The cellular origin of leukotrienes generated by gastrointestinal tissues is not known so far. Release of cysteinyl leukotrienes from chopped vascular tissue of several animal species after stimulation with ionophore A23187 or after antigen challenge has been reported.[91,92] Rings of human abdominal arteries were found to release small amounts of LTC_4, LTD_4, and LTE_4 spontaneously during incubation *in vitro*.[93] Leukotriene formation was significantly stimulated by ionophore A23187.[93] Interestingly, the main source of vascular leukotriene formation stimulated by antigen or ionophore A23187 is the adventitia, while the smooth muscle layer releases considerably less cysteinyl leukotrienes.[91,92] The vascular system thus may not only be an important target organ for leukotriene effects, but also a major site of biosynthesis of these lipoxygenase products. The finding that the vascularly perfused isolated rat stomach releases remarkable amounts of cysteinyl leukotrienes upon stimulation with ionophore A23187[94] may support this hypothesis. In addition, bone marrow-derived cells have been show to synthezise large amounts of lipoxygenase products of arachidonate metabolism.[22] In this context it is of interest that in a recent study glucocorticoids were found to reduce the biosynthetic capacity of rat gastric mucosa for LTC_4 parallel to the reduction in gastric tissue levels of the neutrophilic enzyme myeloperoxidase.[95] Furthermore, treatment of rats with dexamethasone has been reported to result in depletion of mast cells in the gastric mucosa.[96] In mucosal-type mast cells, LTC_4 is the major product of arachidonate metabolism after IgE-dependent activation or

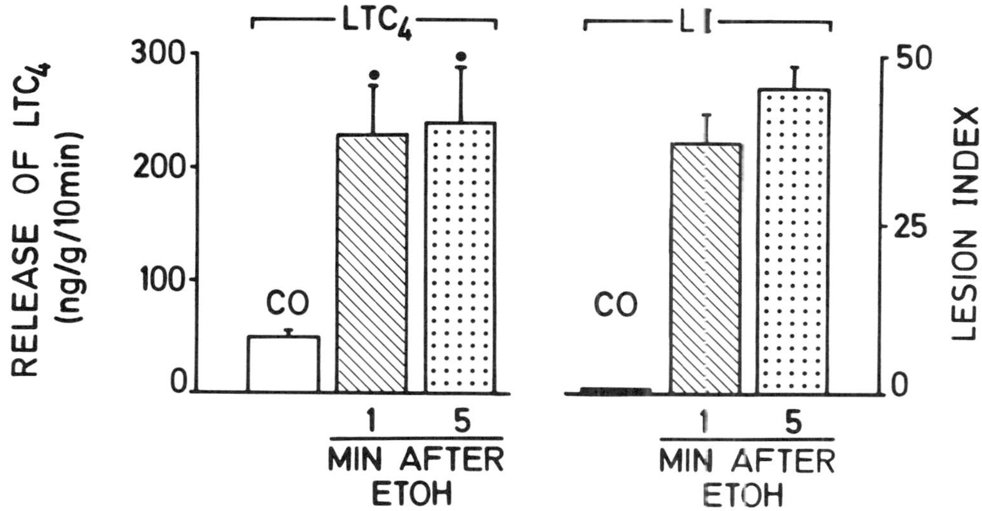

FIGURE 5. Effect of ethanol on gastric lesion production and mucosal formation of LTC_4 in rats. Gastric damage and release of LTC_4 by gastric mucosal fragments incubated *ex vivo* was determined 1 and 5 min, respectively, after intragastric instillation of 1.5 ml ethanol.[105]

ionophore A23187 stimulation.[97] Finally, formation of LTB_4[98] and cysteinyl leukotrienes[99] is increased in the acutely inflamed mucosa of patients with inflammatory bowel diseases. Bone marrow-derived cells may thus contribute significantly to leukotriene production both in normal and inflamed gastrointestinal tissues.

VI. LEUKOTRIENES IN ETHANOL-INDUCED GASTRIC DAMAGE

Microcirculatory changes are a prominent feature of gastric mucosal injury caused by ethanol. Microscopic evaluation of gastric mucosa exposed to ethanol revealed focal accumulations of blood due to hyperemia and hemorrhage.[100] Using a fluorescent *in vivo* microscopy method it was demonstrated that this hyperemia or engorgement is associated with total absence of blood flow.[101] Vascular stasis occurs within less than 1 min after ethanol application[102,103] and clearly precedes the development of necrotic mucosal lesions.[101] In addition, ethanol causes endothelial damage in the capillaries and collecting venules in the superficial mucosa paralleled by increased vascular permeability.[104] Again, these changes occur rapidly and prior to the development of grossly visible mucosal lesions. Agents which protect against mucosal injury such as prostaglandins, cysteamine, or sodium thiosulfate simultaneously prevent the vascular effects of ethanol, although they do not inhibit ethanol-induced necrosis of gastric mucosal surface cells.[103] Taken together, these findings suggest that vascular injury is a crucial pathogenetic factor in the development of gastric hemorrhagic erosions caused by ethanol.

The microcirculatory changes observed after topical ethanol resemble those elicited by exogenous LTC_4.[67] Work performed in our laboratory has demonstrated that intragastric instillation of ethanol stimulates formation of LTC_4 by the gastric mucosa during a subsequent *ex vivo* incubation.[85] The stimulatory action of ethanol on mucosal LTC_4 release is dose-dependent and closely parallels the production of necrotic lesions.[85] As shown in Figure 5 maximal increase in mucosal LTC_4 release can be observed as early as 1 min after exposure to ethanol.[85,105] It is, therefore, conceivable that the microcirculatory events induced by ethanol may be at least partially mediated by vasoactive lipoxygenase products of arachidonate metabolism. Contrary to the marked increase in gastric mucosal release of LTC_4, formation of thromboxane, a potent cyclooxygenase-derived vasoconstrictor,[6] is not stimulated by topical ethanol,[85,106] indicating a selective activation of the 5-lipoxygenase pathway of arachidonate metabolism. As intragastric instillation of ethanol also enhances mucosal release of LTB_4,[86] the activation of the 5-lipoxygenase pathway results either from increased release of the substrate fatty acid or by a stimulatory action on the enzymes involved in the transformation of arachidonic acid to LTA_4.

The precise mechanisms by which leukotrienes could contribute to ethanol-induced mucosal damage are not yet known. LTC_4 is a potent constrictor of gastric submucosal vessels and induces sluggish blood flow and vasocongestion.[67] Cysteinyl leukotrienes have been found to cause extensive plasma leakage in a number of vascular beds.[41,107] Both LTC_4-induced venular constriction and fluid extravasation may aggravate to the decrease in vascular flow caused by ethanol. In rats, LTC_4 reduced gastric mucosal blood flow in a dose-dependent manner.[69] While LTC_4 given alone did not cause damage to the gastric mucosa, subcutaneous infusion of the leukotriene increased dose-dependently the area and number of gastric lesions induced by ethanol, acidified taurocholate, and stress, an effect that was partially prevented by pretreatment with the cysteinyl leukotriene antagonist FPL 55712.[69] Likewise, intraarterial infusion of LTD_4 enhanced the production of gastric mucosal lesions induced by either ethanol or acid.[108] Thus, while cysteinyl leukotrienes do not seem to be ulcerogenic per se, they obviously potentiate the noxious effects of damaging agents. It remains to be investigated whether this potentiation is solely the consequence of the microcirculatory dysfunction caused by the leukotrienes which may decrease the intramucosal clearance of damaging agents and interfere with the delivery of oxygen and nutrients. A similar potentiation of the injurious effects of pro-ulcerogenic agents has been observed with other compounds that reduce gastric mucosal blood flow such as vasopressin.[109] Contrary to the cysteinyl leukotrienes, LTB_4 has no vasoconstrictor activity. Although LTB_4 has been reported to promote plasma leakage by a leukocyte-dependent mechanism,[47] it is unlikely that this 5-lipoxygenase product of arachidonate metabolism plays a major role as mediator of microcirculatory changes in ethanol-induced mucosal damage. Increased formation of LTB_4 may, however, contribute to the migration of inflammatory cells into the gastric mucosa observed in late stages of mucosal damage caused by ethanol. In this context it may be of interest that in patients with active duodenal ulcer peripheral blood monocytes were found to generate more LTB_4 (and less PGE_2) upon zymosan stimulation than normal control subjects.[110] This phenomenon was partially reversed after healing with H_2-antagonists. Whether changes observed in peripheral blood cells are indeed representative of events occurring in the duodenal mucosa should be investigated in more detail and measurements of the production of 5-lipoxygenase products in the gastroduodenal mucosa are necessary to establish or exclude a pathogenetic role of arachidonate lipoxygenase products in human peptic ulcer disease.

VII. EFFECT OF PROTECTIVE DRUGS ON GASTRIC MUCOSAL LEUKOTRIENE FORMATION

A. EFFECT OF LIPOXYGENASE ENZYME INHIBITORS

If increased formation of leukotrienes is involved in gastric mucosal injury caused by ethanol one would expect that drugs that interfere with the enzymatic conversion of arachidonic acid to leukotrienes confer protection. Oral pretreatment of rats with the lipoxygenase inhibitor nordihydroguaiaretic acid (NDGA) inhibited formation of LTC_4 by the gastric mucosa and simultaneously effectively reduced the number and severity of mucosal lesions[85] (Figure 6). Pretreatment with NDGA did not affect mucosal formation of cyclooxygenase-derived arachidonate metabolites.[85] The protective action of NDGA on ethanol-induced gastric damage was confirmed by Quadros and Wilson.[111] These authors found a decrease in gastric juice LTC_4 paralleled by a stimulated PGE_2 release in NDGA-treated rats. Pretreatment with indomethacin

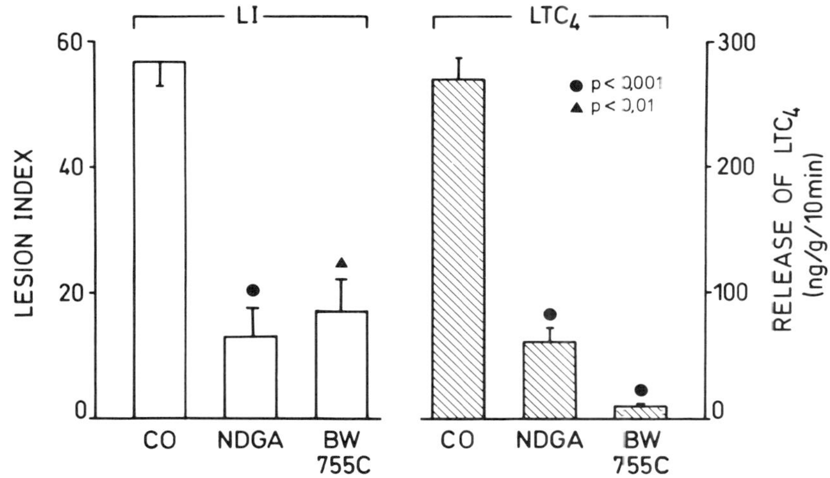

FIGURE 6. Inhibition of ethanol-induced lesion production and gastric mucosal LTC_4 formation by the lipoxygenase inhibitors NDGA and BW755C. Groups of 6 rats were pretreated orally with NDGA (100 mg/kg) or BW755C (50 mg/kg) 30 min prior to intragastric instillation of ethanol. Mucosal damage and *ex vivo* release of LTC_4 from mucosal fragments was determined 5 min later.

prevented the increase in gastric juice prostaglandins, but did not affect the protective action of NDGA, suggesting that the increase in gastric prostaglandin formation observed is not crucial for the protective activity of the drug.

BW755C is an inhibitor of arachidonic acid metabolism via both cyclooxygenase and lipoxygenase pathway in inflammatory exudates.[112] The drug does not, however, inhibit gastric mucosal cyclooxygenase *ex vivo*.[113] Contrary to most nonsteroidal anti-inflammatory compounds such as indomethacin, BW755C given in anti-inflammatory doses failed to induce damage to the gastric mucosa.[113] Oral administration of BW755C significantly reduced the extent of gastric injury caused by intragastric instillation of 40% acidified ethanol or indomethacin.[106] In contrast to the lack of inhibitory action of BW755C on gastric mucosal prostaglandin formation *ex vivo*, the drug inhibits generation of (possibly platelet-derived) thromboxane[106] and LTC_4 (Figure 6) in this tissue; however, as ethanol does not stimulate formation of thromboxane by the gastric mucosa[85,106] and BW755C is also protective against indomethacin-induced mucosal damage, where generation of cyclooxygenase products is practically abolished, it is unlikely that inhibition of gastric thromboxane synthesis or effects on the endogenous prostaglandin system are the mechanism for the protection afforded by BW755C.[106] The marked reduction in gastric mucosal LTC_4 formation observed after treatment with BW755C has been interpreted to support the concept that gastroprotection by BW755C results from its inhibitory action on lipoxygenase enzymes.

Balaa and Goldgar[114] reported that pretreatment of rats with the lipoxygenase enzyme inhibitors diethylcarbamazine or phenidone diminished the damaging effect of intragastric ethanol. Pretreatment with indomethacin did not attenuate the protective effect of carbamazine,[115] indicating again that gastric protection observed with lipoxygenase enzyme inhibitors is not mediated by increased metabolism of the common fatty acid substrate to protective prostaglandins. Further evidence for an involvement of lipoxygenase products in the pathogenesis of ethanol-induced mucosal injury has been suggested by the demonstration of a gastroprotective activity of the recently developed 5-lipoxygenase enzyme inhibitor REV 5901 in this model of experimental ulcer.[116]

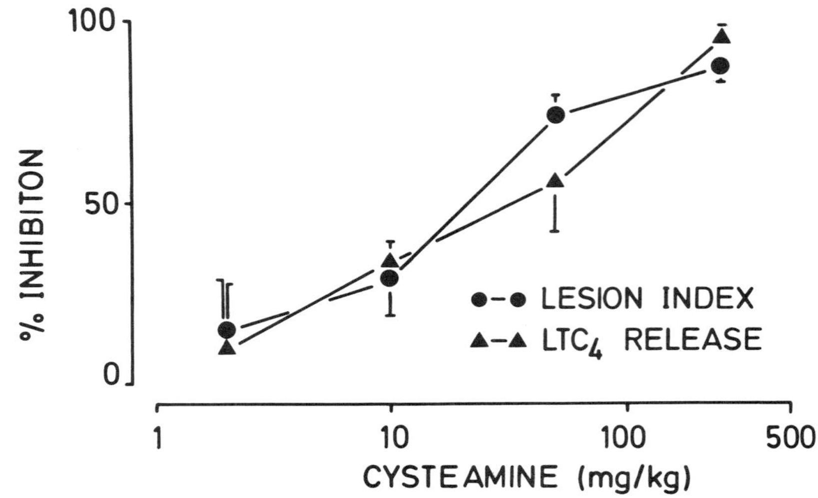

FIGURE 7. Inhibition of ethanol-induced gastric lesion production and LTC_4 release by cysteamine. Rats were pretreated orally with cysteamine 30 min prior to intragastric instillation of ethanol. Gastric damage and *ex vivo* release of LTC_4 from mucosal fragments was determined 5 min later.[122]

B. EFFECT OF AGENTS ALTERING GASTRIC MUCOSAL SULFHYDRYL LEVELS

The gastric mucosa contains particularly high levels of glutathione which comprises the predominant portion of the endogenous nonprotein mucosal sulfhydryls pool.[90] A role of glutathione in protection against hepatic injury is well established. Work by Szabo's group[117,118] has shown that sulfhydryl-containing drugs such as cysteamine or dimercaprol protect rats from ethanol-induced gastric erosions, whereas sulfhydryl-blocking agents counteract the effect of gastroprotective compounds such as $PGF_{2\beta}$, dimercaprol, or cysteamine. From these findings it has been suggested that endogenous nonprotein sulfhydryls play a pivotal role in protection of the gastric mucosa.[117] Additional studies, however, revealed that not only exogenous thiols, but also glutathione-depleting agents such as diethylmaleate[119,120] or cyclohexene-1-one[119] protect the rat gastric mucosa against the injurious effect of ethanol. Furthermore, divalent metals, which decrease the glutathione concentration in the nonprotein fraction of the gastric mucosa, also prevented the necrotizing action of topical ethanol.[121] The mechanism of the protection afforded by sulfhydryl-modulating compounds remained unknown. A mediation by release of endogenous prostaglandins seemed to play a minor role as indomethacin pretreatment attenuated, but not abolished, the protection afforded by some, but not all agents.[119,120] Furthermore, increased formation of mucosal prostaglandins was not a general phenomenon observed after treatment with sulfhydryl-modulating agents.[119,120] As shown in Figures 7 and 8, pretreatment of rats with both the sulfhydryl-containing drug cysteamine and the sulfhydryl-blocking agent diethylmaleate prevented the stimulatory action of ethanol on gastric mucosal LTC_4 formation. Similar findings were found for other agents that either increase or deplete gastric sulfhydryl levels and by various metals[121] (Table 1). The inhibitory action of sulfhydryl-modulating agents on LTC_4 formation by ethanol-challenged gastric mucosa is dose-dependent and closely parallels the protective activity of the compounds.[122,123]

In accordance with previous reports[119,120] pretreatment of rats with sulfhydryl-modulating compounds or metals did not increase formation of protective prostaglandins by rat gastric mucosa. In contrast, with most compounds studied formation of prostaglandins was markedly reduced parallel to the diminished formation of LTC_4.[122,123] Thus, in rats dimercaprol in doses which reduced ethanol-induced lesion production by more than 90% practically abolished the

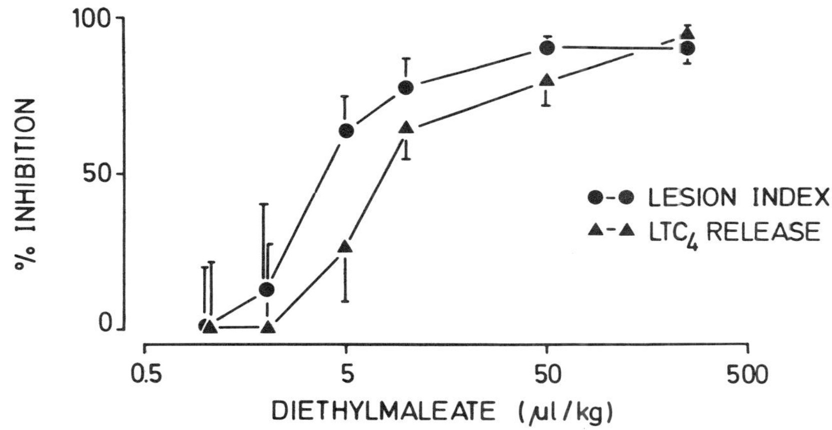

FIGURE 8. Inhibition of ethanol-induced gastric lesion production and LTC_4 release by diethylmaleate. Rats were pretreated orally with diethylmaleate 30 min prior to intragastric instillation of ethanol. Gastric damage and *ex vivo* release of LTC_4 from mucosal fragments was determined 5 min later.[122]

TABLE 1
Effect of Agents Modulating Gastric Mucosal Sulfhydryl (SH) Levels on Gastric Lesion Production and LTC_4 Formation in Rats[123]

Pretreatment	Protection ID_{50} (mg/kg)	LTC_4 formation ID_{50} (mg/kg)
Thiols		
Cysteamine	20	26
L-Cysteine	180	130
N-Acetyl cysteine	290	290
Dimercaprol	15	5
SH-blocking or -depleting agents		
Diethylmaleate	5	9
N-Ethylmaleimide	0.4	2
Iodoacetamide	0.3	10
Metals		
$CdSO_4$	8	25
$ZnCl_2$	7	11
LiCl	4	5
$TeCl_4$	9	23

Note: For methods used, see Figure 7 legend and Reference 122.

synthesizing capacity of the gastric mucosa for prostaglandins.[123] These findings suggest that inhibition of gastric mucosal LTC_4 formation rather than effects on the endogenous prostaglandin system correlates with the protective action of exogenous thiols, agents that block or deplete endogenous mucosal sulfhydryl groups, and metals. Moreover, from these results it is obvious that protection against the necrotizing effect of ethanol does not require an intact gastric cyclooxygenase system and occurs even when mucosal prostaglandin formation is severely suppressed.

C. OTHER DRUGS

Prior to the introduction of the H_2-receptor antagonists carbenoxolone was widely used in the treatment of gastric and duodenal ulcer disease. As carbenoxolone does not inhibit acid secretion,[124] it was the first drug which accelerated ulcer healing by a mechanism relying on mucosa-protective actions. Carbenoxolone inhibits the enzymatic degradation of prostaglandins[125] and increases the release of PGE_2 from human gastric mucosa *in vitro*[126] and *in vivo*.[127] The drug also inhibits formation of thromboxanes by human gastric mucosal tissue *in vitro*.[126] Treatment with carbenoxolone effectively protects against ethanol-induced gastric damage in rats.[128] Contrary to man, in this species *in vitro* effects of carbenoxolone on the gastric mucosal cyclooxygenase system occur at high drug concentrations only and cannot be demonstrated after *in vivo* treatment.[85,129] Carbenoxolone given in protective doses reduced, however, the stimulatory action of intragastric ethanol on LTC_4 release from rat gastric mucosa *ex vivo*.[85] Carbenoxolone also dose-dependently inhibited the calcium ionophore A23187-stimulated formation of LTC_4 and LTB_4 by human gastric mucosa *in vitro*, the IC_{50} being 0.07 mmol/l and 0.2 ml/l, respectively.[130] Tissue concentrations of this order of magnitude are indeed reached in the gastric mucosa after oral administration of therapeutic doses of carbenoxolone in man.[131] Further studies are necessary to elucidate whether the gastroprotection in experimental animals and the ulcer healing action in man afforded by carbenoxolone are directly or indirectly related to inhibition of formation of pro-ulcerogenic lipoxygenase products of arachidonate metabolism.

Similar to carbenoxolone, sulfasalazine, a drug with known benefit in the treatment of inflammatory bowel diseases, has complex actions on the various pathways of arachidonate metabolism. Using a variety of experimental models sulfasalazine was reported to inhibit prostaglandin degrading enzymes, inhibit or stimulate prostaglandin biosynthesis, inhibit thromboxane formation,[132] and inhibit formation of LTB_4[98,133,134] and cysteinyl leukotrienes.[134,135] In rats, subcutaneous injection of sulfasalazine protected against gastric mucosal damage caused by ethanol[136] or cold/immobilization stress.[137] Since sulfasalazine treatment had no significant effect on formation of prostaglandins by the gastric mucosa, it was suggested that the protective mechanism of the drug may rather result from its ability to inhibit the activity of lipoxygenase enzymes.[137]

Mucosal mast cells metabolize arachidonic acid predominantly to LTC_4[97] and may represent a major source of the cysteinyl leukotrienes generated by the gastric mucosa. Mast cells have been implicated in the pathogenesis of acute gastric injury. In rats, restraint stress resulted in both gastric mast cell degranulation and mucosal ulceration.[138] In mice, ethanol caused degranulation and/or disruption of gastric mucosal mast cells and, at certain concentrations of ethanol, mast cell-deficient mice developed less acute gastric injury than control animals.[139] Although mast cell-dependent mechanisms are not a prerequisite for acute mucosal injury, under certain circumstances mast cells have been found to augment the area of ethanol-induced gastric injury.[139] In a recent report, pretreatment of rats with the mast cell stabilizer FPL 52694 was shown to result in marked protection against gastric damage caused by ethanol.[140] Simultaneously, ethanol-stimulated mucosal LTC_4 release was significantly inhibited. From these findings it has been suggested that among other mediators such as histamine, LTC_4 is released from mast cells during ethanol exposure and that mast cell-derived LTC_4 may be involved in the pathogenesis of mucosal damage caused by this irritant.

D. DRUGS ANTAGONIZING LEUKOTRIENE ACTIONS

Only limited data are available on gastroprotection afforded by drugs antagonizing leukotriene effects. In rats, L-649,923, a cysteinyl leukotriene receptor antagonist,[141] significantly reduced the production of gastric lesions after intragastric instillation of ethanol.[105,142] Similarly, the leukotriene receptor antagonist Ly 171,883 was reported to confer protection against ethanol-induced rat gastric damage.[116] The effectiveness of Ly 171,883 was, however, reduced by pretreatment with indomethacin. It remains, therefore, uncertain whether the protection afforded by this drug indeed results from leukotriene receptor antagonism or involves other effects, e.g., on the endogenous gastric prostaglandin system. Finally, intraarterial infusion of FPL 55712 protected rats against gastric ulcers caused by cold/immobilization stress.[143]

Prostaglandins are among the agents that exhibit the most pronounced gastroprotective actions. In rats challenged with ethanol, oral pretreatment with PGE_2 in a dose that reduced gastric mucosal damage by 78% did not inhibit mucosal LTC_4 formation.[122] Similarly, drugs known to stimulate formation of endogenous gastric prostaglandins such as sucralfate[144] or Al-containing antacids[145] conferred marked protection without attenuating the stimulatory effect of ethanol on mucosal LTC_4 synthesis in rats.[146] This implicates that the reduction in mucosal leukotriene formation observed with certain protective drugs is not only the consequence of tissue preservation. PGE_1 and iloprost, a stable PGI_2 analog, have recently been demonstrated to antagonize the vasoconstricting effect of exogenous LTD_4 in the hamster cheek pouch vascular bed.[147] In contrast to the effect of the prostaglandins, the vasoconstriction elicited by LTD_4 was not antagonized by the calcium channel blocking agent nifedipine, indicating that the antagonistic effect is not solely mediated by the vasodilating properties of the compounds.[147] Whether the gastroprotective action of prostaglandins involves a functional antagonism of vascular leukotriene effects remains to be elucidated.

Contrary to natural PGE_2, the synthetic analog 16,16-dimethyl PGE_2 was found to inhibit gastric mucosal LTB_4 release in ethanol-challenged rats.[86] The inhibitory action on leukotriene formation was, however, less pronounced than the gastroprotective activity of the compound. Inhibition of mucosal LTB_4 release by 16,16-dimethyl PGE_2 was only observed when the gastric mucosa was challenged with ethanol *in vivo*, but not when the irritant was applied topically *in vitro*, suggesting that prostaglandin-induced inhibition of leukotriene formation may depend on an intact microcirculation.[86] Unlike PGE_2, 16,16-dimethyl PGE_2 was found to afford some protection to the superficial mucosal cells of the rat gastric mucosa.[148] Further studies are necessary to clarify whether differences in the inhibitory action on gastric leukotriene formation by various types of prostaglandins are related to the extent and/or cellular target of their protective action.

VIII. NONSTEROIDAL ANTI-INFLAMMATORY DRUGS AND THE GASTRIC MUCOSAL-LEUKOTRIENE SYSTEM

Nonsteroidal anti-inflammatory drugs (NSAID) inhibit cyclooxygenase, the enzyme initiating conversion of arachidonate to prostaglandins and thromboxanes.[149] It has been suggested that reduced formation of prostaglandins not only mediates the anti-inflammatory effects of this type of drug, but also their gastrointestinal toxicity.[149] Blockade of the cyclooxygenase pathway could possibly shift the metabolism of arachidonic acid to lipoxygenase-derived products. Increased formation of leukotrienes simultaneously with reduced formation of cyclooxygenase-derived arachidonate metabolites has, in fact, been observed in certain cells and tissues, such as mouse peritoneal marcrophages[150] or inflammatory exudates induced in rats by subcutaneous implantation of carrageenan-soaked sponges.[151] In contrast to these findings, however, oral administration of indomethacin or aspirin inhibited the *ex vivo* sythesizing capacity of the rat gastric mucosa for both prostaglandins and LTC_4.[152,153] Inhibition of gastric mucosal prostaglandin formation was, however, more pronounced than inhibition of leukotriene synthesis after indomethacin or aspirin administration. Thus, oral indomethacin (20 m/kg) inhibited synthesis of PGE_2 by 94% and of LTC_4 by 53% 15 min after dosing. Synthesis of PGE_2 remained reduced to a greater extent than synthesis of LTC_4 for up to 9 h.[152] Similar results were observed after oral administration of aspirin. The mechanism of inhibition of gastric LTC_4 formation by indomethacin and aspirin remains to be elucidated. This inhibition could either by due to indirect actions or to direct effects on the enzymes phospholipase A_2 and/or 5-lipoxygenase. Such enzyme inhibition has, in fact, been observed for high concentrations of indomethacin in rat peritoneal leukocytes.[154] In this context, it is of interest that due to the pharmacokinetics of acidic NSAID, particularly high concentrations of some of these compounds can be reached in the gastric mucosa within short periods of time after oral administration.[155]

The preferential inhibition of rat gastric mucosal cyclooxygenase after administration of nonsteroidal anti-inflammatory compounds results in a relative increase in gastric formation of LTC_4. Furthermore, in the vascularly perfused isolated rat stomach addition of indomethacin to the perfusion medium tended to increase calcium ionophore A23187-induced release of cysteinyl leukotrienes into the perfusate.[94] Contrary to the chopped tissue preparation of rat gastric mucosa (Figure 2), leukotriene release from the perfused isolated rat stomach is stimulated by ionophore A23187.[94] It is thus possible that NSAID inhibit basal gastric LTC_4 release, but increase LTC_4 formation provoked by certain stimuli. The shift in the balance between protective prostaglandins and pro-ulcerogenic cysteinyl leukotrienes caused by NSAID may contribute to the gastric toxicity of these agents. This hypothesis seems to be supported by the protection against NSAID-induced gastric damage afforded by lipoxygenase enzyme inhibitors. In rats, oral administration of BW755C, which effectively inhibits gastric mucosal LTC_4 formation (Figure 6), significantly reduced the extent of gastric damage produced by subcutaneous injection of indomethacin.[106] BW755C treatment did not prevent the inhibitory action of indomethacin on gastric mucosal prostaglandin formation, indicating that the protective action of the drug is not mediated by competition at the site of cyclooxygenase.[106] In addition, leukotriene antagonists have been found to confer protection against indomethacin-induced gastric damage in rats. Thus, oral pretreatment with high doses of L-649,923 or L-660,711, two structurally unrelated cysteinyl leukotriene receptor antagonists, reduced gastric mucosal erosions caused by oral indomethacin.[142]

In mice sensitized with bethanechol oral and/or parenteral administration of NSAID results in severe gastric damage. Using this model it recently has been demonstrated that compounds known to inhibit leukotriene formation such as the 5-lipoxygenase inhibitors REV 5901 and L-651,392 or ferulic and caffeic acids (which have been reported to inhibit LTC_4 synthesis in human neutrophils[156]), as well as the cysteinyl leukotriene receptor antagonists FPL 55712, L-649,923, Wy-44,392, and Ly-171,883, protect against gastric damage caused by subcutaneous indomethacin.[157] With the exception of REV 5901 the compounds also reduced lesions induced by subcutaneously administered piroxicam. Furthermore, the leukotriene antagonists, but not the 5-lipoxygenase inhibitors, studied protected against gastric lesions caused by oral aspirin.[157]

Contrary to aspirin and other NSAID sodium salicylate is not ulcerogenic in rats[113,158] and does not inhibit gastric mucosal prostaglandin formation.[113] Moreover, sodium salicylate was found to protect the gastric mucosa against noxious agents such as ethanol.[159] The mechanism of this protection remained unknown. As pretreatment with indomethacin did not counteract the effect the endogenous prostaglandin system did not seem to play a crucial role in the protection afforded by sodium salicylate. Similar to the lack of effect on the gastric mucosal prostaglandin system[113] oral or subcutaneous administration of sodium salicylate in doses up to 400 mg/kg did not inhibit the basal synthesizing capacity of the rat gastric mucosa for LTC_4. Oral treatment with sodium salicylate prevented, however, the stimulation of gastric mucosal LTC_4 formation caused by topical ethanol.[153] The inhibitory action on ethanol-stimulated gastric LTC_4 formation is dose-dependent and closely parallels the protective activity of the drug against the necrotizing effect of the irritant (Figure 9). Similar to the action of sodium salicylate in rats not challenged with ethanol, the drug had no significant effect on gastric mucosal formation of cyclooxygenase-derived arachidonate metabolites after ethanol exposure.[153]

In contrast to the effect of sodium salicylate, pretreatment with aspirin inhibited gastric mucosal formation of both cyclooxygenase products and LTC_4 in rats challenged with ethanol.[153] Inhibition of formation of cyclooxygenase products was more pronounced than inhibition of LTC_4 release. Thus, while oral pretreatment with aspirin in a dose as low as 1.6 mg/kg

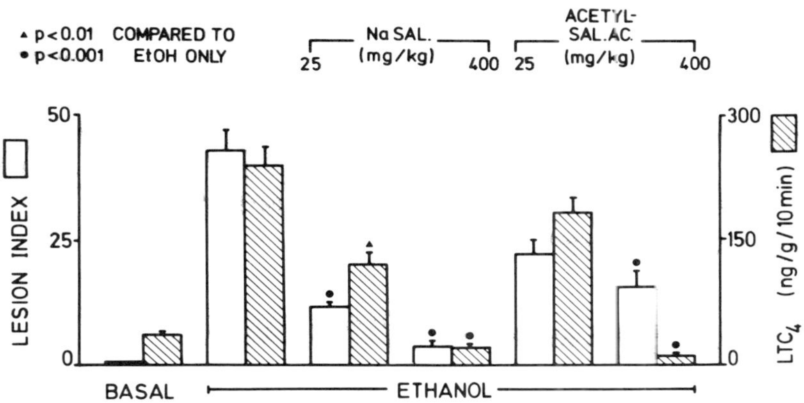

FIGURE 9. Effect of sodium salicylate and acetylsalicylic acid on ethanol-induced gastric lesion production and mucosal LTC_4 release in rats. Gastric damage and stimulation of mucosal LTC_4 formation caused by ethanol are dose-dependently inhibited by oral pretreatment (30 min) with sodium salicylate. While a low dose of acetylsalicylic acid does not inhibit LTC_4 release, a high dose prevents the stimulation of mucosal LTC_4 formation and simultaneously protects against gastric damage caused by ethanol.

significantly reduced formation of cyclooxygenase-derived arachidonate metabolites by ethanol-challenged gastric mucosa, only doses above 100 mg/kg inhibited ethanol-stimulated LTC_4 release. Interestingly, aspirin given in doses that reduced gastric mucosal LTC_4 formation also protected against the necrotizing effect of ethanol (Figure 9). In contrast, oral pretreatment with indomethacin in doses that reduced gastric mucosal LTC_4 formation in rats not treated with ethanol did not overcome the stimulatory action of topical ethanol on gastric LTC_4 formation. Simultaneously, indomethacin did not protect against ethanol-induced gastric damage.[153]

The mechanism of the inhibitory action of sodium salicylate on the activation of the gastric mucosal cysteinyl leukotriene system by ethanol remains unknown. From the lack of inhibitory action of the drug on basal mucosal LTC_4 release the effect does not seem to involve direct enzyme inhibition. After oral administration, aspirin is rapidly hydrolyzed in the gastrointestinal tract, liver, and plasma.[160] It seems, therefore, possible that the protective action observed with high doses of aspirin is mediated by its metabolite salicylic acid. Finally, it is noteworthy that similar to the effect of certain agents modulating gastric mucosal sulfhydryl levels such as cysteamine[122] and dimercaprol,[123] protection induced by high doses of aspirin occurs, although synthesis of prostaglandins in the gastric mucosa is severely suppressed. Thus, while inhibition of the formation of protective prostaglandins seems to be an important factor in the development of gastric mucosal ulcerations, an active cyclooxygenase is not required for the protective activity of NSAID-type drugs.[153]

IX. DIETARY MODULATION OF THE GASTRIC LEUKOTRIENE SYSTEM

The ω-3 polyunsaturated fatty acid 5,8,11,14,17-eicosapentaenoic acid which is present in high amounts in certain marine phospholipids can be metabolized via the 5-lipoxygenase pathway to form leukotrienes of the series 5.[161-163] Treatment of rats with eicosapentaenoic acid has recently been reported to protect the gastric mucosa against a variety of noxious agents such as ethanol, acid, alkali, or aspirin.[164] Treatment with eicosapentaenoic acid significantly inhibited gastric mucosal release of LTC_4 in ethanol-challenged rats;[165] however, HPLC analysis revealed that eicosapentaenoic acid is effectively metabolized by gastric 5-lipoxygenase, resulting in formation of equal amounts of LTC_5 and LTC_4 by gastric mucosa of eicosapentaenoic acid-treated rats. The sum of LTC_5 and LTC_4 generated by ethanol-challenged gastric mucosa in rats treated with protective doses of eicosapentaenoic acid was not different from control rats.[165] While the biologic activity of LTB_5 has been found to be considerably reduced compared to LTB_4,[162,163] LTC_5 was reported to be equipotent with LTC_4 in contracting guinea pig pulmonary parenchymal strips and ileal tissues[161] and to be a slightly, but insignificantly, weaker constrictor of the guinea pig coronary vasculature than LTC_4.[166] In order to elucidate whether modulation of the gastric leukotriene system contributes to the protection afforded by eicosapentaenoic acid, it is necessary to clearly define the effects of leukotrienes of the series 5 on gastric functions, particularly regarding actions on the gastric microcirculation.

X. EFFECT OF SELECTIVE 5-LIPOXYGENASE INHIBITORS ON ETHANOL-INDUCED GASTRIC MUCOSAL DAMAGE

Two recent publications have challenged the role of leukotrienes as mediators of ethanol-induced gastric injury. Thus, oral administration of 5, 10, or 30 mg/kg of the selective inhibitor of 5-lipoxygenase L-651,392 dose-dependently inhibited rat gastric mucosal LTC_4 formation. The two higher doses studied completely prevented the stimulatory action of ethanol on gastric mucosal LTC_4 formation; however, only the low dose of 5 mg/kg conferred some protection against the necrotizing effect of ethanol, while the two higher doses had no significant effect.[167] Similarly, Boughton-Smith et al.[168] reported that in rats treatment with BW A4C or BW A137C, two acetohydroxamic acids which selectively inhibit 5-lipoxygenase, did not protect against gastric mucosal damage caused by ethanol, although mucosal LTC_4 formation was near-maximally inhibited. Recent results from our own laboratory confirm that supression of gastric mucosal LTC_4 formation by selective 5-lipoxygenase inhibitors or some other compounds does not necessarily protect against mucosal damage induced by ethanol exposure (unpublished data). The inability of certain compounds which markedly inhibit gastric leukotriene formation to confer protection suggests that these 5-lipoxygenase products may not be the primary or exclusive mediators of ethanol-induced gastric damage. Exposure of the gastric mucosa to ethanol may possibly activate other lipoxygenases in addition to the 5-lipoxygenase which may also lead to formation of pro-ulcerogenic products. Selective inhibition of the 5-lipoxygenase pathway of arachidonic acid metabolism would not affect biosythesis of such additional lipoxygenase products. Alternatively, leukotrienes may be just one type of mediators among others generated in increased amounts after ethanol challenge. Selective inhibition of one mediator may not interrupt the chain of events which finally result in mucosal necrosis.

Further studies are necessary to clarify to what extent the stimulation of gastric mucosal leukotriene biosynthesis by ethanol and its inhibition by certain drugs is related to noxious or protective events.

ACKNOWLEDGMENT

The author wishes to thank Mrs. Inge Schönewolff for excellent secretarial assistance.

REFERENCES

1. **Robert, A.,** Prostaglandins and the gastrointestinal tract, in *Physiology of the Gastrointestinal Tract,* Johnson, L. R., Ed., Raven Press, New York, 1981, 1407.
2. **Johansson, C. and Bergström, S.,** Prostaglandins and protection of the gastroduodenal mucosa, *Scand. J. Gastroenterol. Suppl.,* 77, 21, 1982.

3. **Robert, A.,** Antisecretory, antiulcer, cytoprotective and diarrhaeogenic properties of prostaglandins, in *Advances in Prostaglandin, Thromboxane Research*, Vol. 2, Ramwell, P. and Paoletti, R., Eds., Raven Press, New York, 1976, 507.
4. **Hawkey, C. J. and Rampton, D. S.,** Prostaglandins and the gastrointestinal mucosa: are they important in its function, disease, or treatment?,*Gastroenterology,* 89, 1162, 1985.
5. **Charlet, N., Gallo-Torres, H. E., Buonameneaux, Y., and Wills, R. J.,** Prostaglandins and the protection of the gastroduodenal mucosa in humans: a critical review, *J. Clin. Pharmacol.*, 25, 564, 1985.
6. **Whittle, B. J. R., Kauffman, G. L., and Moncada, S.,** Vasoconstriction with thromboxanes A_2 induces ulceration of the gastric mucosa, *Nature,* 292, 472, 1981.
7. **Hamberg, M. and Samuelsson, B.,** Prostaglandin endoperoxides. Novel transformation of arachidonic acid in human platelets, *Proc. Natl. Acad. Sci. U.S.A.,* 71, 3400, 1974.
8. **Samuelsson, B., Borgeat, P., Hammarström, S., and Murphy, R. C.,** Introduction of a nomenclature: leukotrienes, *Prostaglandins,* 17, 785, 1979.
9. **Nugteren, D. H.,** Arachidonate lipoxygenase in blood platelets, *Biochim. Biophys. Acta,* 380, 299, 1975.
10. **Famaey, J. P.,** Leukotrienes and the lipoxygenase pathways, *Acta Clin. Belg.*, 36, 3, 1981.
11. **Borgeat, B. and Samuelsson, B.,** Transformation of arachidonic acid by rabbit polymorphonuclear leukocytes. Formation of a novel dihydroxyeicosatetraenoic acid, *J. Biol. Chem.*, 254, 2643, 1979.
12. **Radmark, O., Malmsten, C., and Samuelsson, B.,** Leukotriene A: stereochemistry and enzymatic conversion to leukotriene B, *Biochem. Biophys. Res. Commun.*, 92, 954, 1980.
13. **Borgeat, P. and Samuelsson, B.,** Metabolism of arachidonic acid in polymorphonuclear leukocytes. Structural analysis of novel hydroxylated compounds, *J. Biol. Chem.*, 254, 7865, 1979.
14. **Malmsten, C. L., Palmblad, J., Uden, A. M., Radmark, O., Engstedt, L., and Samuelsson, B.,** Leukotriene B_4: a highly potent and stereospecific factor stimulating migration of polymorphonuclear leukocytes, *Acta Physiol. Scand.*, 110, 449, 1980.
15. **Ford-Hutchinson, A. W., Smith, M. J. H., and Bray, M. A.,** Leukotriene B_4 (isomer III): biological activities of synthethic and biologically derived preparations, *J. Pharm. Pharmacol.*, 33, 332, 1981.
16. **Murphy, R. C., Hammarström, S., and Samuelsson, B.,** Leukotriene C: a slow reacting substance from murine mastocytoma cells, *Proc. Natl. Acad. Sci. U.S.A.*, 76, 4275, 1979.
17. **Corey, E. J., Clark, D. A., Goto, G., Marfat, A., Mioskoski, C., Samuelsson, B., and Hammarström, S.,** Stereospecific total synthesis of a "slow-reacting substance of anaphylaxis" (SRS-A), leukotriene C-1, *J. Am. Chem. Soc.*, 102, 1436, 1980.
18. **Samuelsson, B.,** Leukotrienes: mediators of immediate hypersensitivity reaction and inflammation, *Science,* 220, 568, 1983.
19. **Hammarström, S.,** The leukotrienes, in *Biochemical Actions of Hormones*, Vol. 11, Litwack, G., Ed., Academic Press, Orlando, FL, 1984, 1.
20. **Lewis, R. A. and Austen, K. F.,** The biologically active leukotrienes. Biosynthesis, metabolism, receptors, functions and pharmacology, *J. Clin. Invest.*, 73, 889, 1984.
21. **Borgeat, P., Nadeau, M., Salari, H., Poubelle, P., and Fruteau de LaClos, B.,** Leukotrienes: biosynthesis, metabolism and analysis, in *Advances in Lipid Research,* Vol. 21, Paoletti, R. and Kritchevsky, D., Eds., Academic Press, Orlando, FL, 1985, 47.
22. **Stenson, W. F. and Parker, C. W.,** Leukotrienes, in *Advances in Internal Medicine,* Vol. 30, Stollerman, G. H., Ed., Year Book Medical Publishers, Chicago, 1984, 175.
23. **Parker, C. W.,** The lipoxygenases in leukocytes and other mamalian cells, in *The Leukotrienes. Chemistry and Biology,* Chakrin, L. W. and Bailey, D. M., Eds., Academic Press, Orlando, FL, 1984, 125.
24. **Hansson, G., Lindgren, J. A., Dahlen, S. E., Hedqvist, P., and Sammuelsson, B.,** Indentification and biological activity of novel omega-oxidized metabolites of leukotriene B_4 from human leukocytes, *FEBS Lett.,* 130, 107, 1981.
25. **Shak, S. and Goldstein, I. M.,** Leukotriene B_4 omegahydroxylase in human polymorphonuclear leukocytes. Partial purification and identification as a cytochrome P-450, *J. Clin. Invest.*, 76, 1218, 1985.
26. **Maas, R. L., Brash, A. R., and Oates, J. A.,** Novel leukotriene and lipoxygenase products from arachidonic acid, in *Leukotrienes and Other Lipoxygenase Products,* Vol. 9, Samuelsson, B. and Paoletti, R., Eds., Raven Press, New York, 1982, 29.
27. **Powell, W. S.,** Novel pathway for the metabolism of 6-trans leukotriene B_4 in human polymorphonuclear leukocytes, *Biochem. Biophys. Res. Commun.*, 136, 707, 1986.
28. **Orning, L., Hammarström, S., and Samuelsson, B.,** Leukotriene D: a slow reacting substance from rat basophilic leukemia cells, *Proc. Natl. Acad. Sci. U.S.A.*, 7, 2014, 1980.
29. **Lewis, R. A., Austen, K. F., Drazen, J. M., Clark, D. A., Marfat, A., and Corey, E. J.,** Slow reacting substances of anaphylaxis; identification of leukotrienes C-1 and D from human and rat sources. *Proc. Natl. Acad. Sci. U.S.A.*, 77, 3710, 1980.
30. **Lewis, R. A., Drazen, J. M., Austen, K. F., Clark, D. A., and Corey, E. J.,** Identification of the C(6)-S-conjugate of leukotriene A with cysteine as a naturally ocurring slow reacting substance of anaphylaxis. Importance of the 11-cis-geometry for biological activity, *Biochem. Biophys. Res. Commun.*, 96, 271, 1980.

31. **Parker, C. W., Koch, D., Huber, M. M., and Falkenstein, S. F.,** Formation of the cysteinyl form of slow reacting substance of anaphylaxis (leukotriene E) in human plasma, *Biochem. Biophys. Res. Commun.*, 97, 1038, 1980.
32. **Bernström, K. and Hammarström, S.,** A novel leukotriene formed by transpeptidation of leukotriene E, *Biochem. Biophys. Res. Commun.*, 109, 800, 1982.
33. **Bernström, K. and Hammarström, S.,** Metabolism of leukotriene E_4 by rat tissues: formation of N-acetyl leukotriene E_4, *Arch. Biochem. Biophys.*, 244, 486, 1986.
34. **Hammarström, S., Örning, L., and Bernström, K.,** Metabolism of leukotrienes, *Mol. Cell. Biochem.*, 69, 7, 1985.
35. **Lee, C. W., Lewis, R. A., Tauber, A. I., Mehrotra, M., Corey, E. J., and Austen, K. F.,** The myeloperoxydase-dependent metabolism of leukotrienes C_4, D_4, and E_4 to 6-trans-leukotriene B_4 diasterisomers and the subclass-specific diasteroisomeric sulfoxides, *J. Biol. Chem.*, 258, 15004, 1983.
36. **Drazen, J. M. and Austen, K. F.,** Leukotrienes and airway responses, *Am. Rev. Resp. Dis.*, 136, 985, 1987.
37. **Claesson, H. E. and Haeggström, J.,** Metabolism of leukotriene A_4 by human endothelial cells: evidence for leukotriene C_4 and D_4 formation by leukocyte-endothelial cell interaction, in *Advances in Prostaglandin, Thromboxane, and Leukotriene Research*, Vol. 17, Samuelsson, B., Paoletti, R., and Ramwell, P. W., Eds., Raven Press, New York, 1987, 115.
38. **Metz, S., van Rollins, M., Strife, R., Fujimoto, W., and Robertson, R. P.,** Lipoxygenase pathway in islet endocrine cells. Oxidative metabolism of arachidonic acid promotes insulin release, *J. Clin. Invest.*, 71, 1191, 1983.
39. **Ford-Hutchinson, A. W., Bray, M. A., Doig, M. V., Shipley, M. E., and Smith, M. J. H.,** Leukotriene B: a potent chemokinetic and aggregating substance released from polymorphonuclear leukocytes, *Nature*, 286, 264, 1980.
40. **Bray, M. A.,** Leukotrienes in inflammation, *Agents Actions*, 19, 87, 1986.
41. **Dahlen, S. E., Björk, J., Hedqvist, P., Arfors, K. E., Hammarström, S., Lindgren, J. A., and Samuelsson, B.,** Leukotrienes promote plasma leakage and leukocyte adhesion in postcapillary venules: *in vivo* effects with relevance to the acute inflammatory response, *Proc. Natl. Acad. Sci. U.S.A.*, 78, 3887, 1981.
42. **Soter, N. A., Lewis, R. A., Corey, E. J., and Austen, K. F.,** Local effects of synthetic leukotrienes (LTC_4, LTD_4, LTE_4 and LTB_4) in human skin, *J. Invest. Dermatol.*, 80, 115, 1983.
43. **Camp, R., Jones, R. R., Brain, S., Woolard, P., and Greaves, M.,** Production of intraepidermal microabscesses by topical application of leukotriene B_4, *J. Invest. Dermatol.*, 82, 202, 1984.
44. **Serhan, C. N., Rodin, A., Smolen, J. E., Korchak, H., Samuelsson, B., and Weissmann, G.,** Leukotriene B_4 is a complete secretagogue in human neutrophils: a kinetic analysis, *Biochem. Biophys, Res. Commun.*, 107, 1006, 1982.
45. **Showell, H. J., Naccache, P. H., Borgeat, P., Picard, P., Vallerand, P., Becker, E. L., and Shaafi, R. I.,** Characterization of secretory activity of leukotriene B_4 toward rabbit neutrophils, *J. Immunol.*, 128, 811, 1982.
46. **Rollins, T. E., Zanolari, B., Springer, M. S., Guindon, Y., Zamboni, R., Lau, C. K., and Rokach, J.,** Synthetic leukotriene B_4 is a potent chemotaxin but a weak secretagogue for human PMN, *Prostaglandins*, 25, 281, 1983.
47. **Bray, M. A., Cunningham, F. M., Ford-Hutchinson, A. W., and Smith, M. J. H.,** Leukotriene B_4: a mediator of vascular permeability, *Br. J. Pharmacol.*, 72, 483, 1981.
48. **Higgs, G. A., Salmon, J. A., and Spayne, J. A.,** The inflammatory effects of hydroperoxy and hydroxy acid products of arachidonate lipoxygenase in rabbit skin, *Br. J. Pharmacol.*, 74, 429, 1981.
49. **Goetzl, E. J., Payan, D. G., and Goldman, D. W.,** Immunopathogenetic roles of leukotrienes in human diseases, *J. Clin. Immunol.*, 4, 79, 1984.
50. **Rola-Pleszczynski, M.,** Immunoregulation by leukotrienes and other lipoxygenase metabolites, *Immunol. Today*, 6, 302, 1985.
51. **Higgs, G. A., Moncada, S., and Vane, J. R.,** Eicosanoids in inflammation, *Ann. Clin. Res.*, 16, 287, 1984.
52. **Bhattacherjee, P. and Eakins, K. E.,** Lipoxygenase products: mediation of inflammatory responses and inhibition of their formation, in *The Leukotrienes. Chemistry and Biology*, Chakrin, L. W. and Bailey, D. M., Eds., Academic Press, Orlando, FL, 1984, 195.
53. **Goetzl, E. J., Wong, M. Y. S., and Matthay, M. A.,** Leukotrienes in human hypersensitivity and inflammatory diseases, in *Advances in Inflammation Research*, Vol. 11, Otterness, I., Ed., Raven Press, New York, 1986, 47.
54. **Feldberg, W. and Kellaway, C. H.,** Liberation of histamine and formation of lysolecithin-like substances by cobra venom, *J. Physiol.*, 94, 187, 1938.
55. **Chakravarty, N.,** The occurrence of a lipid-soluble smooth-muscle stimulating principle (SRS) in anaphylactic reaction, *Acta Physiol. Scand.*, 48, 167, 1960.
56. **Morris, H. R., Taylor, G. W., Piper, P. J., Samhoun, M. N., and Tippins, J. R.,** Slow reacting substances (SRSs): the structure identification of SRSs from rat basophilic leukemia (RBL-1) cells, *Prostaglandins*, 19, 185, 1980.

57. **Piper, P. J.,** Pharmacology of leukotrienes, *Br. Med. Bull.*, 33, 255, 1983.
58. **Kreutner, W. and Siegel, M. I.,** Biology of leukotrienes, *Annu. Rep. Med. Chem.*, 19, 241, 1984.
59. **Marom, Z., Shelhamer, J. H., Bach, M. K., Morton, D. R., and Kaliner, M.,** Slow-reacting substances, LTC_4, and LTD_4 increase the release of mucus from human airways *in vitro*, *Am. Rev Resp. Dis.*, 126, 449, 1982.
60. **Bisgaard, H., Kristensen, J., and Sondergaard, J.,** The effect of leukotriene C_4 and D_4 on cutaneous blood flow in humans, *Prostaglandins*, 23, 797, 1982.
61. **Ghelani, A. and Holroyde, M. C.,** Unresponsiveness of human gastrointestinal smooth muscle to SRS-A, *Methods Find. Exp. Clin. Pharmacol.*, 3, 385, 1981.
62. **Goldenberg, M. M. and Subers, E. M.,** The reactivity of rat isolated gastrointestinal tissues to leukotrienes, *Eur. J. Pharmacol.*, 78, 463, 1982.
63. **Yusko, P., Hall, R. A., and Ford-Hutchinson, A. W.,** Contraction of guinea pig gall bladder strips by leukotrienes and other agonists, *Prostaglandins*, 25, 397, 1983.
64. **Bloomquist, E. I. and Kream, R. M.,** Leukotriene D_4 acts in part to contract guinea pig ileum smooth muscle by releasing substance P, *J. Pharmacol. Exp. Ther.*, 240, 523, 1987.
65. **Collins, S. M., Daniel, E. E., and Fox, J. E.,** The effect of leukotriene D_4 on gastrointestinal motility, *Gastroenterology*, 90, 1377, 1986.
66. **Montcalm, E. and Shea-Donohue, T.,** Inhibition of leukotrienes stimulates gastric emptying in rhesus monkeys, *Gastroenterology*, 90, 1796, 1986.
67. **Whittle, B. J. R., Oren-Wolman, N., and Guth, P. H.,** Gastric vasoconstrictor actions of leuktriene C_4, $PGF_{2\alpha}$, and thromboxane mimetic U-46619 on rat submucosal microcirculation *in vivo*, *Am. J. Physiol.*, 248, G580, 1985.
68. **Leung, F. W., Robert, A., and Guth, P. H.,** Gastric mucosal blood flow in rats after administration of 16, 16-dimethyl prostaglandin E_2 at a cytoprotective dose, *Gastroenterology*, 88, 1948, 1985.
69. **Konturek, S. J., Brzozowski, T., Drozdowicz, D., Becka, G., and Jendralla, H.,** Role of leukotrienes (LT) in the formation of acute gastric mucosal damage in rats, *Gastroenterology*, 92, 1477, 1987.
70. **Gulati, N., Philpot, M. E., Gulati, O. P., Malmsten, C., and Huggel, H.,** Effects of leukotriene C_4 and prostaglandin E_2 on the rat mesentery *in vitro* and *in vivo*, *Prostaglandins Leukotrienes Med.*, 10, 257, 1983.
71. **Dembinska-Kiec, A., Simmet, T., and Peskar, B. A.,** Release and vasoconstrictor effect of leukotriene C_4-like immunoreactive material in the anaphylactic guinea pig mesenteric vascular bed, *Eur. J. Pharmacol.*, 101, 259, 1984.
72. **Salvati, P. and Whittle, B. J. R.,** Investigation of the vascular actions of arachidonate lipoxygenase and cyclooxygenase products on the isolated perfused stomach of rat and rabbit, *Prostaglandins*, 22, 141, 1981.
73. **Magous, R., Bali, J. P., Rossi, J. C., and Girard, J. P.,** Leukotrienes stimulate acid secretion from isolated gastric parietal cells, *Biochem. Biophys. Res. Commun.*, 114, 897, 1983.
74. **Pendleton, R. G., Shepherd-Rose, A. J., and Stavorski, J. M.,** Leukotriene effects upon the transgastric potential difference and pepsin secretion, *Eur. J. Pharmacol.*, 123, 29, 1986.
75. **Pendleton, R. G. and Stavorski, J. R.,** Evidence for differing leukotriene receptors in gastric mucosa, *Eur. J. Pharmacol.*, 125, 297, 1986.
76. **Konturek, S. J., Bilski, J., Dembinski, A., Warzecha, A., Beck, G., and Jendralla, H.,** Effects of leukotrienes on gastric acid and alkaline secretions, *Gastroenterology*, 92, 1209, 1987.
77. **Konturek, S. J., Pawlik, W., Beck, G., and Jendralla, H.,** Effects of leukotriene (LT) on pancreatic secretion and blood flow in dogs, *Gastroenterology*, 92, 1477, 1987.
78. **Musch, M. W., Miller, R. J., Field, M., and Siegel, M. I.,** Simulation of colonic secretion by lipoxygenase metabolites of arachidonic acid, *Science*, 217, 1255, 1982.
79. **Montzka, D. M., Smith, P. L., and Fondacara, J. D.,** Action of peptidoleukotrienes (PLTs) on electrolyte transport in rat small intestine, *Gastroenterology*, 92, 1803, 1987.
80. **Levendoglu, H., Snopko, R. M., and Dubin, A.,** Effect of leukotriene B_4 on gastric mucus synthesis by rabbit antral mucosa. Correlation with prostaglandin E_2, *Gastroenterology*, 90, 1518, 1986.
81. **Wölbling, R. H., Aehringhaus, W., Peskar, B. A., Morgenroth, K., and Peskar, B. M.,** Release of slow-reacting substance of anaphylaxis and leukotriene C_4-like immunoreactivity from guinea pig colonic tissue, *Prostaglandins*, 25, 809, 1983.
82. **Aehringhaus, U., Weiler, H., Peskar, B. A., and Peskar, B. M.,** Moelcular mechanisms of the gastric toxicity of antirheumatic drugs, *Arch. Toxicol. Suppl.*, 7, 323, 1984.
83. **Dreyling, K. W., Hoppe, U., Kleine, A., Kozuschek, W., and Peskar, B. M.,** Leukotriene formation in the gastrointestinal tract and effects of anti-inflammatory drugs, in *Side-Effects of Anti-inflammatory Drugs*, Rainsford, K. D. and Velo, G. P., Eds., MTP Press, Lancaster, England, 1985, 101.
84. **Peskar, B. M., Kozuschek, W., Morgenroth, K., Hoppe, U., Dreyling, K. W., and Peskar, B. A.,** Leukotriensynthese durch gastrointestinales Gewebe und ihre pharmakologische Beeinflussung, *Wien Klin. Wochenschr.*, 98, 98, 1986.

85. **Peskar, B. M., Lange, K., Hoppe, U., and Peskar, B. A.,** Ethanol stimulates formation of leukotriene C_4 in rat gastric mucosa, *Prostaglandins,* 31, 283, 1986.
86. **Boughton-Smith, N. K. and Whittle, B. J. R.,** Prostaglandin inhibition of ethanol-induced release of gastric mucosal leukotrienes, *Gastroenterology,* 92, 1325, 1987.
87. **Bennett, A., Hensby, C. N., Sanger, G. J., and Stamford, I. F.,** Metabolites of arachidonic acid formed by human gastrointestinal tissues and their actions on the muscle layers, *Br. J. Pharmacol.,* 74, 435, 1981.
88. **Boughton-Smith, N. K., Hawkey, C. J., and Whittle, B. J. R.,** Biosynthesis of lipoxygenase and cyclooxygenase products from (^{14}C)-arachidonic acid human colonic mucosa, *Gut,* 24, 1176, 1983.
89. **Dreyling, K. W., Hoppe, U., Peskar, B. A., Morgenroth, K., Kozuschek, W., and Peskar, B. M.,** Leukotriene synthesis by human gastrointestinal tissues, *Biochim. Biophys. Acta,* 878, 184, 1986.
90. **Boyd, S.C., Susame, H. M., and Boyden, M. R.,** High concentrations of glutathione in glandular stomach: implications for carcinogenesis, *Science,* 205, 1010, 1979.
91. **Wölbling, R. H., Aehringhaus, U., Peskar, B. M., and Peskar, B. A.,** Release of slow-reacting substance of anaphylaxis from layers of guinea pig aorta, *Prostaglandins,* 25, 823, 1983.
92. **Piper, P. J., Letts, L. G., and Galton, S. A.,** Generation of a leukotriene-like substance from procine vascular and other tissues, *Prostaglandins,* 25, 591, 1983.
93. **Wittmann, G., Peskar, B. M., Edelmann, M., Müller, K. M., Simmet, T., and Peskar, B. A.,** Formation of cysteinyl-containing leukotrienes by human arterial tissues, *Prostaglandins,* 33, 591, 1987.
94. **Peskar, B. M., Kleine, A., Pyras, F., and Müller, M. K.,** Gastrointestinal toxicity. Role of prostaglandins and leukotrienes, *Med. Toxicol.,* 1(Suppl. 1), 39, 1986.
95. **Wallace, J. L.,** Glucocorticoid-induced gastric mucosal damage: inhibition of leukotriene, but not prostaglandin biosynthesis, *Prostaglandins,* 34, 311, 1987.
96. **Rasanen, T.,** Mucosal mast cells of rat stomach: influence of ACTH, cortisone and growth hormone, *Gastroenterology,* 38, 70, 1960.
97. **Razin, E., Mencia-Huerta, J. M., Lewis, R. A., Corey, E. J., and Austen, K. F.,** Generation of leukotriene C_4 from a subclass of mast cells differentiated *in vitro* from mouse bone marrow, *Proc. Natl. Acad. Sci. U.S.A.,* 79, 4665, 1982.
98. **Sharon, P. and Stenson, W. F.,** Enhanced synthesis of leukotriene B_4 by colonic mucosa in inflammatory bowel disease, *Gastroenterology,* 86, 453, 1984.
99. **Peskar, B. M., Dreyling, K. W., Peskar, B. A., May, B., and Goebell, H.,** Enhanced formation of sulfidopeptide-leukotrienes in ulcerative colitis and Crohn's disease: inhibition by sulfasalazine and 5-aminosalicylic acid, *Agents Actions,* 18, 381, 1986.
100. **Lacy, E. R., and Ito, S.,** Microscopic analysis of ethanol damage to rat gastric mucosa after treatment with a prostaglandin, *Gastroenterology,* 83, 619, 1982.
101. **Guth, P. H.,** Gastric blood flow in ethanol injury and prostaglandin cytoprotection, *Scand. J. Gastroenterol.,* 21(Suppl. 125), 86, 1986.
102. **Guth, P. H., Paulsen, G., and Nagata, H.,** Histologic and microcirculatory changes in alcohol-induced gastric lesions in the rat: effect of prostaglandin cytoprotection, *Gastroenterology,* 87, 1083, 1984.
103. **Pihan, G., Majzoubi, D., Haudenschild, C., Trier, J. S., and Szabo, S.,** Early microcirculatory stasis in acute gastric mucosal injury in the rat and prevention by 16,16-dimethyl prostaglandin E_2 or sodium thiosulfate, *Gastroenterology,* 91, 1415, 1986.
104. **Szabo, S., Trier, J. S., Brown, A., and Schnoor, J.,** Early vascular injury and increased vascular permeability in gastric mucosal injury caused by ethanol in the rat, *Gastroenterology,* 88, 228, 1985.
105. **Peskar, B. M.,** Role of leukotrienes in gastric mucosal damage and protection, in *Prostaglandins and Leukotrienes in Gastrointestinal Diseases,* Domschke, W., Dammann, H. G., Peskar, B. M., and Holtenmüller, K. H., Eds., Springer-Verlag, Heidelberg, 1988, 89.
106. **Wallace, J. L. and Whittle, B. J. R.,** Role of prostanoids in the protective actions of BW755C on the gastric mucosa, *Eur. J. Pharmacol.,* 115, 45, 1985.
107. **Hua, X. Y., Dahlen, S. E., Lundberg, J. M., Hammarström, S. and Hedqvist, P.,** Leukotrienes C_4, D_4 and E_4 cause wide-spread and extensive plasma extravasation in the guinea pig, *Naunyn-Schmiedeberg's Arch. Pharmacol.,* 330, 136, 1985.
108. **Pihan, G. and Szabo, S.,** Leukotriene (LTD_4) enhances gastric mucosal lesions induced by ethanol or HCl, *Dig. Dis. Sci.,* 31, 57S, 1986.
109. **Ritchie, W. P.,** Acute gastric mucosal damage induced by bile salts, acid and ischemia, *Gastroenterology,* 68, 699, 1975.
110. **Walsh, J. P., Bloomfield, F. J., Maxwell, W. J., Hogan, F. P., Kelleher, D., and Keeling, P. W. N.,** Effect of H_2 receptor antagonists on prostaglandin E_2 and leukotriene B_4 production in duodenal ulcer disease, *Gut,* 26, A1119, 1985.
111. **Quadros, E. and Wilson, D. E.,** Nordihydroguaiaretic acid (NDGA) prevents ethanol-induced gastric mucosal damage: role of arachidonic acid lipoxygenase pathway metabolites, *Gastroenterology,* 92, 1584, 1987.

112. **Salmon, J. A., Simmons, P. M., and Moncada, S.,** The effects of BW755C and other anti-inflammatory drugs on eicosanoid concentrations and leukocyte accumlation in experimentally-induced acute inflammation, *J. Pharm. Pharmacol.*, 35, 808, 1983.
113. **Whittle, B. J. R., Higgs, G. A., Eakins, K. E., Moncada, S., and Vane, J. R.,** Selective inhibition of prostaglandin production in inflammatory exudates and gastric mucosa, *Nature*, 284, 271, 1980.
114. **Balaa, M. A. and Goldgar, D. E.,** Lipoxygenase enzyme inhibitors diminish ethanol damage to the rat stomach, *Clin Res.*, 34, 436A, 1986.
115. **Balaa, M. A., Kahlon, R., and Subramony, C.,** Diethylcarbamazine: an inhibitor of lipoxygenase enzyme diminishes ethanol damage to the rat stomach, *Gastroenterology*, 90, 1334, 1986.
116. **Nielsen, S. T., Beninati, L., and Chang, J.,** REV 5901 and Ly 171,883 protect rat gastric mucosa against ethanol-induced damage. *Agents Actions*, 21, 320, 1987.
117. **Szabo, S., Trier, J. S., and Frankel, P. W.,** Sulfhydryl compounds may mediate gastric cytoprotection, *Science*, 214, 200, 1981.
118. **Szabo, S., Maull, E. A., and Movahedi, S.,** Sulfhdryl drugs: a new type of gastric cytoprotective agents, *Gastroenterology*, 80, 1298, 1981.
119. **Robert, A., Eberle, D., and Kaplowitz, N.,** Role of glutathione in gastric mucosal cytoprotection, *Am. J. Physiol.*, 247, G296, 1984.
120. **Konturek, S. J., Brzozowski, T., Piastucki, I., Radecki, T., Dupuy, D., and Szabo, S.,** Gastric mucosal protection by agents altering gastric mucosal sulfhydryls, *Digestion*, 37, 65, 1987.
121. **Dupuy, D. and Szabo, S.,** Protection by metals against ethanol-induced gastric mucosal injury in the rat. Comparative biochemical and pharmacologic studies implicate protein sulfhydryls, *Gastroenterology*, 91, 966, 1986.
122. **Lange, K., Peskar, B. A., and Peskar, B. M.,** Stimulation of rat gastric mucosal leukotriene C_4 formation by ethanol and effect of gastric protective drugs, in *Advances in Prostaglandin, Thromboxane, and Leukotriene Research*, Vol. 17, Samuelsson, B., Paoletti, R., and Ramwell, P. W., Eds., Raven Press, New York, 1987, 299.
123. **Peskar, B. M. and Lange, K.,** Role of leukotriene C_4 in gastric protection by sulfhydryl-modulating agents and metals in the rat, *Gastroenterology*, 92, 1573, 1987.
124. **Baron, J. H.,** Effect of carbenoxolone sodium on human gastric acid secretion, *Gut*, 18, 721, 1977.
125. **Peskar, B. M., Holland, A., and Peskar, B. A.,** Effect of carbenoxolone on prostaglandin synthesis and degradation, *J. Pharm. Pharmacol.*, 28, 146, 1976.
126. **Peskar, B. M.,** Effects of carbenoxolone on the gastric mucosal prostaglandin and thromboxane system, *Acta Gastro-ent. Belg.*, 46, 429, 1983.
127. **Rask-Madsen, J., Bukhave, K., Madsen, P. E. R., and Bekker, C.,** Effect of carbenoxolone ongastric prostaglandin E_2 levels in patients with peptic ulcer disease following vagal and pentagastrin stimulation, *Eur. J. Clin. Invest.*, 131, 351, 1983.
128. **Derelanko, M. J. and Long, J. F.,** Carbenoxolone sodium protects rat gastric mucosa against ethanol-induced necrosis, *Proc. Soc. Exp. Biol. Med.*, 166, 394, 1981.
129. **Bennett, A., Melhuish, P. B., and Stamford, I. F.,** Carbenoxolone and deglycyrrhized liquorice have little or no effect on prostanoid synthesis by rat gastric mucosa ex vivo, *Br. J. Pharmacol.*, 86, 693, 1985.
130. **Dreyling, K. W., Lange, K., Peskar, B. A., and Peskar, B. M.,** Release of leukotrienes by rat and human gastric mucosa and its pharmacological modification, *Br. J. Pharmacol.*, 88, 236P, 1986.
131. **Peskar, B. M.,** Effect of carbenoxolone on prostaglandin synthesizing and metabolizing enzymes and correlation with gastric mucosal carbenoxolone concentrations, *Scand. J. Gastroenterol.*, 15(Suppl. 65), 109, 1980.
132. **Hoult, J. R. S.,** Pharmacological and biochemical actions of sulphasalazine, *Drugs*, 32 (Suppl. 1), 18, 1986.
133. **Stenson, W. F. and Lobos, E.,** Sulfasalazine inhibits the synthesis of chemotactic lipids by neutrophils, *J. Clin. Invest.*, 69, 494, 1982.
134. **Dreyling, K. W., Hoppe, U., Peskar, B. A., Schaarschmidt, K., and Peskar, B. M.,** Leukotrienes in Crohn's disease: effect of sulfasalazine and 5-aminosalicylic acid, in *Advances in Prostaglandin, Thromboxane, and Leukotriene Research*, Vol. 17, Samuelsson, B., Paoletti, R., and Ramwell, P. W., Eds., Raven Press, New York, 1987, 339.
135. **Bach, M. K. Brashler, J. R., and Johnson, M. A.,** Inhibition by sulfasalazine of LTC synthetase and of rat liver glutathione S-transferases, *Biochem. Pharmacol.*, 34, 2695, 1985.
136. **Cho, C. H., Ogle, C. W., and Sevilla, E. L.,** The protective effects of sulphasalzine against ethanol-induced gastric damage in rats, *Br. J. Pharmacol.*, 92, 31, 1987.
137. **Ogle, C. W., Cho, C. H., and Dai, S.,** Sulphasalazine and experimental stress ulcers, *Agents Actions*, 17, 153, 1985.
138. **Guth, P. H. and Hall, P.,** Microcirculatory and mast cell changes in restraint-induced gastric ulcer, *Gastroenterology*, 50, 562, 1966.
139. **Galli, S. J., Wershil, B. K., Bose, R., Walker, P. A., and Szabo, S.,** Ethanol-induced acute gastric injury in mast cell-deficient and congenic normal mice. Evidence that mast cells can augment the area of damage, *Am. J. Pathol.*, 128, 131, 1987.

140. **Beck, P. L., Morris, G. P., and Wallace, J. L.,** Inhibition of ethanol-induced gastric damage and leukotriene synthesis by a mast cell stabilizer, *Gastroenterology,* 92, 1797, 1987.
141. **Jones, T. R., Young, R., Champion, E., Charette, L., Denis, D., Ford-Hutchinson, A. W., Frenette, R., Gauthier, J. Y., Guindon, Y., Kakushima, M., Masson, P., McFarlane, C., Piechuta, H., Rokach, J., and Zamboni, R.,** L-649,923, sodium (βS*, γR*)-4-(3-(4-acetyl-3-hydroxy-2-propylphenoxy)-propylthio)-γ-hydroxy-β-methyl-benzene-butanoate, a selective orally active leukotriene receptor antagonist, *Can. J. Physiol. Pharmacol.,* 64, 1068, 1986.
142. **Peskar, B. M.,** Cysteinyl-leukotriene receptor antagonists protect against ethanol- and indomethacin-induced gastric mucosal damage in rats, *Gastroenterology,* 94, A351, 1988.
143. **Ogle, C. W. and Cho, C. H.,** FLP 55712, a leukotriene receptor antagonist, protects against stress-induced gastric ulcers in rats, *IRCS Med. Sci.,* 14, 114, 1986.
144. **Hollander, W., Tarnawski, A., Gergeley, H., and Zipser, R. D.,** Sulcralfate protection of the gastric mucosa against ethanol-induced injury: a prostaglandin-mediated process?, *Scand J. Gastroenterol.,* 19(Suppl. 101), 97, 1984.
145. **Szeleny, I., Postius, S., and Engler, H.,** Evidence for a functional cytoprotective effect produced by antacids in the rat stomach, *Eur. J. Pharmacol.,* 88, 403, 1983.
146. **Lange, K., Peskar, B. A., and Peskar, B. M.,** Inhibition of leukotriene formation as a mode of action of gastroprotective drugs, in *Prostaglandins in Clinical Research,* Sinzinger, H. and Schrör, K., Eds., Alan R. Liss, New York, 1987, 283.
147. **Müller, B. and Schmidtke, M.,** Microvascular effects of iloprost in the hamster cheek pouch, in *Advances in Prostaglandin, Thromboxane, and Leukotriene Research,* Vol. 17, Samuelsson, B., Paoletti, R., and Ramwell, P. W., Eds., Raven Press, New York, 1987, 455.
148. **Whittle, B. J. R., Steel, G., and Wallace, J. L.,** Assessment of the actions of prostanoids in the protection and repair of the gastric mucosa, *Scand. J. Gastroenterol.,* 21(Suppl. 125), 128, 1986.
149. **Vane, J. R.,** Inhibition of prostaglandin synthesis as a mechanism of action for aspirin-like drugs, *Nature, (London) New Biol.,* 231, 232, 1971.
150. **Brune, K., Aehringhaus, U., and Peskar, B. A.,** Pharmacological control of leukotriene and prostaglandin production from mouse peritoneal macrophages, *Agents Actions,* 14, 729, 1984.
151. **Hoppe, U., Peskar, B. A., and Peskar, B. M.,** Effect of indomethacin on prostaglandin and leukotriene formation in rat gastric mucosa and inflammatory exudate, *Naunyn-Schmiedeberg's Arch. Pharmacol.,* 335(Suppl.), R41, 1987.
152. **Peskar, B. M., Hoppe, U., Lange, K., and Peskar, B. A.,** Effect of non-steroidal anti-inflammatory drugs (NSAID) on rat gastric leukotriene formation, *Gastroenterology,* 92, 1573, 1987.
153. **Peskar, B. M., Hoppe, U., Lange, K., and Peskar B. A.,** Effects of non-steroidal anti-inflammatory drugs on rat gastric mucosal leukotriene C_4 and prostanoid release: relation to ethanol-induced injury, *Br. J. Pharmacol.,* 93, 937, 1988.
154. **Ahnfelt-Ronne, I. and Arrigoni-Martelli, E.,** Multiple effects of a new anti-inflammatory agent, timegadine, on arachidonic acid release and metabolism in neutrophils and platelets, *Biochem. Pharmacol.,* 31, 2619, 1982.
155. **Brune, K. and Lanz, R.,** Pharmacokinetics of non-steroidal anti-inflammatory drugs, in *Handbook of Inflammation,* Vol. 5, *The Pharmacology of Inflammation,* Bonta, I. L., Bray, M. A., and Parnham, M. J., Eds., Elsevier, Amsterdam, 1985, 413.
156. **Leung, K. H.,** Selective inhibition of leukotriene C_4 synthesis in human neutrophils by ethacrynic acid, *Biochem. Biophys. Res. Commun.,* 137, 195, 1986.
157. **Rainsford, K. D.,** The effects of 5-lipoxygenase inhibitors and leukotriene antagonists on the development of gastric lesions induced by nonsteroidal antiinflammatory drugs in mice, *Agents Actions,* 21, 316, 1987.
158. **Glenn, E. M., Bowman, B. J., and Rohloff, N. A.,** Anomalous biological effects of salicylates and prostaglandins, *Agents Actions,* 9, 257, 1979.
159. **Robert, A.,** Gastric cytoprotection by sodium salicylate, *Prostaglandins,* 21(Suppl.) , 39, 1981.
160. **Flower, R. J., Moncada, S., and Vane, J. R.,** Analgesic-antipyretics and anti-inflammatory agents: drugs employed in the treatment of gout, in *The Pharmacological Basis of Therapeutics,* Goodman-Gilman, A., Goodman, L. S., Rall, T. W., and Murad, F., Eds., Macmillan, New York, 1985, 674.
161. **Hammarström, S.,** Leukotriene C_5: a slow reacting substance derived from eicosapentaenoic acid, *J. Biol. Chem.,* 255, 7093, 1980.
162. **Terano, T., Salmon, J. A., and Moncada, S.,** Biosynthesis and biologic activity of leukotriene B_5, *Prostaglandins,* 27, 217, 1984.
163. **Leitch, A. G., Lee, T. H., Ringel, E. W., Prickett, J. D., Robinson, D. R., Pyne, S. G., Corey, E. J., Drazen, J. M., Austen, K. F., and Lewis, R. A.,** Immunologically induced generation of tetraene and pentaene leukotrienes in the peritoneal cavities of menhaden-fed rats, *J. Immunol.,* 132, 2559, 1984.

164. **Rogers, C., Pihan, G., Raza, A., and Szabo, S.,** Possible participation of leukotrienes (LT) in the pathogenesis of gastric mucosal lesions and vascular injury induced by ethanol, HCl, NaOH, or aspirin (ASA) in the rat. Effect of eicosapentaenoic acid (EPA) or a lipoxygenase inhibitor L-651,392, *Gastroenterology*, 92, 1808, 1987.
165. **Trautmann, M. and Peskar, B. M.,** Gastroprotektion durch Eicosapentaensäure: Rolle des endogenen Leukotrien- und Prostaglandin-Systems, *Z. Gastroenterol.*, 25, 578, 1987.
166. **Juan, H., Peskar, B. A., and Simmet, T.,** Effect of exogenous 5,8,11,14,17-eicosapentaenoic acid on cardiac anaphylaxis, *Br. J. Pharmacol.*, 90, 315, 1987.
167. **Wallace, J. L., Beck, L., and Morris, G. P.,** Is there a role for leukotrienes as mediators of ethanol-induced gastric mucosal damage? *Am. J. Physiol.*, 254, G117, 1988.
168. **Boughton-Smith, N. K. and Whittle, B. J. R.,** Failure of the inhibition of rat gastric mucosal 5-lipoxygenase by novel acetohydroxamic acids to prevent ethanol-induced damage, *Br. J. Pharmacol.*, 95, 155, 1988.

Chapter 8

PLATELET-ACTIVATING FACTOR: ITS ROLE AS A MEDIATOR OF GASTROINTESTINAL DAMAGE

John L. Wallace

TABLE OF CONTENTS

I. INTRODUCTION

Platelet-activating factor (PAF) was first described by Benveniste et al.[1] as a platelet-stimulating factor found in buffy coats of blood samples from antigen-challenged rabbits. Its structure was confirmed by Demopoulos et al.[2] in 1979 as 1-*O*-alkyl-2-*O*-acetyl-*sn*-glycero-3-phosphocholine. PAF has been reported to be released from several types of cells *in vitro,* including basophils, neutrophils, mast cells, macrophages, monocytes, endothelial cells, platelets, and eosinophils.[3-9]

PAF biosynthesis proceeds via two main steps, both of which are calcium dependent. The stable precursor of PAF, 1-*O*-álkyl-2-acyl-glycero-3-phosphocholine (lyso-PAF), can be released from alkyl-phospholipids in the plasma membrane via the action of phospholipase A_2.[5] Conversion of lyso-PAF to PAF is catalyzed by a unique acetyl CoA transferase, which acetylates the 2′ position of the phosphocholine molecule (see Figure 1). Acetyl CoA transferase is the rate-limiting step in the formation of PAF. Catabolism of PAF can also be catalyzed by two enzymes. In the plasma, PAF is rapidly hydrolyzed by an acid labile enzyme, acetyl hydrolase, giving rise to lyso-PAF.[10-12] This enzyme can also be found in the cytosol of some cells. Phospholipase A_2 can also cleave the 2′ acetyl group, converting PAF back to lyso-PAF. Lyso-PAF can be reacylated into the form of an alkyl-glycero-phosphocholine and stored in cell membranes. Lyso-PAF, therefore, is the intermediate in both PAF biosynthesis and catabolism.

A wide range of biological actions of PAF have also been reported, which include peripheral vasodilation, stimulation of platelet aggregation, stimulation of neutrophil aggregation and degranulation, activation of eosinophils, increase in vascular permeability (probably as a consequence of endothelial dysjunction), and stimulation of lysosomal enzyme release into the circulation.[13-21] It was these actions of PAF which first implicated it as a possible mediator of acute inflammation and anaphylaxis.[22] PAF has also been shown to be a potent bronchoconstrictor[13] and an ulcerogenic agent in the gastrointestinal tract.[16,22,23]

The observation of Heymans et al.[24] that only the naturally occurring stereoisomer (R) was biologically active suggested that PAF acted via a specific receptor. High-affinity binding sites for PAF have now been identified on human and rat platelets, human neutrophils, human lung membranes, rat retina, rat liver, and guinea pig endothelial cells.[25] Interestingly, rat platelets do not have binding sites for PAF.[26] Over the past decade, several specific PAF receptor antagonists have been developed which have proven to be useful tools in the dissection of the role of PAF in several diseases. The properties and development of such antagonists have been reviewed in detail by Braquet et al.,[25] and only their actions pertaining to the role of PAF in gastrointestinal diseases are discussed in this chapter.

II. ULCEROGENIC ACTIONS OF PLATELET-ACTIVATING FACTOR

The ulcer promoting actions of PAF in the gastrointestinal tract were first reported by Bessin et al.,[16] who noted intestinal infarct following administration of PAF to dogs at doses causing acute circulatory collapse. Gonzalez-Crussi and Hsueh[22] reported that bolus administration of high doses of PAF (~4 to 10 μg/kg) concomitantly with endotoxin led to necrosis in the small bowel of the rat. Based on these data, they proposed a role for PAF in necrotizing enterocolitis. The gastric ulcerogenic actions of PAF were first described in detail by Rosam et al.[23] Intravenous infusion of PAF to rats at doses of 10 to 100 ng/kg/min over 20 min led to extensive focal hyperemia and hemorrhagic necrosis in the gastric mucosa (Figure 2). Histologically, the damage was characterized by vascular congestion involving the entire mucosal layer in the involved regions (Figure 3) and focal necrosis. Aggregates of neutrophils were frequently present in submucosal and mucosal venules. Even at doses of PAF not causing macroscopically

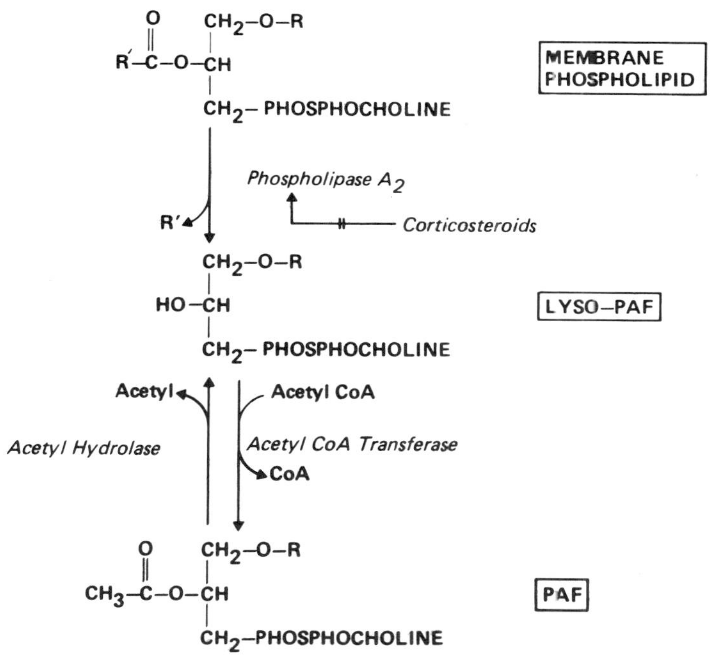

FIGURE 1. Schematic diagram of the biosynthetic pathway for platelet-activating factor (PAF). R and R′ indicate fatty acids. As indicated, the action of phospholipase A_2 can be inhibited by corticosteroids leading to inhibition of PAF synthesis.[5] Note that lyso-PAF is the intermediate in both the anabolism and catabolism of PAF. In neutrophils, R′ is usually arachidonic acid.[124]

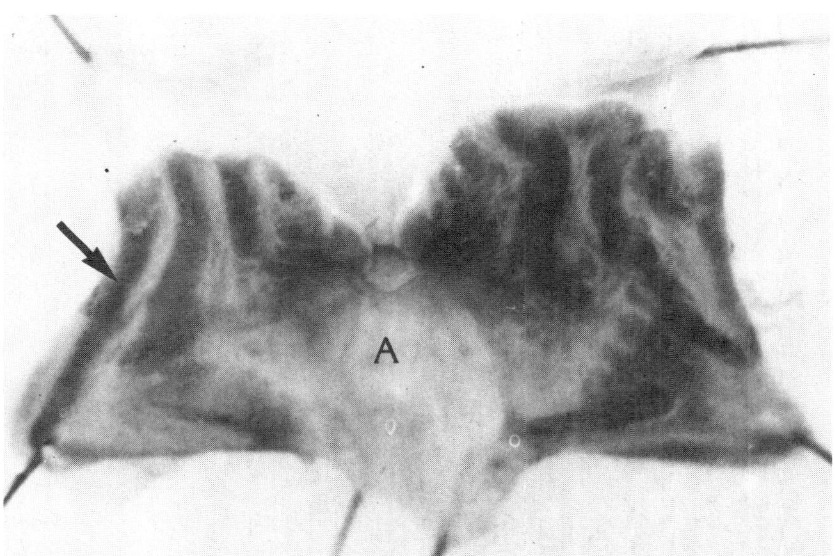

FIGURE 2. Photograph of the mucosal surface of a rat stomach following a 20-min i.v. infusion of PAF at a dose of 100 ng/kg/min. Note the extensive erythematous bands (arrow) in the corpus region. The antral region (A) appears relatively normal.

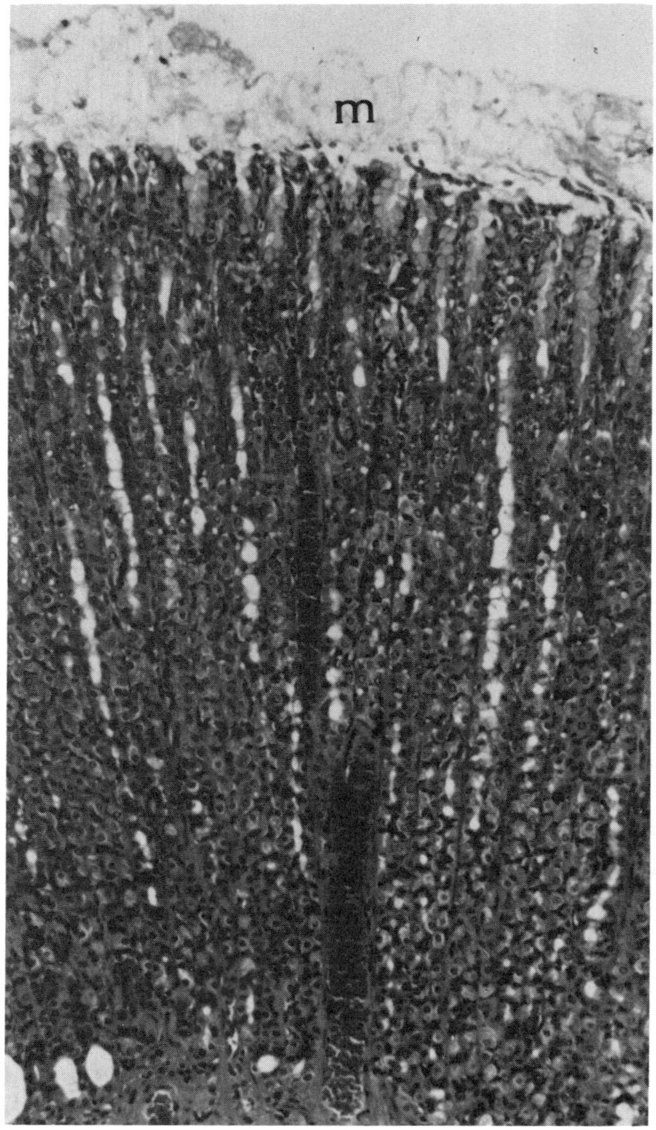

FIGURE 3. Light micrograph of the gastric mucosa of a rat following a 20-min i.v. infusion of PAF at a dose of 100 ng/kg/min. Note the vasocongestion, particularly in the large collecting venules, which extends throughout the depth of the mucosa. Exfoliation of surface epithelial cells and release of mucus (m) onto the luminal surface is evident. (H & E. Magnification × 125.)

visible gastric damage, there was histological evidence of disturbed gastric mucosal blood flow. Indeed, congestion of subepithelial venules was noted in 75% of the rats treated with PAF at a dose of 10 ng/kg/min. To assess the possibility that these low doses of PAF predisposed the gastric mucosa to damage, *ex vivo* gastric chamber studies were performed in which the effects of PAF on the resistance of the gastric mucosa to damage by a topical irritant was assessed.[27] PAF was administered intravenously for 5 min at doses of 0.3 to 100 ng/kg/min. Two minutes after beginning the infusion of PAF, the chambered gastric mucosa was "challenged" with 20%

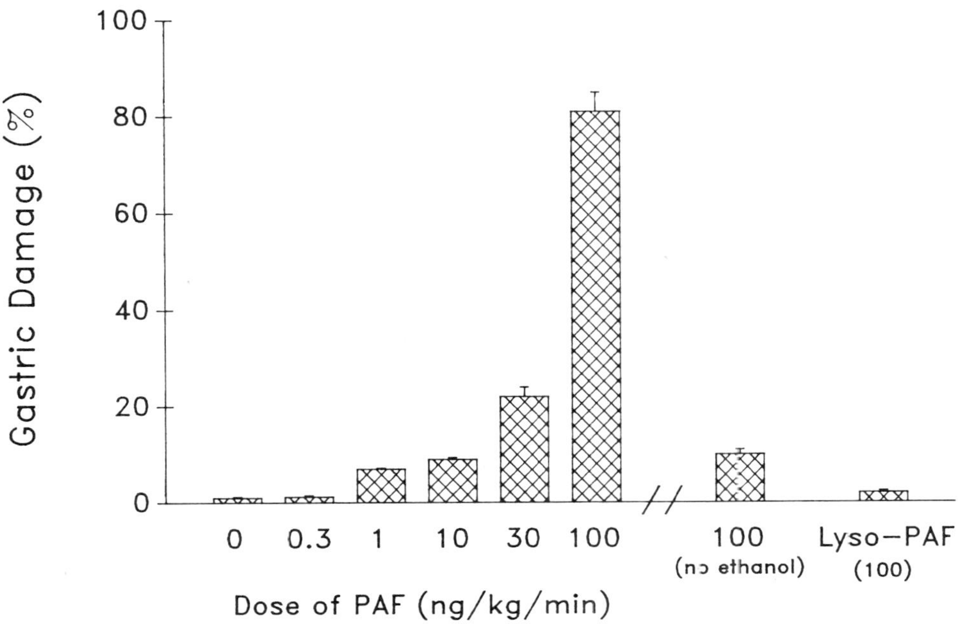

FIGURE 4. Effects of a 5-min i.v. infusion of PAF on the susceptibility of the chambered rat stomach to damage induced by topical application of 20% ethanol. PAF caused a dose-dependent increase in the extent of gastric damage induced by the ethanol. Note that the highest dose of PAF (100 ng/kg/min) produced only a low level of damage when 20% ethanol was not applied to the mucosa. Also note that lyso-PAF did not augment the damage induced by 20% ethanol. (Adapted from Reference 27.)

ethanol (applied topically). As can be seen in Figure 4, application of 20% ethanol without PAF infusion caused minimal gastric damage. The damaging effects of 20% ethanol were not significantly altered by concomitant intravenous administration of lyso-PAF (100 ng/kg/min); however, intravenous administration of PAF caused a dose-dependent increase in 20% ethanol-induced damage. Even at a dose as low as 1 ng/kg/min, the extent of 20% ethanol-induced damage was significantly augmented. The synergistic interaction of PAF with a topical irritant was not limited to 20% ethanol. Topical application of the bile acid, sodium taurocholate (2 m*M*), caused hemorrhagic damage to 3% of the glandular mucosa (Figure 5). The extent of hemorrhagic damage was increased to 29% when PAF was infused intravenously (100 ng/kg/min) during the challenge with sodium taurocholate. These studies therefore suggest that release of PAF under some circumstances (such as during septic shock), could significantly predispose the gastric mucosa to damage induced by endogenous substances (such as bile salts), the presence of which the gastric mucosa would normally tolerate.

Infusion of PAF to rats also leads to extensive necrosis and hemorrhage in the small bowel. Using release of acid phosphatase as an enzyme marker of cell death, we[28] demonstrated that the duodenum, jejunum, and to a lesser extent, the terminal ileum were extensively damaged following a 10-min intravenous infusion of PAF. Conversely, the distal colon did not appear to be susceptible to PAF-induced damage at the dose tested.

PAF-induced gastrointestinal damage has also been reported in other laboratory animals. As mentioned earlier, Bessin et al.[16] noted extensive vascular congestion in the gastrointestinal tract of dogs following intravenous infusion of PAF. Lees et al.[29] reported that intravenous administration of PAF to anesthetized cats resulted in gastric damage characterized by vascular congestion, edema, epithelial exfoliation, and hemorrhage. Using an *ex vivo* gastric chamber model in dog, Whittle et al.[30] and Soybel et al.[31] both reported that local intraarterial infusion of PAF caused alterations in mucosal appearance. Both of these groups reported that shortly after

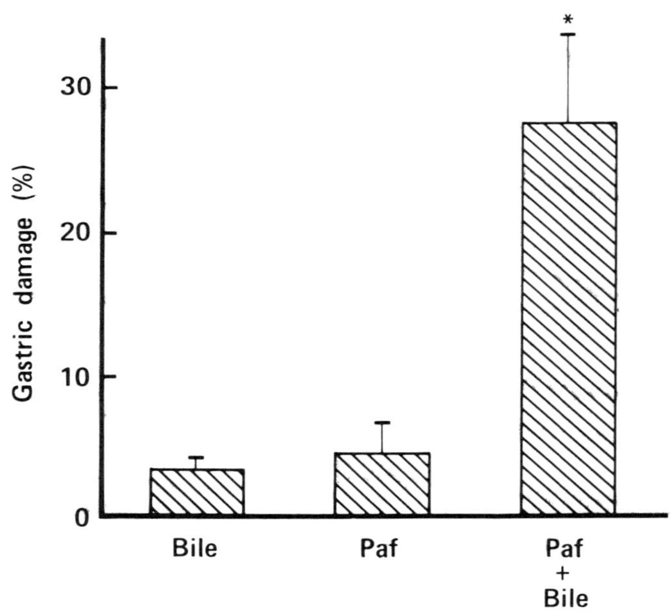

FIGURE 5. Synergistic interaction of i.v. PAF (100 ng/kg/min for 5 min) and topically applied bile salt (sodium taurocholate in 50 m*M* HCl). $^{*}p$ <0.01 compared to the bile or PAF groups. (Adapted from Reference 27.)

beginning the infusion of PAF, mucosal coloration changed from a uniform pink to a more "mottled" appearance. Whittle et al.[30] used histological assessment to confirm that the mucosa was indeed damaged. As in the rat, PAF caused marked subepithelial edema, congestion of the microvasculature (particularly the collecting venules), hemorrhage, and, in some cases, necrosis. Soybel et al.[31] noted significant increases in sodium and potassium ion efflux, as well as marked outpouring of fluid into the lumen of the stomach during the infusion of PAF. They interpreted these changes as being indicative of an increase in mucosal permeability to extracellular fluid, probably subsequent to edema formation in the lamina propria and submucosa. Interestingly, Soybel and associates did not observe any significant changes in mucosal permeability to hydrogen ions during the infusion of PAF.

III. MECHANISM OF ULCEROGENIC ACTIONS OF PAF

A. SYSTEMIC HYPOTENSION

As mentioned above, PAF is a potent peripheral vasodilator. During infusion of PAF at doses causing gastrointestinal damage, marked systemic hypotension is observed. Arterial blood pressure remains depressed throughout the period of the infusion of PAF, after which it gradually recovers toward resting levels.[32] Such changes in arterial pressure might result in reduced gastrointestinal blood flow and thereby predispose these tissues to damage. Indeed, hemorrhagic shock increases the susceptibility of the gastrointestinal tract to damage and has been used as an animal model for gastric[33,34] (see Chapter 9) and small intestinal[35] ulceration. This hypothesis, at least as it pertains to PAF-induced damage in the stomach, has been tested in several ways. First, Rosam et al.[23] demonstrated that intravenous infusions of either prostacyclin, isoproterenol, or nitroprusside at doses eliciting a decrease in systemic arterial blood pressure of similar magnitude to that induced by an ulcerogenic dose (50 ng/kg/min) of PAF caused little or no damage (Table 1). Second, Wallace and Whittle[27] noted a poor correlation between the dose-response curves for the effect of PAF on blood pressure and the

TABLE 1
Comparison of Ulcerogenic Effects of PAF with Other Hypotensive Agents

Compound	Dose (μg/kg/min)	Damage score (0-3)	% with Hemorrhage	Change in blood pressure (mmHg)
Vehicle	—	0.5 ± 0.2[a]	0	1 ± 2
Prostacyclin	0.5	0.6 ± 0.2[a]	0	-55 ± 4
Isoproterenol	0.5	0.3 ± 0.2[a]	0	-50 ± 3
Nitroprusside	10.0	1.4 ± 0.4[a]	0	-72 ± 2
PAF	0.05	2.6 ± 0.2	75	-62 ± 4

Note: All drugs (or the vehicle) were infused i.v. for 20 min. Gastric damage was scored by an observer unaware of the treatment on a 0 (normal) to 3 (severe) scale. Change in blood pressure refers to the difference between the resting mean arterial pressure and that at the end of the infusion period (a negative sign indicates a decrease in pressure). The % with hemorrhage was determined histologically. For further details of these experiments, see Reference 23.

[a]Denote a significant difference (p <0.05) in the damage score when compared to the group treated with PAF.

effect of PAF on the susceptibility of the gastric mucosa to damage induced by topically applied 20% ethanol. Furthermore, we demonstrated that if the topical irritant was not applied to the stomach until after the PAF-induced hypotension had dissipated, significant augmentation of damage was still observed. Third, and most convincingly, Whittle et al.[30] and Soybel et al.[31] each demonstrated that local arterial infusion of PAF at doses not affecting systemic blood pressure still caused significant gastric damage.

Experiments such as these have not been performed to assess the role of hypotension in PAF-induced damage in the small bowel. It remains possible, therefore, that reduced intestinal perfusion as a consequence of systemic hypotension could be a contributing factor to intestinal damage induced by PAF.

B. PLATELET ACTIVATION

As the name suggests, PAF can stimulate the activation of platelets leading to aggregation,[1] thrombus formation,[18] and a state of thrombocytopenia.[13] The mechanism by which PAF activates platelets remains unclear and controversial.[25] PAF-induced thrombus formation could play a role in the production of gastrointestinal damage by occluding small blood vessels in the mucosa and thereby causing ischemia. The only studies which have been performed to assess the contribution of platelet activation/aggregation to PAF-induced gastrointestinal damage are those of Rosam et al.[23] in the rat. They demonstrated that rats made thrombocytopenic by treatment with an antiplatelet serum (raised in rabbits) were still susceptible to gastric damage induced by PAF (Figure 6). The report of Inarrea et al.[36] that rat platelets do not have binding sites for PAF suggested that platelet activation would not play an important role in ulcerogenesis; however, it was possible that platelet aggregation might be stimulated by a second mediator, such as thromboxane A_2(TXA_2) released in response to PAF (see Section F).

Unfortunately, no similar studies on the ulcerogenic actions of PAF have been performed using animals with PAF-sensitive platelets. It remains possible that thrombus formation plays an important role in the development of gastrointestinal damage induced by PAF. Indeed, the ability of dog and cat platelets to bind PAF may explain the greater sensitivity of these animals to PAF-induced gastrointestinal damage when compared to rats.[30]

C. NEUTROPHIL AGGREGATION/DEGRANULATION

As mentioned in the Introduction, specific binding sites for PAF have been identified on human neutrophils.[37] PAF has been shown to cause aggregation of neutrophils *in vitro* at concentrations as low as 100 pM.[6] Following intradermal injections of PAF in the rabbit,

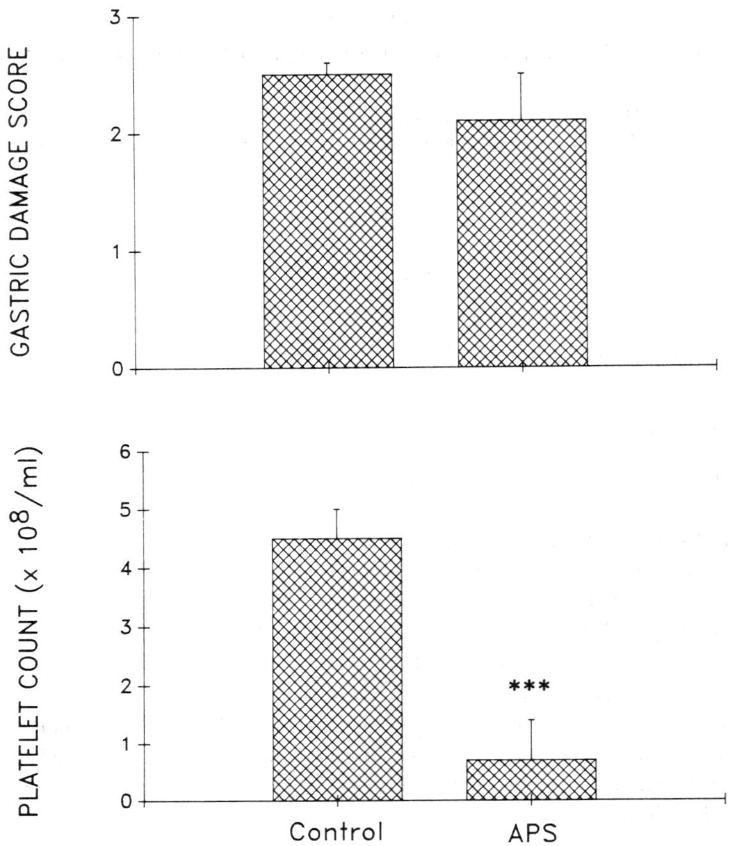

FIGURE 6. Effects of treatment with antiplatelet serum (APS) on circulating platelet numbers and susceptibility to PAF-induced gastric damage. Note that APS-induced thrombocytopenia did not alter the susceptibility of the stomach to damage induced by PAF. $^{***}p < 0.001$ compared to the control group. (Adapted from Reference 23.)

neutrophils were observed accumulating at the injection site within 5 min.[15] Using *in vivo* microscopy techniques, Bjork et al.[21] observed adherence of neutrophils to postcapillary venular endothelium within 5 min of administration of PAF in a hamster cheek pouch preparation. Subsequently, aggregates of neutrophils and platelets were observed within the lumen of the venules. Bjork et al. noted that these aggregates were eventually swept away by the flow of blood. They suggested that the aggregates would eventually become lodged in the lung. Indeed, Camussi et al.[7] noted numerous neutrophil aggregates in the rabbit lung following administration of PAF. It is possible that the trapping of neutrophil aggregates in the lung might account for the marked neutropenia which has been noted following PAF administration,[10] as well as contributing to the pulmonary hypertension induced by PAF.[7]

Neutrophil aggregates have also been observed in postcapillary venules in the stomach following administration of PAF[27] (Figure 7). We postulated that these aggregates may restrict the drainage of blood from the mucosa and thereby predispose it to damage induced by a topical irritant. In support of this hypothesis, Whittle et al.[38] noted marked erythrocyte sludging following application of PAF to an *in vivo* rat submucosa preparation. Whittle et al. also noted margination of neutrophils and reduced gastric mucosal blood flow. The reduced blood flow and sludging appeared to be a consequence of the neutrophil margination, since effects of PAF on

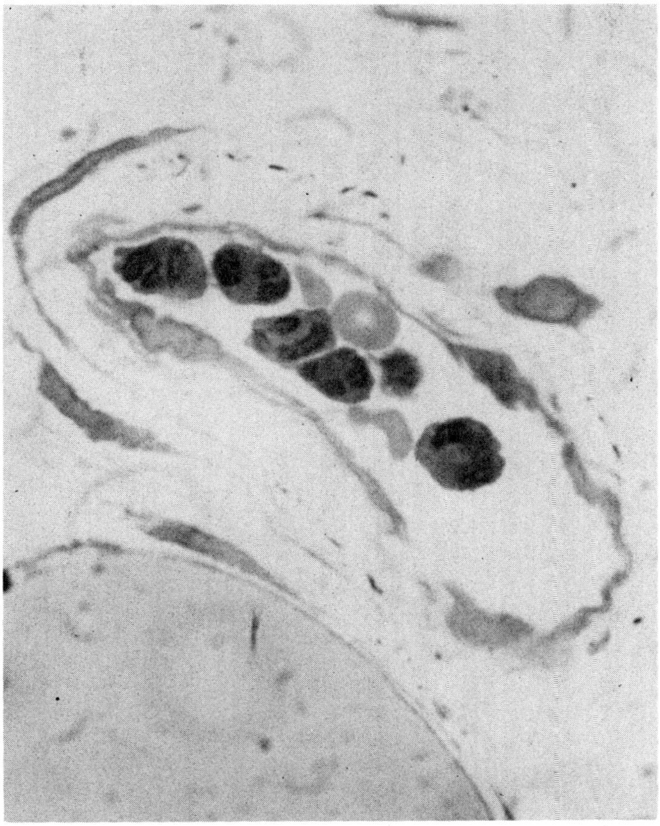

FIGURE 7. Light micrograph showing accumulation of neutrophils in a venule in the gastric submucosa following i.v. infusion of PAF. (Toluidine blue. Magnification ×3700.)

microvascular diameter were not observed. Further evidence that PAF causes accumulation of neutrophil aggregates in the stomach is the observation that PAF administration results in a significant increase in myeloperoxidase activity in the stomach[39] (see Figure 8). Myeloperoxidase is an enzyme found predominantly in azurophilic granules of neutrophils, and has been widely used as a marker of neutrophil infiltration and acute inflammation.[40-43]

In addition to causing a reduction of gastrointestinal blood flow, aggregation of neutrophils would likely be accompanied by the release of several factors which might contribute to gastrointestinal damage. For instance, neutrophils contain several lysosomal enzymes, as well as myeloperoxidase, which could contribute to tissue necrosis. Doebber et al.[14] noted significant increases in plasma levels of lysosomal hydrolase following PAF administration, and suggested that this enzyme might contribute to some of the damaging effects of PAF. Neutrophils also release several free radicals when stimulated. As covered extensively in Chapter 9, neutrophil-derived free radicals may play an important role in gastrointestinal ulceration. Neutrophils also release several metabolites of arachidonic acid, such as TXA_2[44] and leukotrienes,[45] which have been shown to have pro-ulcerogenic actions in the stomach.[46,47] The possible mediation of PAF-induced gastrointestinal damage by these substances and others is discussed more fully later in this chapter.

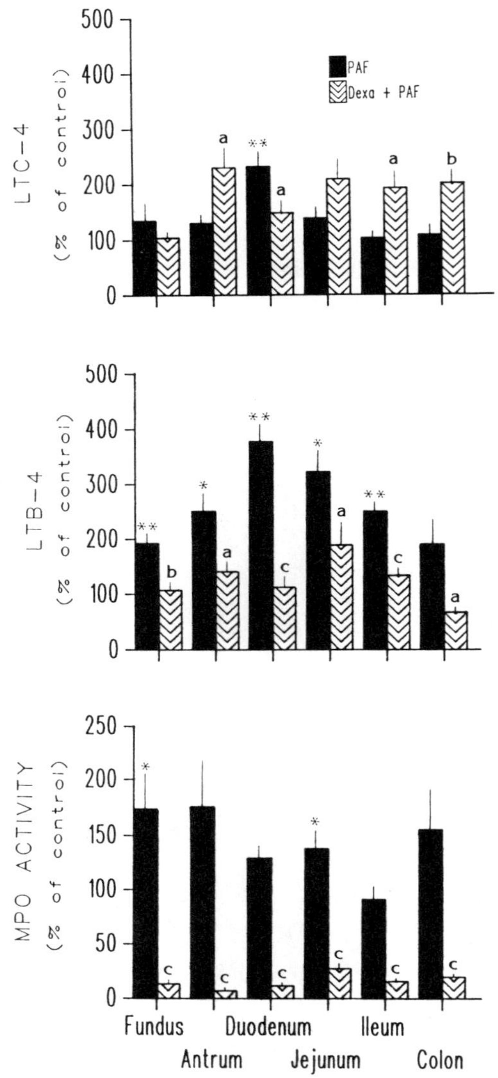

FIGURE 8. Effects of a 10-min i.v. infusion of PAF on gastric LTB_4 synthesis, LTC_4 synthesis, and myeloperoxidase (MPO) activity. Data are presented as a percent of control studies in which saline was infused i.v. in place of PAF. Also shown is the effect of pretreatment with dexamethasone (Dexa; 4 mg/kg at -6 and -30 h) on the response to PAF. $^{*}p$ <0.05, $^{**}p$ <0.01 compared to controls. $^{(a)}p$ <0.05, $^{(b)}p$ <0.01, $^{(c)}p$ <0.001 compared to the PAF group.

D. EFFECTS ON VASCULAR PERMEABILITY

Administration of PAF to laboratory animals has been shown to cause and increase in vascular permeability[21,48-50] and marked systemic hemoconcentration.[32,51-53] The increase in vascular permeability appears to be due to direct effects of PAF on the endothelium, although in some species such effects may be mediated through neutrophils and/or platelets.[53] Such effects of PAF do not appear to be confined solely to laboratory animals. Guinot et al.[54] recently noted a wheal and flare reaction in man following intradermal injections of PAF. These effects could be blocked by pretreatment with a specific PAF antagonist. Increased vascular permeability has also been observed in the gastrointestinal tract following intravenous infusions of PAF.[55-57] PAF caused marked leakage of labeled albumin into the lumen of the stomach and small intestine, but not the distal colon. Furthermore, a significant increase in interstitial levels of plasma protein in samples of stomach and small intestine was observed in these studies. Using a similar technique, Guarner et al.[58] noted the appearance of plasma proteins in the peritoneal cavity of rats following PAF infusion. Interestingly, the volume of peritoneal fluid (ascites) accounted for approximately 80% of the total loss of plasma from the intravascular space.

Increased vascular permeability could contribute to PAF-induced gastrointestinal damage in two ways: (1) accumulation of plasma in the lamina propria could result in stretching of the epithelium, which could eventually lead to rupture and (2) the loss of plasma from the intravascular space gives rise to hemoconcentration. As the hematocrit increases, the rheological properties of blood changes such that blood flow is markedly reduced, especially through the postcapillary venules. Thus, the increased vascular permeability could result in decreased gastrointestinal blood flow. The resulting reduction in the supply of nutrients and oxygen to the epithelium would render it more susceptible to damage.

There is some experimental evidence suggesting that PAF-induced hemoconcentration is important in the mechanism of ulcerogenesis, although it is clearly not the only important factor. For instance, reduction of PAF-induced gastric damage by pretreatment with BW755c was also accompanied by a significant reduction of PAF-induced hemoconcentration.[32] Whether these two events are epiphenomena is unclear. We recently demonstrated that PAF-induced hemoconcentration could be significantly reduced by pretreatment with dexamethasone.[39] This drug had no effect on the severity of PAF-induced gastric damage, but did significantly reduce the damage induced by PAF in the small intestine. Thus, it would appear that hemoconcentration is not an important factor in the production of damage in the stomach, but may be important in the mechanism of action of PAF in the small bowel.

E. EFFECTS ON MOTILITY

The ability of PAF to induce contraction of gastrointestinal smooth muscle has been demonstrated in several species of laboratory animals.[59-61] These studies all suggested that there were specific binding sites for PAF on gastrointestinal smooth muscle. Bardon and Deragnaucourt[62] demonstrated that intraperitoneal injection of PAF markedly altered the interdigestive motility pattern in rats and postulated that there was a "possible role for PAF in the digestive motor function changes observed during gastrointestinal or general inflammatory and allergic states".

Mersereau and Hinchey[63-65] demonstrated that hypercontractility of the stomach was a feature of a number of animal models of gastric ulceration. For instance, exposure to cold-restraint stress resulted in gastric hypercontractility (frequent, high amplitude contractions), which could be blocked by vagotomy. They postulated that the contraction of the stomach gave rise to regions along the base of rugal folds which, because of compression, had reduced mucosal blood flow. These regions were also the regions where necrosis was most often observed.

Esplugues and Whittle[66,67] recently tested the hypothesis that PAF might also stimulate hypercontractility of the stomach. They found that local intraarterial infusion of PAF led to a significant increase in intragastric pressure. Upon cessation of the PAF infusion, a further increase in intragastric pressure was observed. The changes in intragastric pressure induced by PAF were not affected by pretreatment with atropine, dexamethasone, BW755c, indomethacin, or the thromboxane synthetase inhibitor, benzylimidazole;[66] however, pretreatment with cimetidine or tetrodotoxin did appear to reduce PAF-induced changes in gastric motility, suggesting a role for histamine and the enteric nervous system in the mediation of these actions of PAF.[67] Whether these effects on gastric motility are important in the production of damage by PAF has not yet been determined.

Another interesting, albeit anecdotal, observation supporting a role for motility in the pathogenesis of PAF-induced gastrointestinal damage was the observation of Tokumura et al.[61] that PAF produced a completely different profile of motility effects in the colon than it did in the duodenum, jejunum, or ileum. This is interesting in light of the observation that PAF infusion resulted in severe damage to the duodenum, jejunum, and ileum, but not the colon.[28]

F. RELEASE OF OTHER MEDIATORS

The gastric damage observed following an intravenous infusion of PAF may be a consequence of the release of other pro-ulcerogenic substances. Since PAF-induced gastric damage was characterized by mucosal vasocongestion, Rosam et al.[23] tested the hypothesis that such damage might be caused by other vasoactive mediators, in particular histamine and norepinephrine. They found that pretreatment with the histamine antagonists mepyramine (H_1) and cimetidine (H_2), or the α-adrenergic antagonist, phentolamine, did not significantly alter the susceptibility of the rat stomach to damage induced by PAF. Several eicosanoids have been implicated as mediators of gastrointestinal damage and their synthesis has been shown to be increased following administration of PAF. For instance, TXA_2 is a potent stimulator of platelet aggregation and a vasoconstrictor which has been shown to increase gastric damage induced by such agents as bile salts[46] (see Chapter 6). Furthermore, inhibition of thromboxane synthesis has been shown to reduce gastric damage induced by agents such as ethanol.[68] Whether TXA_2 acts as a mediator of PAF-induced gastrointestinal damage in species other than the rat is not known; however, we demonstrated that pretreatment with the cyclooxygenase inhibitors acetylsalicylic acid or indomethacin, or the thromboxane synthetase inhibitor 1-benzylimidazole (BZI), did not significantly effect PAF-induced gastric damage or systemic hypotension in the rat.[32]

There is ample evidence supporting a role for leukotrienes as intermediates of some of the actions of PAF. As reviewed in Chapter 7, leukotrienes have been implicated in the pathogenesis of ethanol-induced gastric damage, as well as in inflammatory bowel disease. Leukotrienes are potent chemotactic and chemokinetic substances, some of which also increase vascular permeability.[69-71] Whittle et al.[47] demonstrated that leukotriene C_4 (LTC_4) had potent vasoconstrictor actions in the rat submucosa and suggested that such actions were consistent with a role for this substance in the production of gastric damage. Peskar et al.[72] demonstrated that following oral administration of ethanol to rats, gastric LTC_4 synthesis was markedly increased. Furthermore, pretreatment with the 5-lipoxygenase inhibitor nordihydroguauretic acid (NDGA) prevented the increase in LTC_4 synthesis and gastric damage induced by ethanol. Wallace and Whittle[32] had previously demonstrated that the dual cyclooxygenase/5-lipoxygenase inhibitor, BW755c, could dose-dependently reduce the extent of gastric damage induced by ethanol or indomethacin in the rat.

There is also reason to believe that PAF infusion would lead to enhanced synthesis of leukotrienes by the gastrointestinal tract. Various groups have demonstrated that PAF activates the 5-lipoxygenase pathway in neutrophils[73-77] (a primary source of LTB_4[45]). In a study using rats, PAF-induced gastric damage and hemoconcentration was shown to be significantly reduced by the dual cyclooxygenase/5-lipoxygenase inhibitor BW755c.[32] Furthermore, Young et al.[78] demonstrated that PAF-induced mortality in mice could be significantly reduced by several inhibitors of 5-lipoxygenase, while Myers et al.,[79] using a similar model, showed that glucocorticoids protected against PAF-induced mortality. Glucocorticoids are believed to inhibit leukotriene (and prostaglandin) synthesis by inhibiting phospholipase A_2.[80]

Recently, Hsueh et al.[81] demonstrated that administration of PAF into the superior mesenteric artery *in vitro* resulted in the appearance of a substance in the venous effluent of the intestine with biological activity similar to LTC_4. Furthermore, this LTC_4-like substance had the same retention time as authentic LTC_4 when the venous effluent was analyzed by high-performance liquid chromatography (HPLC). Pretreatment of the intestinal segment with a leukotriene receptor antagonist (FPL 55712) prevented the marked vasoconstriction they noted shortly after administering PAF.

To further examine the role of leukotrienes as mediators of PAF-induced damage, we examined the effects of pretreatment with dexamethasone on gastrointestinal leukotriene synthesis and the susceptibility of the gastrointestinal tract to PAF-induced damage.[39] Intravenous infusion of PAF to rats produced significant increases in LTB_4 synthesis in all regions of the stomach and small intestine examined (see Figure 8). LTC_4 synthesis was significantly elevated in the stomach and duodenum. Thus, these results from an *in vivo* study confirm the previous *in vitro* results of Hsueh et al.[81] Pretreatment with dexamethasone 30 and 6 h prior to the infusion of PAF resulted in significant inhibition of LTB_4 synthesis in all regions studied, while only significantly reducing LTC_4 synthesis in the duodenum. This pretreatment with dexamethasone did not significantly alter the susceptibility of the stomach to damage induced by PAF, but did significantly reduce PAF-induced damage in the small intestine and PAF-induced hemoconcentration. These results, therefore, suggest that PAF-induced damage in the stomach and small intestine may occur through different mechanisms. The data also suggest that leukotrienes may play a role in mediating the effects of PAF on vascular permeability. Such a conclusion was also reached when reduction of gastric leukotriene synthesis was produced by feeding rats a diet in which the sole source of lipid was cod liver oil.[82] Fish oils are rich in the precursors of eicosapentaenoic acid (EPA), which like arachidonic acid, is a precursor of prostaglandins and leukotrienes; however, the biological activity of the prostaglandins and leukotrienes derived from EPA differs markedly from that of the eicosanoids derived from arachidonic acid. Gastric LTB_4 synthesis in the group of rats fed the cod liver oil was approximately 50% lower than in control rats which received sunflower oil as their dietary source of lipid. Despite the reduced gastric LTB_4 synthesis, susceptibility to damage induced by intravenously administered PAF did not change; however, as with the dexamethasone treatment, PAF-induced hemoconcentration was significantly reduced in rats fed the diet supplemented with cod liver oil.

G. SUMMARY

The possible mechanisms of action of PAF in the gastrointestinal tract are numerous, and there are likely additional ones to those listed above. Based on data presently available, it is impossible to say which, if any, of the proposed mechanisms is the most important. It is likely that several actions of PAF act in concert to produce hemorrhage and necrosis in the gastrointestinal tract. Figure 9 summarizes some of the cellular sites of action of PAF, and the consequences in the gastrointestinal mucosa that these actions would produce. As shown in the figure, a common event of several of these proposed sites of action is a reduction of mucosal blood flow. Such an effect would result in a reduced supply of oxygen and nutrients to the cells of the mucosa, and thereby predispose them to damage induced by a luminal irritant or a blood-borne agent. In the cases of the stomach and duodenum, reduced mucosal blood flow would also reduce the ability of the mucosa to buffer intraluminal acid. The resistance of gastric epithelial cells to damage by acid is very much dependent on the flow of blood rich in bicarbonate ("the alkaline tide").

The assumption that PAF produces damage to the various regions of the gastrointestinal tract through a common mechanism may not be valid. As discussed above, there is some evidence that PAF-induced damage to the small intestine can be prevented by agents which do not affect PAF-induced damage in the stomach. It is difficult, however, to determine if such differences are related to different mechanisms of action, or are purely a consequence or regional variations in the susceptibility to damage.

Another complicating factor in considering the mechanism of action of PAF is the interspe-

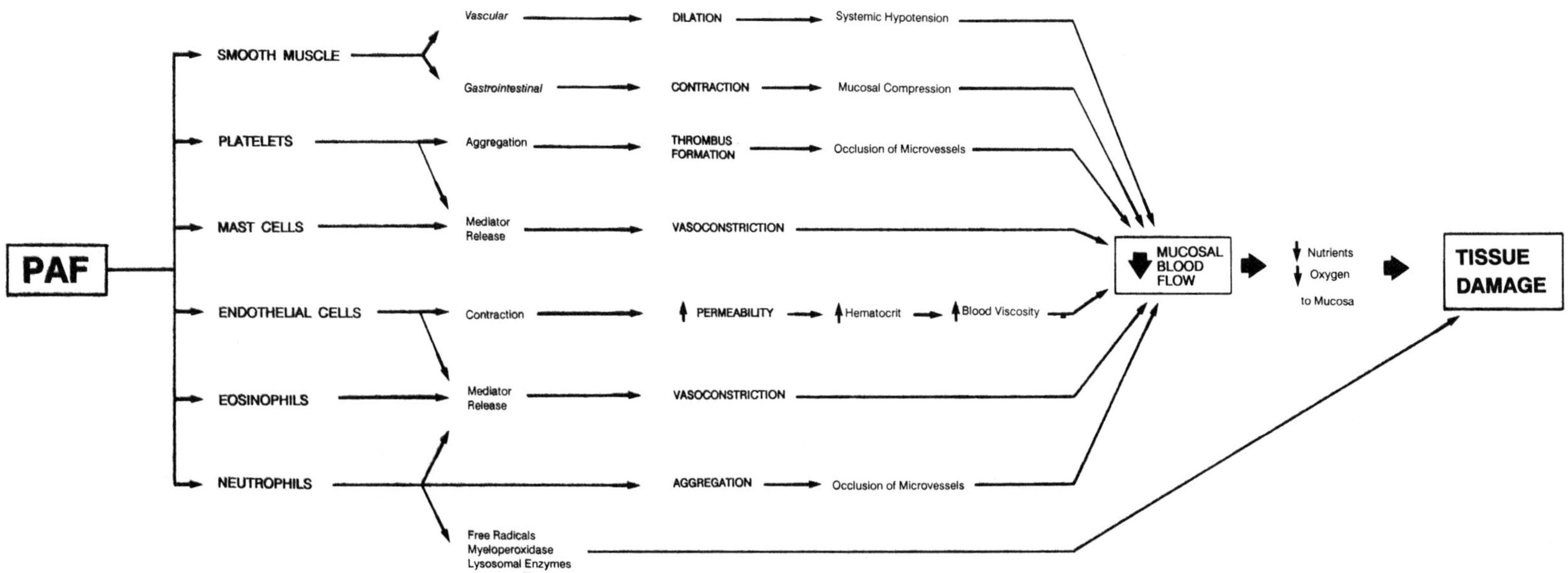

FIGURE 9. Schematic diagram summarizing some of the possible mechanisms involved in PAF-induced hemorrhage and necrosis in the gastrointestinal tract. Note that through several actions, PAF could cause a reduction in mucosal blood flow. The resulting decrease in the supply of oxygen and nutrients to the mucosa may increase its susceptibility to damage by luminal agents, or directly cause cell necrosis. Undoubtedly, several other factors than are shown on this figure play important roles in the mechanism of action of PAF.

cies variation. As discussed earlier in this chapter, there is considerable variation between species in terms of the sensitivity of platelets to PAF. Furthermore, there is also variation between species in terms of sensitivity to the actions of other mediators, the release of which is triggered by PAF. For instance, PAF-induced mortality in rabbits has been shown to be related to thromboxane release,[83] whereas PAF-induced mortality in mice is unaffected by inhibition of thromboxane synthesis.[78,79]

IV. ROLE OF PAF IN MEDIATING GASTROINTESTINAL DAMAGE AND INFLAMMATION

A. GASTROINTESTINAL NECROSIS AND HEMORRHAGE IN SEPTIC SHOCK

Septic shock is a major risk factor for gastrointestinal hemorrhage.[84] It is usually encountered following gastrointestinal or urogenital tract surgery[85] and is characterized by such symptoms as systemic hypotension, stimulation of blood clotting cascades, and increased vascular permeability. Mortality associated with septic shock ranges from 10 to 70%.[86,87] Despite extensive research into the pathogenesis of septic shock, the mechanism through which these effects are mediated is poorly understood. Laboratory studies on septic shock have utilized animal models in which bacterial endotoxins are injected intravenously (endotoxic shock). Using such models, several chemical mediators have been shown to play a role in producing the symptoms of endotoxic shock. In recent years, substantial evidence has accumulated supporting a role for PAF in the mechanism of action of endotoxin. Studies on the role of PAF in endotoxic shock were first stimulated by the similarity between the effects of administration of endotoxin or PAF to laboratory animals.[88]

The evidence supporting a role for PAF as a mediator of the gastrointestinal damage associated with septic or endotoxic shock falls into three main categories:

1. PAF administration produces gastrointestinal damage and systemic effects similar to those seen in endotoxic shock.
2. Administration of endotoxin to laboratory animals results in the stimulation of PAF release.
3. The gastrointestinal and systemic effects of endotoxin administration can be abrogated by pretreatment with a receptor antagonist for PAF.

The effects of PAF administration have been described in detail earlier in this chapter. To reiterate, PAF produces hemorrhagic damage in the stomach and small intestine, but not the descending colon. A similar pattern of damage has been observed in a rat model of endotoxic shock.[56] The histological characteristics of gastrointestinal necrosis induced by PAF or endotoxin are indistinguishable.[55] Both agents also produce profound plasma protein leakage into the gastrointestinal tract, with a similar pattern of severity in terms of the tissues most affected.[55] As mentioned above, the systemic effects of PAF, including hypotension and hemoconcentration, are similar to those observed in endotoxic or septic shock.

Studies on the release of PAF following endotoxin administration are hampered by the technical difficulty of measuring PAF release *in vivo*. As mentioned above, the half-life of PAF in plasma is extremely short (<30 s[10]), so meaningful plasma concentrations of PAF are difficult to obtain. A similar difficulty in the measurement of unstable eicosanoids, such as TXA_2, is overcome by measuring plasma levels of the stable catabolite, TXB_2. Measurement of a catabolite of PAF as an index of PAF biosynthesis is complicated by the fact that the breakdown product of PAF (lyso-PAF) is also the precursor for PAF. Measurement of PAF biosynthesis is also complicated by the absence of simple assay procedures, such as radioimmunoassay. Hence, assays of PAF rely primarily upon its physiochemical[89] or biological[90-96] properties, or a combination of the two.

Despite the above-mentioned difficulties, a few groups have been able to detect PAF in blood and have studied the effects of endotoxin administration on PAF biosynthesis. Doebber et al.[90] reported that PAF was not detectable in samples of rat blood under basal conditions. Furthermore, PAF was not detectable in blood 1.5 min after intravenous administration of endotoxin; however, in samples of blood collected 10 min after endotoxin administration, PAF was present in concentrations of up to 4.7 n*M*. Doebber et al.[90] calculated that such plasma levels of PAF could be achieved by intravenous administration of 300 pmol/kg body weight. Interestingly, Rosam et al.[23] used doses in that range in their study demonstrating the ulcerogenic properties of PAF in the stomach.

Release of PAF from gastrointestinal tissues has also been demonstrated following endotoxin administration to rats. By studying the release of PAF *in vitro* from tissue samples, the problems associated with the rapid catabolism of PAF by plasma acetyl hydrolase are avoided. Lagente et al.[97] and Whittle et al.[91] demonstrated that release of PAF from samples of jejunum taken from endotoxin-treated rats were up to 17-fold higher than that from control samples (see Figure 10).

As yet, there are no published reports of increased PAF synthesis in patients with septic shock. It is interesting, however, that Gram-negative sepsis is accompanied by highly significant increases in the circulating plasma levels of phospholipase A_2 and lyso-phosphatidylcholines.[98]

With the development of specific receptor antagonists, the role of PAF in endotoxic shock has been more clearly elucidated. Terashita et al.[99] demonstrated that the structural analog of PAF, CV-3988, significantly reduced the early hypotensive effects of administration of endotoxin to rats. Similar findings were reported by Doebber et al.[90] using another antagonist, kadsurenone. A PAF-antagonist derived from the leaves of *Ginkgo biloba* (BN-52021) was shown to inhibit anaphylaxis in the guinea pig[100] and to reduce the hypotension and thrombocytopenia induced by endotoxin in the rat[101] and guinea pig.[102] Inhibition of endotoxin-induced gastrointestinal damage was first demonstrated by Wallace and Whittle[103] using CV-3988. We later demonstrated that the hypotension and gastrointestinal damage induced by endotoxin could also be inhibited by BN-52021 and Ro-193704, at doses shown to inhibit PAF-induced hypotension and gastrointestinal damage[55] (Figures 11 and 12). In addition to reducing the endotoxin-induced gastrointestinal necrosis and hemorrhage which was macroscopically visible, PAF antagonists also significantly reduced PAF- and endotoxin-induced plasma protein leakage into lumen of the stomach and gut,[55-57] as well as systemic hemoconcentration (Figure 13).

Unfortunately, there have yet to be any reports of specific inhibitors of PAF biosynthesis. Such agents would provide further information on the role of PAF in gastrointestinal damage associated with endotoxic or septic shock. It is known that corticosteroids can prevent endotoxic shock in several species of laboratory animals,[104] and for many years, corticosteroids were widely recommended for the treatment of septic shock in man[87,105] (their use is now somewhat controversial). Whether the beneficial effects of corticosteroids in animal models of endotoxic shock are related to the reported ability of these agents to inhibit PAF biosynthesis[5,94,95] is not yet clear.

It is interesting that prostaglandins can reduce the gastrointestinal damage and some of the systemic effects of endotoxin,[56,106,107] but do not appear to block such effects induced by intravenous administration of PAF.[108] It is possible that the protective actions of prostaglandins in endotoxic shock are related to inhibition of PAF release. Indeed, Camussi et al.[6] demonstrated that prostacyclin (PGI_2) significantly reduced PAF release from neutrophils *in vitro*.

Two excellent reviews on PAF antagonists and the role of platelet-activating factor in shock have recently been published.[109,110]

B. ACUTE GASTRIC DAMAGE BY ETHANOL AND ASPIRIN

Since PAF is a potent ulcerogenic agent in the stomach which can be released under certain circumstances, it is possible that it might play a role in the production of gastric hemorrhage and necrosis following oral administration of such agents as ethanol and aspirin. This hypothesis has

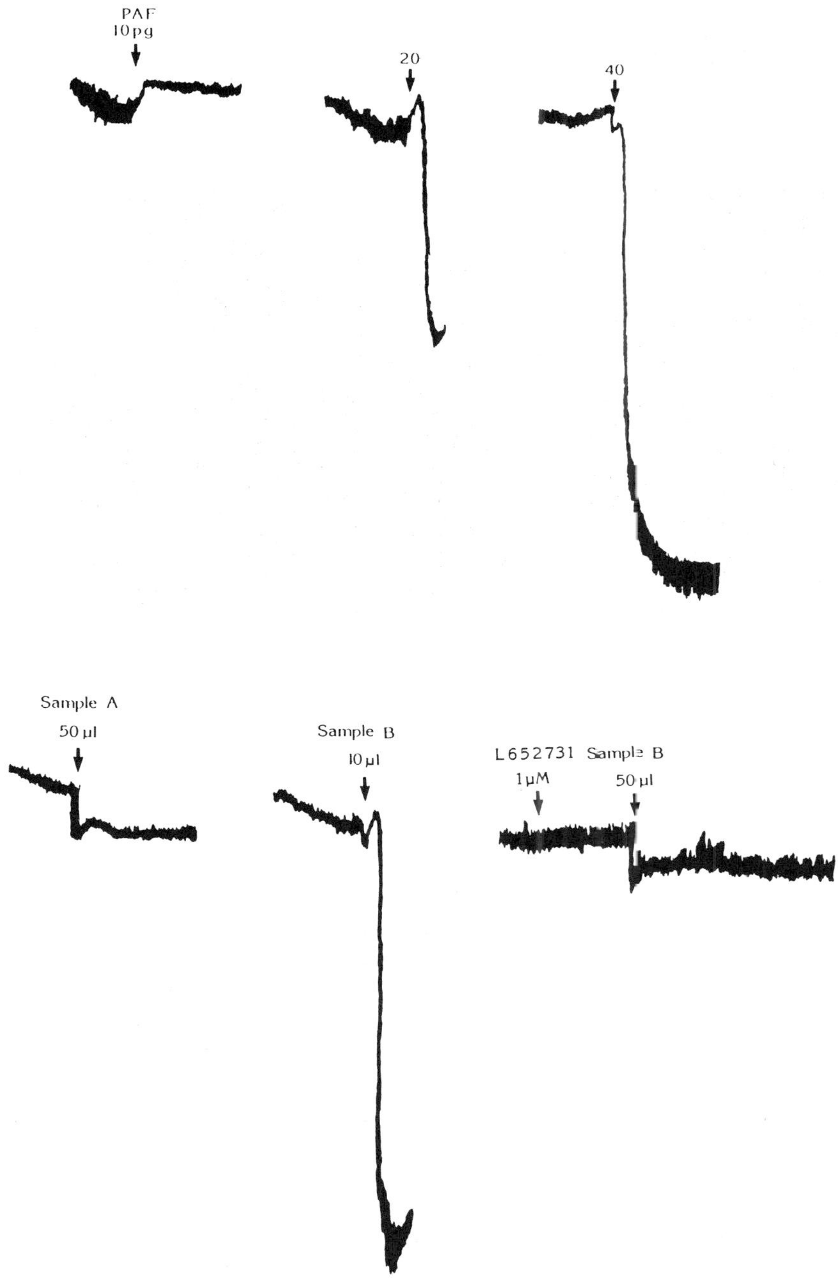

FIGURE 10. Representative traces from a platelet aggregometer. PAF-like activity in tissue incubates was measured using a bioassay based on the ability of PAF to stimulate aggregation of washed[125] rabbit platelets. A downward deflection of the pen is indicative of platelet aggregation. (Top) By testing graded quantities of authentic PAF, a standard curve of % aggregation vs. concentration of PAF could be constructed. (Bottom) Samples of jejunal tissue were excised from a rat following administration of endotoxin or vehicle (control). Following incubation in an appropriate medium, extraction, and purification by thin-layer chromatography, the samples were tested for PAF-like activity. Sample A is from a control rat. Sample B is from an endotoxin-treated rat. Note that the aggregation induced by Sample B could be blocked by pretreating the platelets with L652731, a specific PAF antagonist. See Whittle et al.[91] for further details of these experiments.

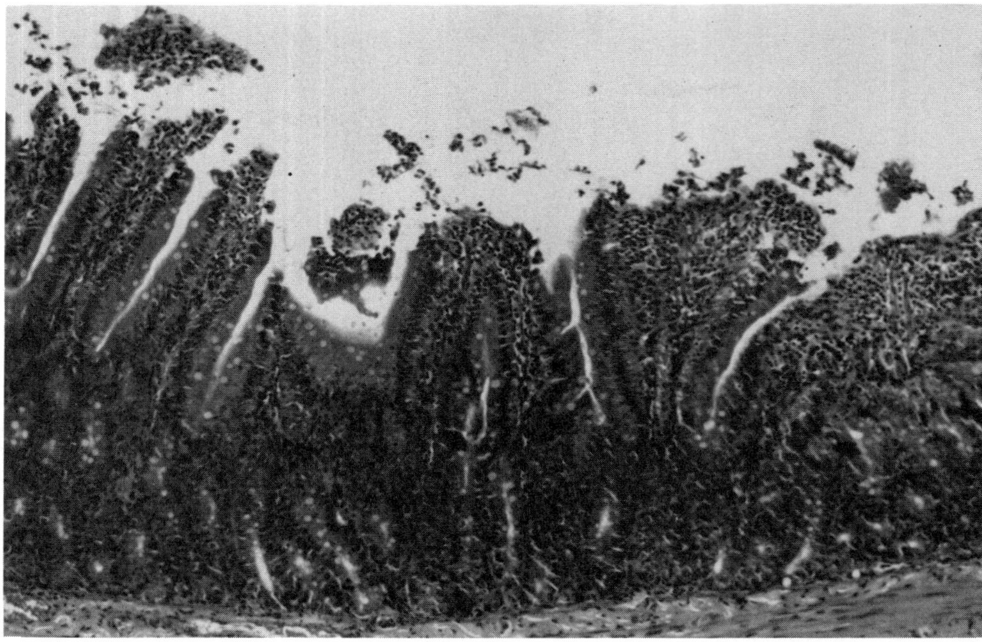

FIGURE 11. Light micrographs of sections of rat duodenum. (A) Rat treated with *E. coli* endotoxin (25 mg/kg). Note extensive necrosis of the mucosa with cellular debris present in the lumen. (H & E. Original magnification× 110.) (B) Rat treated with BN-52021 (20 mg/kg) 5 min prior to receiving endotoxin (as in A). Villus structure is intact. Some subepithelial edema is evident at the villus tip (arrow). (H & E. Original magnification ×110.)

been tested by assessing the effects of pretreatment with specific PAF antagonists on the development of gastric damage following administration of these agents. Pretreatment with BN-52021 or Ro-193704 at doses shown to block PAF-induced gastric damage did not significantly alter the susceptibility of the gastric mucosa to damage induced by oral administration of absolute ethanol[55] (see Figure 14); however, pretreatment with CV-3988 did cause a significant reduction in ethanol-induced damage. This effect was thought to be due to an action of this compound unrelated to antagonism of PAF receptors, since the other two PAF antagonists did not exhibit a similar action. Rainsford[111] demonstrated that another PAF antagonist, kadsurenone, failed to significantly alter the susceptibility of the gastric mucosa to damage induced by oral administration of acidified 50% ethanol or aspirin (200 mg/kg). The results of these two studies therefore suggest that PAF does not play an important role in the production of gastric damage by ethanol or aspirin.

C. INFLAMMATORY BOWEL DISEASE

Inflammatory bowel disease is a term which is used to describe two distinct diseases, Crohn's disease and ulcerative colitis. Both diseases have unknown etiology and are characterized by chronic inflammation and ulceration in the gastrointestinal tract. Because PAF is a potent ulcerogenic agent as well as having several pro-inflammatory actions, it has been implicated as a mediator in inflammatory bowel disease. Wengrower et al.[112] recently reported that samples of colon from a control population of patients released little or no PAF when incubated *in vitro;* however, when biopsies from patients with active ulcerative colitis were used, significant PAF release was detected. Furthermore, Wengrower et al. demonstrated that *in vitro* incubation of the tissue samples with corticosteroids or sulfasalazine (the drugs-of-choice in inflammatory bowel disease), PAF release could be dose-dependently inhibited. Thus, these authors suggested that

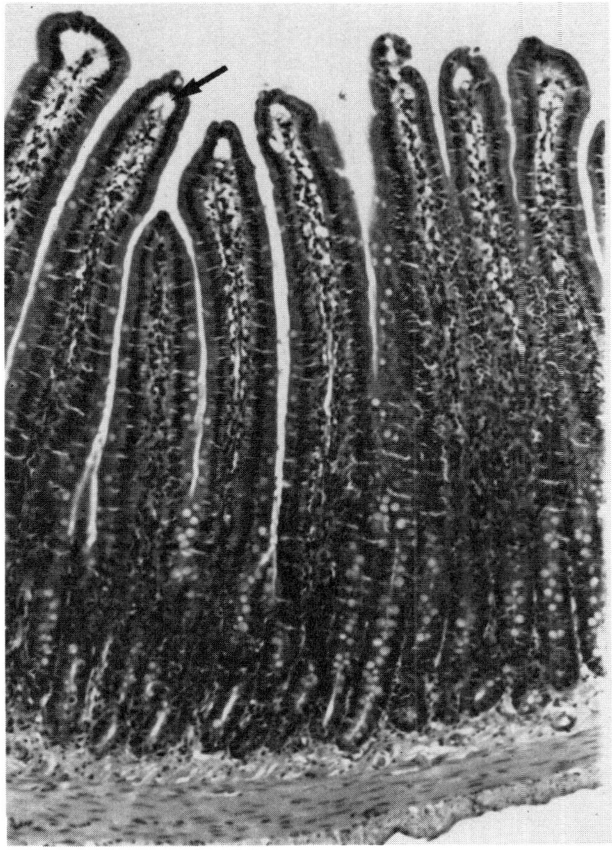

FIGURE 11B.

inhibition of PAF synthesis could be an important mechanism of action of two of the major drugs used in the treatment of inflammatory bowel disease.

Using a recently described animal model for chronic colitis,[113] we demonstrated that PAF biosynthesis was significantly elevated in samples of inflamed colon.[114] Interestingly, PAF biosynthesis was increased during the chronic, but not the acute phase of the inflammation in this model (Figure 15). A role for PAF in chronic colitis was further supported by the demonstration that oral treatment with a PAF antagonist (BN-52021) significantly reduced the colonic inflammation and ulceration in this animal model.[114]

D. CIRRHOSIS AND ASCITES FORMATION

A number of recent studies have implicated PAF as an important mediator of some of the circulatory disturbances, such as peripheral vasodilation and hypotension,[115] associated with cirrhosis of the liver. For instance, Villamediana et al.[116] demonstrated that infusion of PAF to rats produced similar cardiovascular effects as were observed in a rat model of cirrhosis, and that cirrhotic rats had significantly elevated plasma levels of PAF when compared to controls. Caramelo et al.[117] demonstrated that PAF levels in the blood of cirrhotic patients were significantly elevated above those of controls. As discussed above, PAF has been suggested to play an important role as a mediator of the hypotension, hemoconcentration, and gastrointestinal damage associated with endotoxic shock. This is relevant to a role for PAF in cirrhosis and ascites formation, since there is a very high incidence of bacterial infection associated with

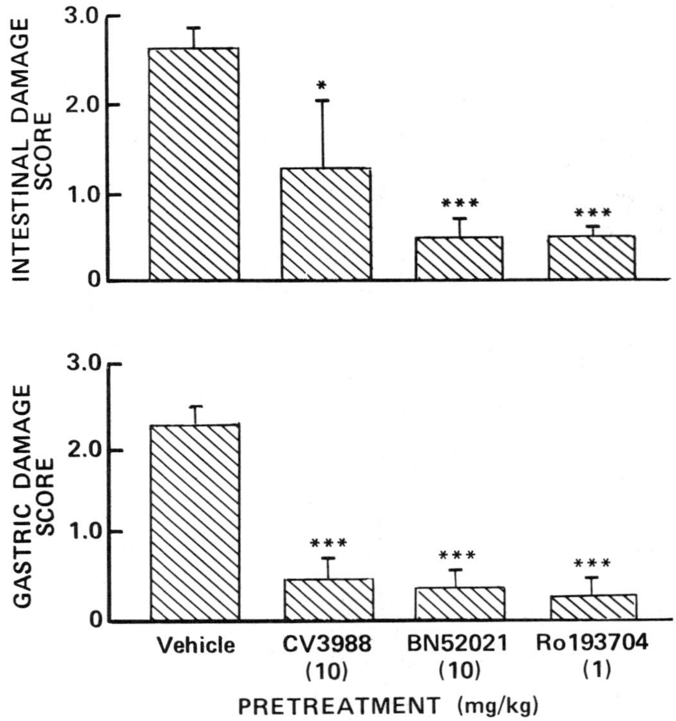

FIGURE 12. Histological scores of damage in the small intestine (top) and in stomach (bottom) induced by intravenous administration of endotoxin from *E. coli*. Rats were pretreated with a PAF-antagonist or the vehicle. Damage was scored on a 0 (normal) to 3 (severe) scale by an observer unaware of the treatment. $^{*}p<0.05$, $^{**}p<0.01$, $^{***}p<0.001$ compared to the vehicle-treated group.

cirrhosis.[118] Interestingly, Caramelo et al.[117] noted the highest plasma levels of PAF in those patients who had ascites and bacterial infection. Since marked changes in vascular permeability, leading to hemoconcentration, have been observed following administration of endotoxin or PAF to rats, it is possible that PAF may play a role in the accumulation of fluid in the peritoneal cavity (ascites) in cirrhotic patients. This hypothesis is supported by the finding of Guarner et al.[58] that endotoxin administration to rats resulted in the accumulation of fluid in the peritoneum. Similar ascites formation could be induced by infusion of PAF. Furthermore, endotoxin-induced ascites formation could be significantly reduced by pretreatment with a specific PAF antagonist.

Very little is known about the actions of PAF on the liver. Specific binding sites for PAF have recently been identified on rat liver plasma membranes,[119] and synthesis of PAF by Kupffer cells has been demonstrated.[120] It is therefore possible that PAF-induced ascites formation is a result of a direct action of PAF on the liver, giving rise to increased plasma leakage from the hepatic microcirculation. Another possibly more feasible explanation is that the reduced capacity of the Kupffer cells to clear endotoxin in the cirrhotic liver, as well as the increased permeability of the gut[119] may lead to higher circulating levels of endotoxin. As shown by several groups, endotoxin can stimulate PAF release into the blood, and its production in several organs, including the liver and gastrointestinal tract.[58] The circulating levels of PAF might then be responsible for the ascites formation observed in cirrhosis. It is noteworthy that there is a high incidence of bleeding in the upper gastrointestinal tract of cirrhotic patients,[121] possibly another phenomenon mediated by endotoxin-induced PAF release.

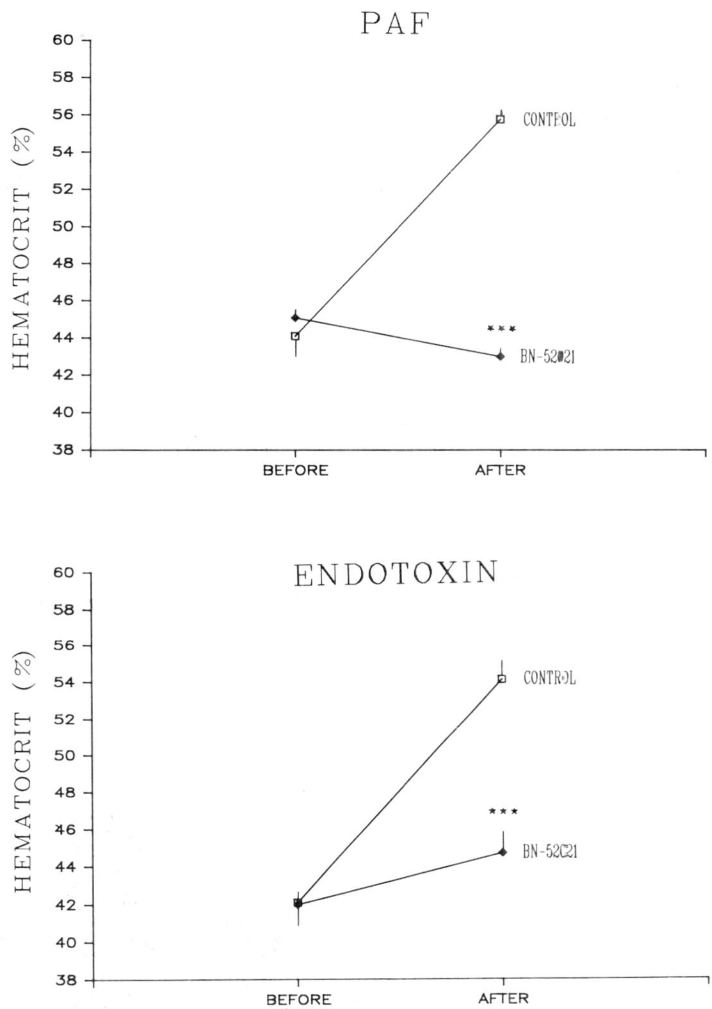

FIGURE 13. Effects of pretreatment with the PAF-antagonist BN-52021 (20 mg/kg i.v.) on hemoconcentration induced by intravenous PAF (top) or *S. typhosa* endotoxin (bottom). Lines connect the mean ± SEM hematocrit values for samples taken before and 20 min after administration of the PAF or endotoxin.

V. SUMMARY AND FUTURE PERSPECTIVES

Taking into account the potent pro-ulcerogenic actions of PAF and the evidence of its release and involvement in several animal models of gastrointestinal disease, it seems very likely that PAF is an important mediator of damage processes in the gastrointestinal tract. With the highly specific receptor antagonists for PAF now available, assessment of the role of PAF in several diseases in man are certainly a possibility. Improvements in assay procedures are required to make possible the meaningful and inexpensive determinations of plasma levels of PAF in patients with various maladies (including septic shock, inflammatory bowel disease, and cirrhosis). The development of specific inhibitors of PAF biosynthesis which are effective *in vivo* will further improve our ability to study the pathophysiological role of PAF.

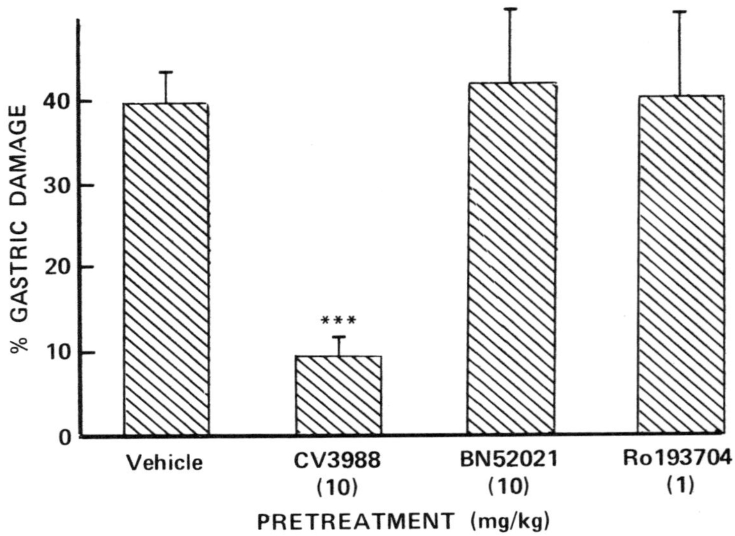

FIGURE 14. Effects of pretreatment with PAF antagonists on the extent of gastric damage induced by oral administration of absolute ethanol. Gastric damage was quantified planimetrically. Note that only CV3988 produced a significant (p <0.001) reduction of macroscopically visible ethanol-induced damage.

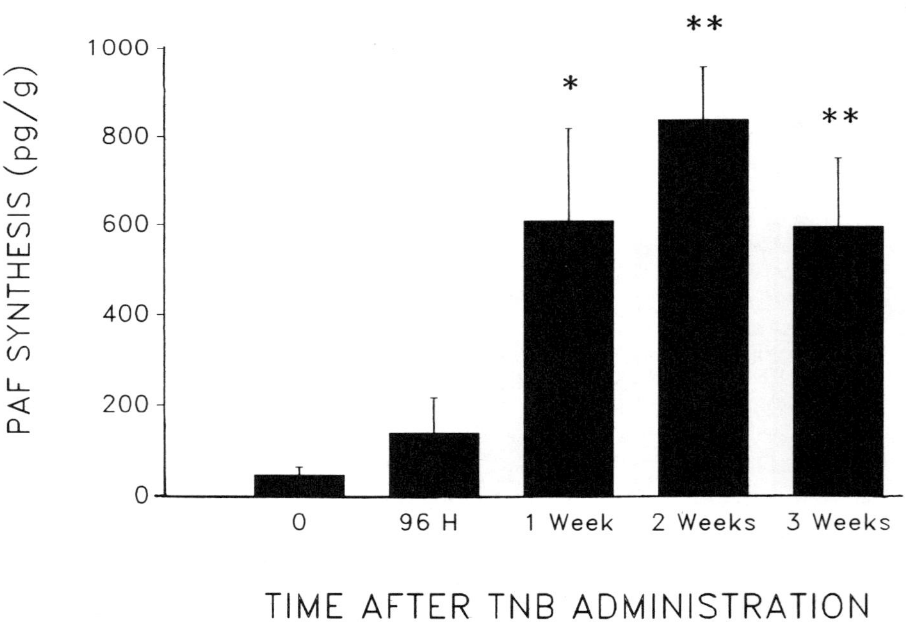

FIGURE 15. Release of platelet-activating factor by samples of inflamed colonic tissue taken 96 h to 3 weeks after induction of colitis by intracolonic administration of trinitrobenzene sulfonic acid (TNB). PAF release was significantly ($^{*}p$ <0.05, $^{**}p$ <0.01) higher than control (untreated) levels only during the chronic phase of the inflammation (PAF was not detectable 24 or 72 h after TNB administration). See Reference 114 for further details of these experiments.

As mentioned earlier in this chapter, the mechanism of action of PAF in the gastrointestinal tract is not yet clearly understood. There are several possible modes of action in addition to those reviewed in this chapter. For instance, PAF may stimulate the generation of free radicals, which have been shown to have potent damaging actions on various tissues (see Chapter 9). Indeed, a role for PAF in postischemic gastric injury, a model in which free radicals have been shown to play an important role, has recently been suggested.[122]

Another recent finding which will undoubtedly be further explored in the future is the action of PAF in the central nervous system. Cucala et al.[123] recently demonstrated that intracerebroventricular injections of PAF at doses devoid of systemic hypotensive effects caused inhibition of pentagastrin-stimulated gastric acid secretion.

Finally, the interaction between PAF and other inflammatory mediators is not well understood. It is conceivable that PAF and other inflammatory mediators, such as eicosanoids, act in concert to produce some effects and may also regulate the biosynthesis of one another. As reviewed earlier in this chapter, PAF can stimulate the 5-lipoxygenase pathway of arachidonic acid metabolism in some cell types. Little is known of the effects of pharmacological modulation of one pathway on the activity of another. Since eicosanoids and PAF arise from similar membrane phospholipids, a better understanding of the regulation of phospholipase A_2 activity, and the effects of dietary manipulation of membrane phospholipid pools on the synthesis of these substances is required.

REFERENCES

1. **Benveniste, J., Henson, P. M., and Cochrane, C. G.,** Leukocyte-dependent histamine release from rabbit platelets. The role for IgE, basophils and platelet-activating factor, *J. Exp. Med.*, 136, 1356, 1972.
2. **Demopoulos, C. A., Pinckard, R. N., and Hanahan, D. J.,** Platelet-activating factor. Evidence for 1-*O*-alkyl-2-acetyl-*sn*-glyceryl-3-phosphorylcholine as the active component (a new class of lipid chemical mediators), *J. Biol. Chem.*, 254, 9355, 1979.
3. **Lynch, J. M. and Henson, P. M.,** The intracellular retention of newly synthesized platelet-activating factor, *J. Immunol.*, 137, 2653, 1986.
4. **Chignard, M., LeCouedic, J.-P., Tence, M., Vargaftig, B. B., and Benveniste, J.,** The role of PAF in platelet aggregation, *Nature*, 279, 799, 1979.
5. **Mencia-Huerta, J. M. and Benveniste, J.,** Platelet-activating factor and macrophages. I. Evidence for the release from rat and mouse peritoneal macrophages and not from mastocytes, *Eur. J. Immunol.*, 9, 409, 1979.
6. **Camussi, G., Tetta, C., Segoloni, G., Deregibus, M. C., and Bussolino, F.,** Neutropenia induced by platelet-activating factor (PAF-acether) released from neutrophils: the inhibitory effect of prostacyclin (PGI_2), *Agents Actions*, 11, 550, 1981.
7. **Camussi, G., Tetta, C., and Bussolino, F.,** Inhibitory effect of prostacyclin (PGI_2) on neutropenia induced by intravenous injection of platelet-activating-factor (PAF) in the rabbit, *Prostaglandins*, 25, 343, 1983.
8. **Benveniste, J.,** PAF — a new mediator of anaphylaxis and immune complex deposition from rabbit and human basophils, *Nature*, 249, 581, 1974.
9. **Prescott, S. M., Zimmerman, G. A., and McIntyre, T. M.,** Human endothelial cells in culture produce platelet-activating factor (1-alkyl-2-acetyl-*sn*-glycero-3-phosphocholine) when stimulated with thrombin, *Proc. Natl. Acad. Sci. U.S.A.*, 81, 3534, 1984.
10. **McManus, L. M., Hanahan, D. J., Demopoulos, C. A., and Pinckard, R. N.,** Pathobiology of the intravenous infusion of acetyl glyceryl ether phosphorylcholine (AGEPC), a synthetic platelet-activating factor (PAF), in the rabbit, *J. Immunol.*, 124, 2919, 1980.
11. **Stafforini, D. M., Prescott, S. M., and McIntyre, T. M.,** Human plasma platelet-activating factor acetylhydrolase. Purification and properties, *J. Biol. Chem.*, 262, 4223, 1987.
12. **Stafforini, D. M., McIntyre, T. M., Carter, M. E., and Prescott, S. M.,** Human plasma platelet-activating factor acetylhydrolase. Association with lipoprotein particles and role in degradation of platelet-activating factor, *J. Biol. Chem.*, 262, 4215, 1987.
13. **Vargaftig, B. B., Chignard, M., Benveniste, J., Lefort, J., and Wal, F.,** Background and present studies of research on platelet-activating factor (PAF-acether), *Ann. N. Y. Acad. Sci.*, 3710, 119, 1981.

14. **Doebber, T. W., Wu, M. S., and Shen, T. Y.,** Platelet activating factor intravenous infusion in rats stimulates vascular lysosomal hydrolase secretion independent of blood neutrophils, *Biochem. Biophys. Res. Commun.*, 125, 980, 1984.
15. **Humphrey, D. M., Hanahan, D. J., and Pinckard, R. N.,** Induction of leukocytic infiltrates in rabbit skin by acetyl glyceryl ether phosphorylcholine, *Lab. Invest.*, 47, 227, 1982.
16. **Bessin, P., Bonnet, J., Thibaudeau, D., Agier, B., Beaudet, Y., and Gilet, F.,** Pathophysiology of shock states caused by PAF-acether in dogs and rats, in *Platelet-Activating Factor - INSERM Symposium No. 23*, Benveniste, J. and Arnoux, B., Eds., Elsevier, Amsterdam, 1983, 343.
17. **Issekutz, A. C. and Szpejda, M.,** Evidence that platelet activating factor may mediate some acute inflammatory responses, *Lab. Invest.*, 54, 275, 1986.
18. **Bourgain, R. H., Maes, L., Braquet, P., Andries, R., Touqui, L., and Braquet, M.,** The effect of 1-*O*-alkyl-2-acetyl-*sn*-glycero-3-phosphocholine (PAF-acether) on the arterial wall, *Prostaglandins*, 30, 185, 1985.
19. **Bjork, J. and Smedegard, G.,** Acute microvascular effects of PAF-acether, as studied by intravital microscopy, *Eur. J. Pharmacol.*, 96, 87, 1983.
20. **Shaw, J. O., Pinkard, R. N., Ferrigni, K. S., McManus, L. M. and Hanahan, D. J.,** Activation of human neutrophils with 1-*O*-hexadecyl/octadecyl-2-acetyl-*sn*-glyceryl-3-phosphorylcholine (platelet activating factor), *J. Immunol.*, 127, 1250, 1981.
21. **Bjork, J., Lindbom, L., Gerdin, B., Smedegard, G., Arfors, K., and Benveniste, J.,** Paf-acether (platelet-activating factor) increases microvascular permeability and affects endothelium-granulocyte interaction in microvascular beds, *Acta Physiol. Scand.*, 119, 305, 1983.
22. **Gonzalez-Crussi, F. and Hsueh, W.,** Experimental model of ischemic bowel necrosis. The role of platelet-activating factor and endotoxin, *Am. J. Pathol.*, 112, 127, 1983.
23. **Rosam, A.-C., Wallace, J. L., and Whittle, B. J. R.,** Potent ulcerogenic actions of platelet-activating factor on the stomach, *Nature*, 319, 54, 1986.
24. **Heymans, F., Michel, E., Borrel, M., Wichrowski, B., Godfroid, J., Convert, O., Coeffier, E., Tence, M., and Benveniste, J.,** New total synthesis and high resolution ^{1}H NMR spectrum of platelet-activating factor, its enantiomer and racemic mixtures, *Biochim. Biophys. Acta*, 666, 230, 1981.
25. **Braquet, P., Touqui, L., Shen, T. Y., and Vargaftig, B. B.,** Perspectives in platelet activating factor research, *Pharmacol. Rev.*, 39, 97, 1987.
26. **Inarrea, P., Gomez-Cambronero, J., Pascual, J., del Carmen Ponte, M., Hernando, L., and Sanchez-Crespo, M.,** Synthesis of PAF-acether and blood volume changes in gram-negative sepsis, *Immunopharmacology*, 9, 45, 1985.
27. **Wallace, J. L. and Whittle, B. J. R.,** Picomole doses of platelet-activating factor predispose the gastric mucosa to damage by topical irritants, *Prostaglandins*, 31, 989, 1986.
28. **Wallace, J. L. and Whittle, B. J. R.,** Profile of gastrointestinal damage induced by platelet-activating factor, *Prostaglandins*, 32, 137, 1986.
29. **Lees, I. W., Payne, A. N., Wallace, J. L., and Whittle, B. J. R.,** Cardiopulmonary and gastric effects of intravenous PAF in anaesthetized cats, *Br. J. Pharmacol.*, 89, 504P, 1986.
30. **Whittle, B. J. R., Kauffman, G. L., and Wallace, J. L.,** Gastric vascular and mucosal damaging actions of platelet activating factor in the canine stomach, in *Advances in Prostaglandin, Thromboxane, and Leukotriene Research*, Vol. 17A, Samuelsson, B., Paoletti, R., and Ramwell, P. W., Eds., Raven Press, New York, 1987, 285.
31. **Soybel, D. I., Ashley, S. W., and Cheung, L. Y.,** Effects of platelet-activating factor (PAF) on canine gastric mucosal blood flow and permeability to luminal acid, *Am. J. Surg.*, 155, 180, 1988.
32. **Wallace, J. L. and Whittle, B. J. R.,** Effects of inhibitors of arachidonic acid metabolism on PAF-induced gastric mucosal damage and haemoconcentration, *Br. J. Pharmacol.*, 89, 415, 1986.
33. **Mersereau, W. A. and Hinchey, E. J.,** Effects of gastric acidity on gastric ulceration induced by haemorrhage in the rat, utilizing a gastric chamber technique, *Gastroenterology*, 64, 1130, 1973.
34. **Itoh, M. and Guth, P. H.,** Role of oxygen-derived free radicals in hemorrhagic shock-induced gastric lesions in the rat, *Gastroenterology*, 88, 1162, 1985.
35. **Parks, D. A. and Granger, D. N.,** Role of hydrogen peroxide in ischemic injury to the small intestine, *Gastroenterology*, 84, 1207, 1984.
36. **Inarrea, P., Gomez-Cambronero, J., Nieto, M., and Crespo, M. S.,** Characteristics of the binding of platelet-activating factor to platelets of different animal species, *Eur. J. Pharmacol.*, 105, 309, 1984.
37. **Valone, F. H. and Goetzl, E. J.,** Specific binding by human polymorphonuclear leucocytes of the immunological mediator 1-*O*-hexadecyl/octadecyl-2-acetyl-*sn*-glycero-3-phosphorylcholine, *Immunology*, 48, 141, 1983.
38. **Whittle, B. J. R., Morishita, T., Ohya, Y., Leung, F. W., and Guth, P. H.,** Microvascular actions of platelet-activating factor on rat gastric mucosa and submucosa, *Am. J. Physiol.*, 251, G772, 1986.

39. **Wallace, J. L. and MacNaughton, W. K.,** Gastrointestinal damage induced by platelet-activating factor: role of leukotrienes, *Eur. J. Pharmacol.*, 151, 43, 1988.
40. **Bradley, P. P., Priebat, D. A., Christensen, R. D., and Rothstein, G.,** Measurement of cutaneous inflammation: estimation of neutrophil content with an enzyme marker, *J. Invest. Dermatol.*, 78, 206, 1982.
41. **Krawicz, J. E., Sharon, P., and Stenson, W. F.,** Assessment of inflammation in rat and hamster models, *Gastroenterology*, 87, 1344, 1984.
42. **Mullane, K. M., Kraemar, R., and Smith, B.,** Myeloperoxidase activity as a quantitative assessment of neutrophil infiltration into ischemic myocardium, *J. Pharmacol. Methods*, 14, 157, 1985.
43. **Wallace, J. L.,** Glucocorticoid-induced gastric mucosal damage: inhibition of leukotriene, but not prostaglandin biosynthesis, *Prostaglandins*, 34, 311, 1987.
44. **Higgs, G. A., Moncada, S., Salmon, J. A., and Seager, K.,** The source of thromboxane and prostaglandins in experimental inflammation, *Br. J. Pharmacol.*, 79, 863, 1983.
45. **Borgeat, P. and Samuelsson, B.,** Transformation of arachidonic acid by rabbit polymorphonuclear leukocytes, *J. Biol. Chem.*, 254, 2643, 1979.
46. **Whittle, B. J. R., Kauffman, G. L., and Moncada, S.,** Vasoconstriction with thromboxane A_2 induces ulceration of the gastric mucosa, *Nature*, 292, 472, 1981.
47. **Whittle, B. J. R., Oren-Wolman, N., and Guth, P. H.,** Gastric vasoconstrictor actions of leukotriene C_4, $PGF_{2\alpha}$, and thromboxane mimetic U-46619 on rat submucosal microcirculation *in vivo*, *Am. J. Physiol.*, 248, G580, 1985.
48. **Archer, C. B., Page, C. P., Paul, W., Morley, J., and McDonald, D. A.,** Inflammatory characteristics of platelet-activating factor (PAF-acether) in human skin, *Br. J. Dermatol.*, 110, 45, 1983.
49. **Morley, J., Page, C. P., and Paul, W.,** Inflammatory actions of platelet-activating factor (PAF-acether) in guinea-pig skin, *Br. J. Pharmacol.*, 80, 503, 1983.
50. **Paul, W. and Page, C. P.,** Cutaneous responses to synthetic platelet activating factor (PAF-acether) in the guinea pig, *Agents Actions*, 13, 455, 1983.
51. **Handley, D. A., Lee, M. L., and Saunders, R. N.,** Evidence for a direct effect on vascular permeability of platelet-activating factor induced hemoconcentration in the guinea pig, *Thromb. Haemostasis*. 54, 756, 1985.
52. **Handley, D. A., Van Valen, R. G., Melden, M. K., and Saunders, R. N.,** Evaluation of dose and route effects of platelet activating factor-induced extravasation in the guinea pig, *Thromb. Haemostasis*, 51, 2431, 1984.
53. **Handley, D. A., Arbeeny, C. M., Lee, M. L., Van Valen, R. G., and Saunders, R. N.,** Effects of platelet activating factor on endothelial permeability to plasma macromolecules, *Immunopharmacology*, 8, 137, 1984.
54. **Guinot, P., Braquet, P., Duchier, J., and Cournot, A.,** Inhibition of PAF-acether induced weal and flare reaction in man by a specific PAF antagonist, *Prostaglandins*, 32, 160, 1986.
55. **Wallace, J. L., Steel, G., Whittle, B. J. R., Lagente, V., and Vargaftig, B.,** Evidence supporting a role for platelet-activating factor (PAF) as a mediator of endotoxin-induced gastrointestinal damage in the rat. Effects of three PAF antagonists, *Gastroenterology*, 93, 765, 1987.
56. **Wallace, J. L., Steel, G., and Whittle, B. J. R.,** Gastrointestinal plasma leakage in endotoxic shock. Inhibition by prostaglandin E_2 and by a platelet-activating factor antagonist, *Can. J. Physiol. Pharmacol.*, 65, 1428, 1987.
57. **Wallace, J. L.,** PAF- and endotoxin-induced gastrointestinal ulceration: inhibitory effects of BN52021, *Methods Find. Exp. Clin. Pharmacol.*, in press.
58. **Guarner, F., MacNaughton, W. K., and Wallace, J. L.,** Induction of ascites formation by platelet-activating factor, *Proc. Taipei Conf. Prostaglandins*, in press.
59. **Hwang, S.-B., Lee, C. C., Cheak, M. J., and Shen, T. Y.,** Specific receptor sites for 1-*O*-alkyl-2-acetyl-*sn*-glycero-3-phosphocholine (platelet activating factor) on rabbit and guinea pig smooth muscle membranes, *Biochemistry*, 22, 4756, 1983.
60. **Findlay, S. R., Lichtenstein, L. M., Hanahan, D. J., and Pinckard, R. N.,** Contraction of guinea pig ileal smooth muscle by acetyl glyceryl ether phosphorylcholine, *Am. J. Physiol.*, 241 C130, 1981.
61. **Tokumura, A., Fukuzawa, K., and Tseukatani, H.,** Contractile effect of 1-*O*-hexadecyl-2-*O*-acetyl-*sn*-glycero-3-phosphocholine on strips of isolated rat intestine, *J. Pharm. Pharmacol.*, 36, 210, 1984.
62. **Bardon, T. and Deragnaucourt, J.,** Effects of platelet activating factor (PAF) on the digestive motility in the conscious rat, *Dig. Dis. Sci.*, 30, 758, 1985.
63. **Mersereau, W. A. and Hinchey, E. J.,** Hypothermia-induced gastric hypercontractility in the genesis of the restraint ulcer, *Can. J. Surg.*, 24, 622, 1981.
64. **Mersereau, W. A. and Hinchey, E. J.,** Synergism between acid and gastric contractile activity in the genesis of ulceration and hemorrhage in the phenylbutazone-treated rat, *Surgery*, 90, 516, 1981.
65. **Mersereau, W. A. and Hinchey, E. J.,** Role of gastric mucosal folds in formation of focal ulcers in the rat, *Surgery*, 91, 150, 1982.
66. **Esplugues, J. V. and Whittle, B. J. R.,** PAF and thromboxane mimetic stimulate rat gastric contractility after local arterial infusion, *Br. J. Pharmacol.*, 92, 620P.

67. **Esplugues, J. V. and Whittle, B. J. R.,** Mechanisms underlying PAF-induced rat gastric motility *in vivo*, *J. Physiol.*, 395, 115P, 1987.
68. **Whittle, B. J. R.,** Cellular mediators in gastric damage: actions of thromboxane A_2 and its inhibitors, in *Mechanisms of Mucosal Protection in the Upper Gastrointestinal Tract*, Allen, A., Flemstrom, G., Garner, A., Silen, W., and Turnberg, L. A., Eds., Raven Press, New York, 1984, 295.
69. **Ford-Hutchinson, A. W., Bray, M. A., Doig, M. V., Shipley, M. E., and Smith, J. H.,** Leukotriene B_4, a potent chemotactic and aggregating substance released from polymorphonuclear leukocytes, *Nature*, 266, 264, 1980.
70. **Dahlen, S. E., Bjork, J., Hedqvist, P., Arfors, K.-E., Hammarström, S., Lindgren, J. A., and Samuelsson, B.,** Leukotrienes promote plasma leakage and leukocyte adhesion in postcapillary venules: *in vivo* effects with relevance to the acute inflammatory response, *Proc. Natl. Acad. Sci. U.S.A.*, 78, 3887, 1981.
71. **Lewis, R. A. and Austen, K. F.,** The biologically active leukotrienes. Biosynthesis, functions, and pharmacology, *J. Clin. Invest.*, 73, 889, 1983.
72. **Peskar, B. M., Lange, K., and Peskar, B. A.,** Ethanol stimulates formation of leukotriene C_4 in rat gastric mucosa, *Prostaglandins*, 31, 283, 1986.
73. **Voelkel, N. F., Worthen, S., Reeves, J. T., Henson, P. M., and Murphy, R. C.,** Non-immunological production of leukotrienes induced by platelet-activating factor, *Science*, 281, 286, 1980.
74. **Chilton, F. H., O'Flaherty, J. T., Walsh, C. E., Thomas, M. J., Wykle, R. L., DeChatelet, L. R., and Waite, B. M.,** Stimulation of the lipoxygenase pathway in polymorphonuclear leukocytes by 1-*O*-alkyl-2-*O*-*sn*-glycero-3-phosphocholine, *J. Biol. Chem.*, 257, 5402, 1982.
75. **Smith, R. J. and Bowman, B. J.,** Stimulation of human neutrophil degranulation with 1-*O*-octadecyl-2-*O*-acetyl-*sn*-glyceryl-3-phosphorylcholine: modulation by inhibitors of arachidonic acid metabolism, *Biochem. Biophys. Res. Commun.*, 104, 1495, 1982.
76. **Lin, A. H., Morton, D. R., and Gorman, R. R.,** Acetyl glyceryl ether phosphorylcholine stimulates leukotriene B_4 synthesis in human polymorphonuclear leukocytes, *J. Clin. Invest.*, 70, 1058, 1982.
77. **Bonnet, J., Thibaudeau, D., and Bessin, P.,** Dependency of the paf-acether induced bronchospasm on the lipoxygenase pathway in the guinea-pig, *Prostaglandins*, 26, 457, 1983.
78. **Young, J. M., Maloney, P. J., Jubb, S. N., and Clark, J. S.,** Pharmacological investigation of the mechanisms of platelet-activating factor induced mortality in the mouse, *Prostaglandins*, 30, 545, 1985.
79. **Myers, A., Ramey, E., and Ramwell, P.,** Glucocorticoid protection against PAF-acether toxicity in mice, *Br. J. Pharmacol.*, 79, 595, 1983.
80. **Flower, R. J. and Blackwell, G. J.,** Anti-inflammatory steroids induce biosynthesis of a phospholipase A_2 inhibitor which prevents prostaglandin generation, *Nature*, 278, 456, 1979.
81. **Hsueh, W., Gonzalez-Crussi, F., and Arroyave, J. L.,** Release of leukotriene C_4 by isolated, perfused rat small intestine in response to platelet-activating factor, *J. Clin. Invest.*, 78, 108, 1986.
82. **Wallace, J. L., MacNaughton, W. K., Guarner, F., Rodriguez, R., and Malagelada, J. R.,** Role of leukotrienes as mediators of gastric damage and hemoconcentration induced by platelet-activating factor, *Gastroenterology*, in press.
83. **Lefer, A. M., Muller, H. F., and Smith, J. B.,** Pathophysiological mechanisms of sudden death induced by platelet activating factor, *Br. J. Pharmacol.*, 83, 125, 1984.
84. **Skillman, J. J., Gould, S. M., Chung, R. S. K., and Silen, W.,** The gastric mucosal barrier: clinical and experimental studies in critically ill and normal man, and in the rabbit, *Ann. Surg.*, 172, 564, 1970.
85. **Litton, A.,** Gram-negative septicaemia in surgical practice, *Br. J. Surg.*, 62, 773, 1975.
86. **McCabe, W. R.,** Endotoxin and bacteraemia due to gram-negative organisms, *N. Engl. J. Med.*, 283, 1342, 1970.
87. **Lundberg, D., Alestig, K., Haglund, U., and Hellman, A.,** Intensive care treatment in septic shock, *Scand. J. Infect. Dis.*, Suppl. 41, 187, 1983.
88. **Wallace, J. L.,** Platelet-activating factor: an endogenous mediator of gastrointestinal ulceration in endotoxic shock?, *Bull. Inst. Pasteur*, 85, 345, 1987.
89. **Murphy, R. C. and Clay, K. L.,** Measurement of platelet-activating factor by physiochemical techniques, *Am. Rev. Resp. Dis.*, 136, 207, 1987.
90. **Doebber, T. W., Wu, M. S., Robbins, J. C., Choy, B. M., Chang, M. N., and Shen, T. Y.,** Platelet activating factor (PAF) involvement in endotoxin-induced hypotension in rats. Studies with PAF-receptor antagonist kadsurenone, *Biochem. Biophys. Res. Commun.*, 127, 799, 1985.
91. **Whittle, B. J. R., Boughton-Smith, N. K., Esplugues, J. V., Hutcheson, I., and Wallace, J. L.,** Increased intestinal formation of platelet-activating factor following endotoxin-induced damage, *Br. J. Pharmacol.*, 92, 3, 1987.
92. **Chang, S., Feddersen, C. O., Henson, P. M., and Voelkel, N. F.,** Platelet-activating factor mediates hemodynamic changes and lung injury in endotoxin-treated rats, *J. Clin. Invest.*, 79, 1498, 1987.
93. **Parente, L., Fitzgerald, M., De Nucci, G., and Moncada, S.,** The release of lyso-PAF from guinea-pig lungs, *Eur. J. Pharmacol.*, 112, 281, 1985.

94. **Parente, L., Fitzgerald, M. F., Flower, R. J., and De Nucci, G.,** The effect of glucocorticoids on lyso-PAF formation *in vitro* and *in vivo*, *Agents Actions,* 17, 312, 1985.
95. **Parente, L. and Flower, R. J.,** Hydrocortisone and 'macrocortin' inhibit the zymosan-induced release of lyso-PAF from rat peritoneal leucocytes, *Life Sci.,* 36, 1225, 1985.
96. **Fitzgerald, M. F., Moncada, S., and Parente, L.,** The anaphylactic release of platelet-activating factor from perfused guinea-pig lungs, *Br. J. Pharmacol.,* 88, 149, 1986.
97. **Lagente, V., Lidbury, P., Steel, G., Vargaftig, B. B., Wallace, J. L., and Whittle, B. J. R.,** Role of PAF as a mediator of endotoxin-induced gastrointestinal damage, *Br. J. Pharmacol.,* 90, 114P, 1987.
98. **Vadas, P.,** Elevated plasma phospholipase A_2 levels: correlation with the hemodynamic and pulmonary changes in gram-negative septic shock, *J. Lab. Clin. Med.,* 104, 873, 1984
99. **Terashita, Z., Imura, Y., Nishikawa, K., and Sumida, S.,** Is platelet activating factor (PAF) a mediator of endotoxin shock?, *Eur. J. Pharmacol.,* 109, 257, 1985.
100. **Vilain, B., Lagente, V., Touvay, C., Desquand, S., Randon, J., Lefort, F., Braquet, B., and Vargaftig, B. B.,** Pharmacological control of the *in vivo* passive anaphylactic shock by the PAF-acether antagonist compound BN 52021, *Pharmacol. Res. Commun.,* 18 (Suppl.), 119, 1986.
101. **Etienne, A., Hecquet, F., Soulard, C., Spinnewyn, B., Clostre, F., and Braquet, P.,** *In vivo* inhibition of plasma protein leakage and salmonella enteritidis-induced mortality in the rat by a specific paf-acether antagonist: BN 52021, *Agents Actions,* 17, 368, 1985.
102. **Adnot, S., Lefort, J., Braquet, P., and Vargaftig, B. B.,** Interference of the PAF-acether antagonist BN 52021 with endotoxin-induced hypotension in the guinea-pig, *Prostaglandins,* 32, 791, 1986.
103. **Wallace, J. L. and Whittle, B. J. R.,** Prevention of endotoxin-induced gastrointestinal damage by CV-3988, an antagonist of platelet-activating factor, *Eur. J. Pharmacol.,* 124, 209, 1986.
104. **Nicholson, D. P.,** Glucocorticoids in the treatment of shock and the adult respiratory distress syndrome, *Clin. Chest Med.,* 3, 121, 1982.
105. **Shumer, W.,** Septic shock, *JAMA,* 242, 1906, 1979.
106. **Arvidsson, S., Falt, K., and Haglund, O.,** Gastric mucosal damage in sepsis — effects of pretreatment with a synthetic prostaglandin E_1 analogue, *Gut,* 26, 1025, 1985.
107. **Odonkor, P., Mowat, C., and Himal, H.,** Prevention of sepsis-induced gastric lesions in dogs by cimetidine via inhibition of gastric secretion and prostaglandin via cytoprotection, *Gastroenterology,* 80, 375, 1981.
108. **Steel, G., Wallace, J. L., and Whittle, B. J. R.,** Failure of prostaglandin E_2 and its 16,16-dimethyl analogue to prevent the gastric mucosal damage induced by PAF, *Br. J. Pharmacol.,* 90, 365, 1987.
109. **Saunders, R. N. and Handley, D. A.,** Platelet-activating factor antagonists, in *Annual Review of Pharmacology and Toxicology,* Vol. 27, George, R., Okun, R. and Cho, A. K. Eds., Annual Reviews, Palo Alto, CA, 1987, 237.
110. **Feuerstein, G. and Hallenbeck, J. M.,** Prostaglandins, leukotrienes, and platelet-activating factor in shock, in *Annual Review of Pharmacology and Toxicology,* Vol. 27, George, R., Okun, R., and Cho, A. K., Eds., Annual Reviews, Palo Alto, CA, 1987, 237.
111. **Rainsford, K. D.,** Relative roles of leukotrienes and platelet activating factor in experimentally-induced gastric ulceration, *Pharmacol. Res. Commun.,* 18, 209, 1986.
112. **Wengrower, D., Eliakim, R., Karmeli, F., Razin, E., and Rachmilewitz, D.,** Pathogenesis of ulcerative colitis (UC): enhanced colonic formation of inositol phosphates (IP) and platelet activating factor (PAF), *Gastroenterology,* 92, 1691, 1987.
113. **Morris, G. P., Beck, P. L., Herridge, M. S., Szewczuk, M., Depew, W., and Wallace, J. L.,** A hapten-induced model for chronic inflammation of the rat colon, *Gastroenterology,* 94, in press.
114. **Wallace, J. L.,** Release of platelet-activating factor (PAF) and accelerated healing induced by a PAF-antagonist in an animal model of chronic colitis, *Can. J. Physiol. Pharmacol.,* 66, 422, 1988.
115. **Mashford, M. L., Mahon, W. A., and Chalmors, T. C.,** Studies of the cardiovascular system in the hypotension of liver failure, *N. Engl. J. Med.,* 267, 1071, 1962.
116. **Villamediana, L. M., Sanz, E., Fernandez-Gallardo, S., Caramelo, C., Sanchez, M., Braquet, P., and Lopez-Novoa, J. M.,** Effects of the platelet-activating factor antagonist BN 52021 on the hemodynamics of rats with experimental cirrhosis of the liver, *Life Sci.,* 39, 201, 1986.
117. **Caramelo, C., Fernandez-Gallardo, S., Santos, J. C., Inarrea, P., Sanchez-Crespo, M., Lopez-Novoa, J. M., and Hernando, L.,** Increased levels of platelet-activating factor in blood from patients with cirrhosis of the liver, *Eur. J. Clin. Invest.,* 17, 7, 1987.
118. **Wyke, R. J.,** Problems of bacterial infection in patients with liver disease, *Gut,* 28, 623, 1987.
119. **Hwang, S.-B.,** Specific receptor sites for platelet-activating factor on rat liver plasma membranes, *Arch. Biochem. Biophys.,* 257, 339, 1987.
120. **Buxton, D. P., Hanahan, D. J., and Olson, M. L.,** Stimulation of glycogenolysis and platelet-activating factor production by heat aggregated immunoglobulin perfused liver, *J. Biol. Chem.,* 259, 13758, 1984.
121. **Teres, J., Bordas, J. M., Bru, C., Diaz, F., Bruguera, M., and Rodes, J.,** Upper gastrointestinal bleeding in cirrhosis: clinical and endoscopic correlations, *Gut,* 17, 37, 1976.

122. **Droy-Lefaix, M. T., Braquet, P., and Drouet, Y.,** Involvement of platelet-activating factor (PAF-acether) in post ischemic gastric lesions in the rat, *Gastroenterology,* 92, 1375, 1987.
123. **Cucala, M., Wallace, J. L., Guarner, F., Rodriguez, R., Salas, A., and Malagelada, J. R.,** Central regulation of gastric acid secretion by platelet activating factor (PAF), *Gastroenterology,* 94, A81, 1988.
124. **Swendsen, C. L., Ellio, J. M., Chilton, F. H., O'Flaherty, J. T., and Wykle, R. L.,** 1-*O*-Alkyl-2-acetyl-*sn*-glycero-3-phosphocholine. A novel source of arachidonic acid in neutrophils stimulated by the Ca^{2+} ionophore A23187, *Biochem. Biophys. Res. Commun.,* 113, 72, 1983.
125. **Radomski, M. and Moncada, S.,** An improved method for washing of human platelets with prostacyclin, *Thromb. Res.,* 30, 383, 1983.

Chapter 9

ROLE OF OXYGEN-DERIVED FREE RADICALS IN LESION FORMATION IN THE UPPER GASTROINTESTINAL TRACT

Naoji Yasue and Paul H. Guth

TABLE OF CONTENTS

I. INTRODUCTION

Since the discovery of superoxide dismutase (SOD) by McCord and Fridovich,[1] studies concerned with free radicals have increased markedly. In the field of medical research, a great deal of evidence has been accumulated demonstrating the important physiological and pathophysiological role of free radicals, such as their role in the bacteriocidal effect of human leukocytes and their participation in diseases of the heart, lung, kidney, and brain.[2-8] In recent years there have been many reports suggesting a role for oxygen-derived free radicals (oxyradicals) in the pathogenesis of microcirculatory disturbances and parenchymal damage in the gastrointestinal tract, mainly relating to ischemia-reperfusion injury. In this chapter, the authors present an overview of recent reports concerning the injurious effects of oxygen-derived free radicals in the upper gastrointestinal tract and prospects for research in this field.

II. SPECIES OF OXYGEN-DERIVED FREE RADICALS AND HOW THEY ARE GENERATED IN THE LIVING BODY

O_2 has two unpaired electrons in its outer orbital (it exists in biradical form). O_2 itself is a strong oxidant, but its reactivity is not high because of its particular electron configuration of unpaired electrons with parallel spins. O_2 is eventually metabolized to H_2O by accepting four electrons, but in this process, it can produce a reactive oxygen metabolite in each univalent step. Univalent reduction of molecular oxygen generated the superoxide anion (O_2^-), divalent reduction results in hydrogen peroxide (H_2O_2) generation, and the hydroxyl radical ($OH^•$) is a product of the reduction of H_2O_2 and O_2^-. These metabolites, including singlet oxygen ($^1O_2$), are considered oxygen-derived free radicals in general. Hydrogen peroxide is not truly an oxyradical because it does not have an unpaired electron. Singlet oxygen exists in two forms ($^1\Delta g$ and $^1\Sigma^+g$). The $^1\Delta g$ form is thought to be dominant in living bodies. The $^1\Delta g$ form does not have an unpaired electron. Nevertheless, these are usually included in this category because of their cytoxicity as oxygen metabolites. Among the oxygen-derived free radicals, the hydroxyl radical is considered the oxyradical most harmful to biological substrates.

Superoxide is generated via two pathways in the cell body. One is spontaneous dismutation by itself and by transitional metal complexes, ascorbic acid, quinones or thiols, etc., and the other is enzymatic generation by the oxidative enzymes, such as mitochondrial enzymes and cytochrome oxidase. Once superoxides are generated, hydrogen peroxide and hydroxyl radical are generated in subsequent reactions. Oxyradicals are generated mainly by NAPDH oxidase of blood phagocytes and by xanthine oxidase of the endothelial and parenchymal cells during ischemia-reperfusion in the gastrointestinal tract.

III. OXYGEN-DERIVED FREE RADICALS GENERATED BY THE NADPH OXIDASE SYSTEM OF PHAGOCYTES

A. SUPEROXIDE AND HYDROGEN PEROXIDE

After a specific membrane pertubation, a plasma membrane-associated NADPH oxidase is activated and cytoplasmic NADPH is oxidized to $NADP^+$. Two electrons are donated to two molecules of oxygen in this process, and finally two molecules of superoxide are generated.[9,10]

$$^2O_2 + NADPH \rightarrow {}^2O_2^- + NADP^+ + H^+ \quad (1)$$

O_2^- is the dominant form produced in the physiological pH range of 7.4. In the case of pKa of 4.8, it may be protonated to form the perhydroxyl radical (HO_2^-). This form is a much more powerful oxidant than O_2^-. The generated O_2^- will produce hydrogen peroxide (H_2O_2) via spontaneous dismutation and enzymatic (superoxide dismutase) dismutation:

$$O_2^- + O_2 + 2H^+ \rightarrow H_2O_2 + O_2 \quad (2)$$

H_2O_2 is relatively stable compared to other oxyradicals, and its injurious effect is weaker than other species. Nevertheless, it is still harmful by itself and has an important role in the generation of hydroxyl radicals.

B. HYDROXYL RADICAL

The ability of phagocytes to generate hydroxyl radical ($OH^{\cdot}$) and the mechanism by which this is accomplished is not well confirmed.[9] The cooperation of O_2^-. H_2O_2, and myeloperoxidase seems necessary to generate $OH\cdot$.[11] The following mechanism is postulated[12]

$$O_2 + HOCl + H^+ \xrightarrow{\text{myeloperoxidase}} OH^{\cdot} + Cl^- + O_2 \quad (3)$$

C. SINGLET OXYGEN

Singlet oxygen ($^1O_2$) is also generated via a myeloperoxidase-dependent mechanism:[13]

$$H_2O_2 + Cl^- + H^+ \xrightarrow{\text{myeloperoxidase}} HOCl + H_2O \quad (4)$$

$$H^+ + OCl^- + H_2O_2 \rightarrow {}^1O_2 + H_20 + H^+ Cl^- \quad (5)$$

In addition, $^1O_2$ is generated via the spontaneous dismutation or O_2^- or the Haber-Weiss reaction.[9]

D. HYPOHALOUS ACID

Hypohalous acid is another important oxygen metabolite produced via the H_2O_{2-} myeloperoxidase-halide system in phagocytes, but not by the xanthine oxidase system in other cells. Myeloperoxidase catalyzes the oxidation of the halides (Cl^-, I^-, Br^-) in the presence of H_2O_2 and the corresponding hypohalous acid (hypochlorous acid, HOCl; hypobromous acid, HOBr; hypoiodous acid, HOI) is generated:[10]

$$H_2O_2 + X^- \xrightarrow{\text{myeloperoxidase}} HOX + H_2O \quad (6)$$

From the standpoint of concentration of halides in *in vivo* circumstances, the hypochlorous acid is considered predominant among these hypohalous acids. Because of their strong oxidative ability, they are undoubtedly harmful to biological substrates. Furthermore, HOCI cooperates with phagocytes to chlorinate amines, and yield the long-lived, powerful oxidants, N-chloramines.[14,15]

IV. OXYGEN-DERIVED FREE RADICALS GENERATED BY THE XANTHINE OXIDASE SYSTEM

In recent years, studies by Granger et al.[16-24] of oxyradical generation in the gastrointestinal tract have demonstrated the important role the xanthine oxidase (XOD) system plays in ischemia-reperfusion injury. The gastrointestinal mucosa is rich in xanthine dehydrogenase. During ischemia, xanthine dehydrogenase is converted to its oxidase form (XOD). This conversion requires the presence of protease and calcium ion. [25] In addition, during ischemia, adenosinetriphosphate (ATP) is catabolized to hypoxanthine, which accumulates in the tissue. Hypoxanthine and molecular oxygen, which is delivered to the tissue during reperfusion, are the substrates needed by XOD to generate oxyradicals.

A. SUPEROXIDE AND HYDROGEN PEROXIDE

O_2^- is generated as follows in this system:[9]

$$\text{Hypoxanthine} + H_2O + 2O_2 \xrightarrow{XOD} \text{xanthine} + 2O_2^- + 2H^+ \quad (7)$$

$$\text{Xanthine} + H_2O + 2O_2 \rightarrow \text{uric acid} + 2O_2^- + 2H^+ \quad (8)$$

Hydrogen peroxide is generated via the spontaneous dismutation of O_2^- and via dismutation by SOD:[26]

$$O_2^- + O_2^- + 2H^+ \xrightarrow{SOD} O_2 + H_2O_2 \quad (2)$$

The production of O_2^- and H_2O_2 from the XOD system depends on the reduction state of the enzyme.[27] In the case of 6- and 4-electron reduced enzymes, H_2O_2 generation occurs rapidly via a flavin semiquinone-superoxide complex and $FADH_2$ without releasing O_2^- from the active site, while in the case of 2-electron reduced enzyme, the enzyme causes O_2^- generation.[9,28]

B. HYDROXYL RADICAL

The xanthine-XOD system generates both O_2^- and H_2O_2. These products interact to generate $OH^\bullet$:

$$O_2^- + H_2O_2 \; OH. + OH^- + O_2 \quad (9)$$

This process is known as the Haber-Weiss reaction. The Haber-Weiss reaction is relatively slow compared to the rate of spontaneous dismutation of O_2^-. Therefore, generation of the $OH^\bullet$ via this process was considered unlikely to occur in living bodies;[29] however, in the presence of transition metals (such as Fe) or their chelates, the following reaction occurs rapidly:

$$O_2^- + M^{n+} \rightarrow O_2 + M^{(n-1)} \text{ (Fenton reaction)} \quad (10)$$

$$H_2O_2 + M^{(n-1)} \rightarrow M^{n+} + OH^\cdot + OH^- \quad (11)$$

The metal catalyzes the Haber-Weiss reaction and is responsible for generation of $OH^\bullet$.[30] In addition, the possibility has been suggested that semiquinones react directly with H_2O_2 to generate $OH^\bullet$. In this case, the presence of metals is not necessary.[31]

C. SINGLET OXYGEN

Highly reactive $^1O_2$ also is generated via the Haber-Weiss reaction, as well as by the spontaneous dismutation of O_2^-. The reaction is as follows:[32]

$$H_2O_2 + O_2^- + H^+ \rightarrow OH^- = OH^\cdot + {}^1O_2 \quad (12)$$

Figure 1 shows schematically the generation of oxygen-derived free radicals from xanthine-XOD system during the ischemia-reperfusion period in the gastrointestinal tract.

V. MECHANISM OF CELL DAMAGE BY THE OXYGEN-DERIVED FREE RADICALS

Although oxyradicals attack all biological components, cell membrane phospholipids, enzyme protein, and DNA are the well-documented targets of these oxyradicals. Among these targets, lipid peroxidation by oxyradicals seems most important in terms of gastrointestinal injury. O_2^- and H_2O_2 can cross plasma membranes and gain access to intracellular sites. H_2O_2 can diffuse large distance and cause damage to the tissue far from its site of generation. On the other hand, highly reactive oxidants such as $OH^\bullet$ and $^1O_2$ will react with the targets nearest to where they are generated. Lipid peroxidation can be initiated by a reactive oxygen metabolite,

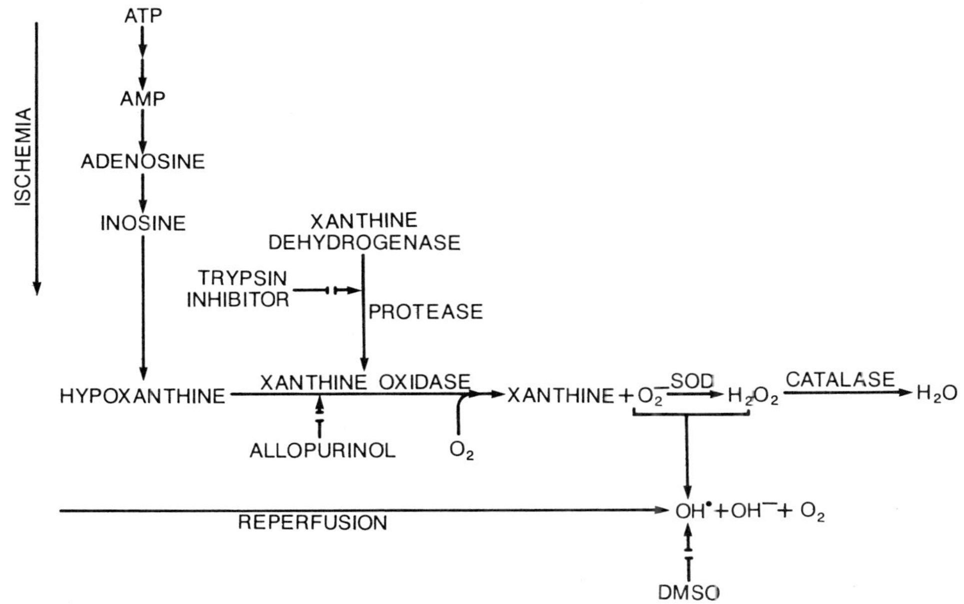

FIGURE 1. Mechanism of oxygen radical production during ischemia-reperfusion period in the gastrointestinal tract.[25]

including iron-oxygen complex and hypohalous acid, as well as the oxyradicals, to generate a lipid-free radical.[9] A lipid-free radical will generate a lipid peroxyradical that will attack an unsaturated fatty acid to generate a hydroperoxide and a lipid-free radical. This chain propogation will continue until termination where the collision of two radicals forms non-radical products. The equation of this chain reaction is as follows:

$$LH + OH^{\cdot} \rightarrow L^{\cdot} + H_2O \tag{13}$$

$$L^{\cdot} + O_2 \rightarrow LOO^{\cdot} \tag{14}$$

$$LOO^{\cdot} + LH \rightarrow LOOH + L^{\cdot} \tag{15}$$

Termination reactions:

$$L^{\cdot} + L^{\cdot}\text{, } LOO^{\cdot} + LOO^{\cdot} \text{ or } LOO^{\cdot} + L^{\cdot} \rightarrow \text{nonradical products} \tag{16}$$

where: LH= unsaturated fatty acid, $L^{\cdot}$ = lipid-free radical, $LOO^{\cdot}$ = lipid peroxyradical, and LOOH = lipid hydroperoxide. Once oxyradicals result in lipid peroxidation and damage of cellular membranes, the release of intracellular components such as lysosomal enzymes, leads to further tissue damage. Another important mechanism of cell damage by oxyradicals, particularly $OH^{\cdot}$, is degradation of hyaluronic acid, which is a principal component of the epithelial basement membrane.[33,34]

VI. SYSTEMS FOR SCAVENGING OXYGEN-DERIVED FREE RADICALS

Oxyradicals are generated constantly in the living body. There are endogenous mechanisms to counteract these deleterious species and to protect the body against serious injury.

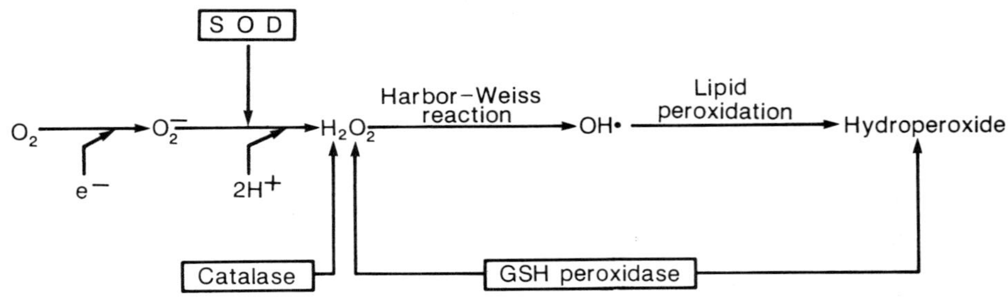

FIGURE 2. Scavenging system of oxygen-derived free radicals.

A. SUPEROXIDE

Superoxide dismutase is a well-studied enzyme that catalyzes the dismutation of O_2^- to H_2O_2:[1,35]

$$O_2^- + O_2^- + sH^+ \xrightarrow{SOD} H_2O_2 + O_2 \quad (2)$$

The enzyme catalyzed dismutation of O_2^- occurs at a much faster rate than does the spontaneous dismutation of O_2^-. Based on its metallic components there are three forms of this enzyme: Cu, Zn-SOD, Mn-SOD and Fe-SOD.

B. HYDROGEN PEROXIDE

Representative scavengers of H_2O_2 are catalase and glutathione peroxidase. The mode of dismutation of H_2O_2 by catalase depends on the H_2O_2 concentration.[9,36] At low concentrations of H_2O_2, catalase acts as follows:

$$AH_2\text{ (electron donor)} + H_2O_2 \xrightarrow{catalase} A + 2H_2O \quad (17)$$

At higher concentrations of H_2O_2,

$$H_2O_2 + H_2O_2 \xrightarrow{catalase} O_2 + 2H_2O \quad (18)$$

Glutathione peroxidase catalyzed H_2O_2 dismutation by the following reaction:

$$H_2O_2 + 2GSH \xrightarrow{GSH\ peroxidase} 2H_2O + GSSG \quad (19)$$

In addition, glutathione peroxidase can reduce hydroperoxide[37] and can stop chain propagation of lipid peroxidation.

C. HYDROXYL RADICAL, SINGLET OXYGEN, AND HYPOHALOUS ACID

There is no specific enzyme or compound in the living body that has the ability to scavenge these species. The scavengers of O_2^- and H_2O_2 can be considered to function like scavengers of these species because they prevent formation of these highly reactive oxygen metabolites by scavenging of O_2^- and H_2O_2. Figure 2 summarizes these scavenging systems.

VII. DISTURBANCE OF MICROCIRCULATION OF OXYRADICALS

Many studies concerning the disturbance of the microcirculation by oxyradicals have been performed in the small intestine, hamster cheek pouch, and mesentery, but not in the upper gastrointestinal tract (stomach and duodenum); however, it is worthwhile to review these studies to clarify the injurious effects of these radicals at the tissue and organ level.

A. VASCULAR PERMEABILITY STUDIES

As described before, XOD, hypoxanthine, and molecular oxygen are implicated in the generation of oxyradicals. They are formed or are supplied during ischemia-reperfusion injury. In addition, the intestine is the richest source of the dehydrogenase form of xanthine oxidase.[38] The ischemia-reperfusion model in the small intestine has therefore proven to be valuable for examining the effect of oxyradicals on vascular permeability as well as tissue injury. Granger et al.[16-24] have reported many studies using this model. They used osmotic reflection coefficient determinations as an indication of vascular permeability. Pretreatment with SOD, dimethylsulfoxide (DMSO, a hydroxyl radical scavenger), or catalase protected against the ischemia-reperfusion induced vascular permeability increase, whereas antihistaminergic agents, indomethacin or methyl prednisolone did not.[17,19,21] Their investigations indicated that oxygen-derived free radicals are responsible for the alteration of vascular permeability, but histamine, prostaglandin, and lysosomal enzymes do not play a role in this change. Further, the finding that both DMSO and catalase provided significant protection against ischemic-reperfusion injury suggests that the highly reactive hydroxyl radical is the primary mediator of the microvascular permeability change.[19,21] They also demonstrated the important role of XOD as a source of oxyradicals by means of pretreatment with allopurinol and folic acid which inhibit XOD, or soybean trypsin inhibitor, which interferes with the conversion of xanthine dehydrogenase to XOD. [18,25] These substances significantly attenuated the ischemia-reperfusion induced increase in vascular permeability. In addition, the direct arterial infusion of hypoxanthine-XOD also increased microvascular permeability in the small intestine. Both SOD and DMSO significantly protected against this change.[22] These findings support the concept that oxygen-derived free radicals are the major mediators of the microvascular permeability change in ischemia-reperfusion intestinal injury. Their source in the small intestine is the enzyme XOD catalyzing the reaction between hypoxanthine and molecular oxygen.

B. *IN VIVO* MICROSCOPIC STUDIES

Incandescent fluorescent *in vivo* microscopic observations of the microcirculatory disturbances caused by oxygen-derived free radicals were performed by Del Maestro et al.[39,40] In the hamster cheek pouch preparation, they observed a significant leak of macromolecules (fluorescein-labeled dextran) from postcapillary venules and larger venules (>20 μm) after the topical application of XOD and hypoxanthine. Macromolecular extravasation was not observed from arteries, arterioles, or capillaries. Arteriolar vasoconstriction was observed after an initial vasodilation. Of interest, there also appeared increased leukocyte rolling in both arterioles and venules, and granulocyte adhesion in postcapillary venules.[33] Concomitant application of SOD, catalase, DMSO, or L-methionine, which is a scavenger of $OH^{\bullet}$ and a quencher of $^1O_2$, with the xanthine oxidase solution resulted in marked prevention of macromolecular extravasation. These results indicate that oxyradicals generated from the xanthine oxidase system, especially $OH^{\bullet}$, are responsible for the microcirculatory changes.

In vivo microscopic observations of the gastric mucosal microcirculation in a rat ischemia-reperfusion model were performed by Morishita and Guth.[41] Gastric acid is an important factor in the pathogenesis of gastric injury. Their observations were done both in the absence and in the presence of HCl to clarify the effect of HCl on the gastric microcirculation during hemorrhagic hypotension and after the reinfusion of shed blood. They found a significant correlation between decreased red blood cell velocity and blood pressure during hypotension with the topical application of either HCl or Krebs solution. There was a significantly greater decrease in red blood cell velocity with the topical application of HCl, however. When the blood pressure was 27% of basal value, red blood cell flow stopped in about 50% of experimental

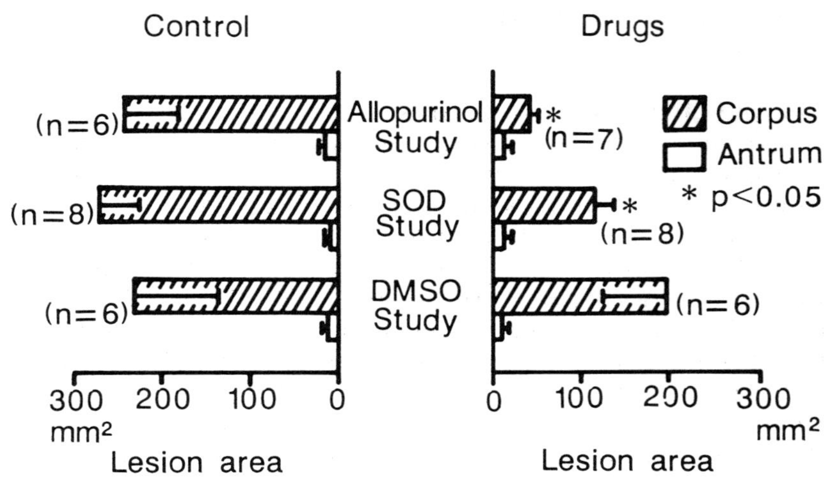

FIGURE 3. Effect of allopurinol, SOD, and DMSO on area of gastric lesions induced by hemorrhagic shock plus HCl. *indicates $p < 0.05$ relative to control (unpaired t test).[42]

animals but red blood cells were always present within the microvessels with Krebs solution application. On the other hand, blood flow stopped in all experimental animals and red blood cells disappeared in over 70% of animals with HCl application. With retransfusion, blood pressure returned to almost basal values in both groups, but red blood cell velocity returned to basal values only in the Krebs solution group. In the HCl group, red blood cell velocity measurement was impossible because of very poor flow of blood cells in the microvessels. Moreover, mucosal bleeding was observed in 75% of rats in the HCl group following retransfusion. Bleeding did not occur in the Krebs' solution group. Their findings indicate that the presence of HCl adds to the pathophysiological features accompanying ischemia due to hemorrhagic hypotension followed by reinfusion of shed blood.

VIII. STUDIES OF GASTRIC MUCOSAL INJURY BY OXYGEN-DERIVED FREE RADICALS

Itoh and Guth[42] demonstrated the important role of oxyradicals in the pathogenesis of gastric mucosal injury in a rat ischemia-reperfusion plus HCl model. In the presence of intragastric instillation of 0.1 *N* HCl, hemorrhagic hypotension to below 30 mmHg arterial pressure followed by retransfusion of shed blood caused marked macroscopic gastric mucosal injury. The simultaneous intravenous infusion of SOD or pretreatment with allopurinol significantly protected against this mucosal injury, but DMSO infusion did not (Figure 3). In another study,[43] however, these investigators noted that the ischemia-induced gastric mucosal injury was the same whether or not the stomach was reperfused. Perry et al.[44] reported that ^{51}Cr-labeled red blood cell leakage was increased in the ischemia-reperfusion plus acid model. They found that allopurinol and SOD, as well as DMSO, significantly reduced the loss of this indicator into the gastric lumen. Smith et al.[45] demonstrated the important role, not only of oxygen-derived free radicals, but also of the iron catalyzed Haber-Weiss reaction in generating hydroxyl radicals in hemorrhagic shock-induced extravasation of red blood cells from the gastric mucosa. Gastric mucosal clearance of ^{51}Cr-labeled red blood cells was measured during a 30-min control period, a 30-min ischemic period (hemorrhage to 25 mmHg arterial pressure), and a 60- to 80-min reperfusion period (reinfusion of shed blood). Control rats showed a dramatic rise in the leakage of ^{51}Cr-labeled red blood cells into the gastric lumen; however, ^{51}Cr-labeled red blood cell leakage was significantly attenuated by treatment with deferoxamine, an iron chelating agent. A similar reduction in red blood cell leakage was also observed in rats receiving SOD and in rats that had been placed on a sodium tungstate diet which results in the inactivation of XOD. On the other hand, tissue injury assessed histologically was not prevented by these treatments. Von Ritter et al.[46] also reported significant protection against gastric mucosal injury by SOD and allopurinol in the baboon ischemia-reperfusion model. The findings of these reports indicate that oxygen-derived free radicals contribute significantly to the ischemia-reperfusion plus acid injury in the stomach.

The findings of Smith et al.[45] indicate that the iron-catalyzed Haber-Weiss reaction generates hydroxyl radicals that, in turn, mediate ischemia-reperfusion induced bleeding. The failure of oxyradical scavenging to prevent histological injury[45] and the finding that the ischemia-induced histological gastric mucosal injury is the same whether the stomach is reperfused,[43] indicates that factors other than oxyradicals mediate the disruption of the gastric mucosa during ischemia and reperfusion.

In an *in vitro* study of monolayer culture of rat fundic mucosa, Hiraishi et al.[47] demonstrated the injurious effect of oxyradicals on the gastric mucosal cells. Application of xanthine and XOD to the monolayer caused marked ^{51}Cr release from prelabeled cells. Catalase, unlike SOD and DMSO, significantly protected ^{51}Cr release from culture cells. They concluded that H_2O_2 was a major mediator of cell injury *in vitro*.

There are only a few preliminary reports demonstrating the role of oxyradicals on gastric lesion formation in other experimental models. Cochran et al.[48] demonstrated that DMSO, either fed over a 5-d period or given as a single-dose gavage, also prevented the mucosal injury induced by cold-restraint stress. Terano et al.[49] reported the role of oxyradicals in ethanol-induced gastric lesions. They found that allopurinol and SOD, as well as DMSO, protected against ethanol-induced mucosal lesions. These results suggest the possibility that oxyradicals are involved in other forms of gastric injury in addition to ischemia-reperfusion injury. Further investigations are needed to confirm these possibilities.

IX. OXYGEN-DERIVED FREE RADICALS — ACID INTERACTION IN GASTRIC LESION FORMATION

The presence of gastric acid is thought to be a prerequisite factor to gastric mucosal lesion formation. In the ischemia-reperfusion model, the animals routinely receive intragastric instillation of HCl. Itoh and Guth[43] compared the extent of histological gastric injury of ischemia alone with that of ischemia plus reperfusion, both in the presence of 0.1 *N* HCl intragastrically. They studied rats subjected to ischemia (hemorrhagic hypotension) for 20 min and reperfusion (reinfusion of shed blood) and then kept for 20 min, or ischemia alone for 40 min. These experimental rats showed significantly more severe damage compared to time-matched controls (no hemorrhage with HCl); however, there was no significant difference in the extent of gastric mucosal histological injury between the ischemia-reperfused rats and the ischemia alone rats. Smith et al.[45] also demonstrated that blocking oxyradical formation or scavenging oxyradicals prevented gastric bleeding but did not alter the histologic gastric mucosal injury. The determination of the pathogenesis of ischemia-reperfusion injury of the gastric mucosa is confounded by the presence of ischemia, intragastric acid, and retransfusion. To clarify these problems, Yasue and Guth [50] investigated the separate effects of HCl, ischemia, and retransfusion on lesion formation in the rat hemorrhagic hypotension model of ischemia-reperfusion. To determine the role of retransfusion, the extent of histologic injury was compared among rats subjected to ischemia plus reperfusion (infusion of shed blood), ischemia alone, and control group (no hypotensive-induced ischemia). All animals received saline intragastrically (no acid). No gross lesions were seen in any rats; however, the extent of histologic damage of the ischemia-

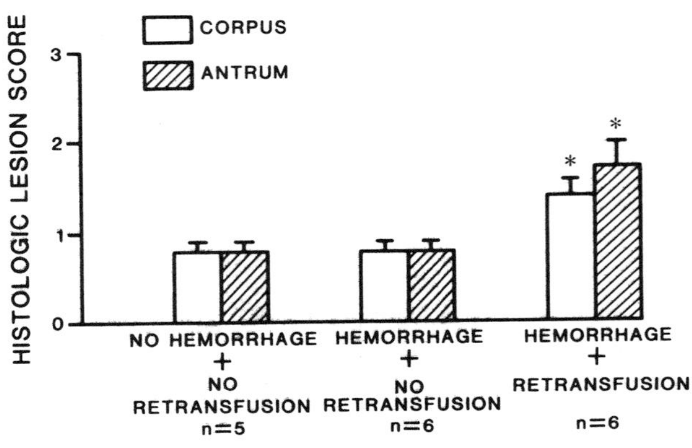

FIGURE 4. Effect of retransfusion of shed blood on the histological lesions scores in the absence of intragastric acid. *Significantly different from no retransfusion groups, $p < 0.05$ (ANOVA with contrasts).[50]

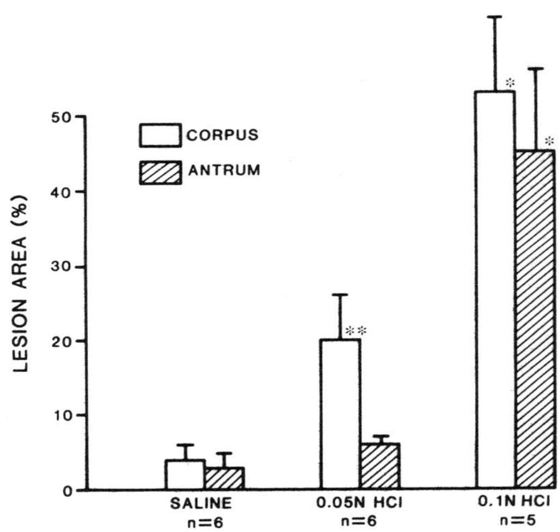

FIGURE 5. Effect of exogenous acid on area of gastric lesions induced by hemorrhagic shock. *Significantly different from 0.05 *N* HCl and saline groups, $p < 0.02$, and ** significantly different from saline group, $p < 0.05$ (ANOVA with contrasts).

reperfusion group was significantly greater than both the ischemia-alone group and the control group (Figure 4). This result indicates that ischemia followed by infusion of shed blood causes histologic mucosal injury in the corpus and antrum, even in the absence of intragastric HCl. The effect of intragastric HCl on lesion formation was studied. Saline, 0.05 *N* HCl, or 0.1 *N* HCl, was instilled intragastrically. The rats were then subjected to hemorrhagic hypotension (<30 mmHg arterial pressure) for 20 min, followed by infusion of shed blood and maintenance for another 20 min.

Intragastric HCl increased gastric mucosal lesions formation (both grossly and histologically) in a dose-dependent manner (Figures 5 and 6). These results suggest that while oxyradicals formed during reperfusion do cause some histologic injury, HCl greatly potentiates this damage. A possible explanation of why the ischemia alone plus HCl model showed the same extent of histologic damage as the ischemia-reperfusion plus HCl model[43] may be that ischemia

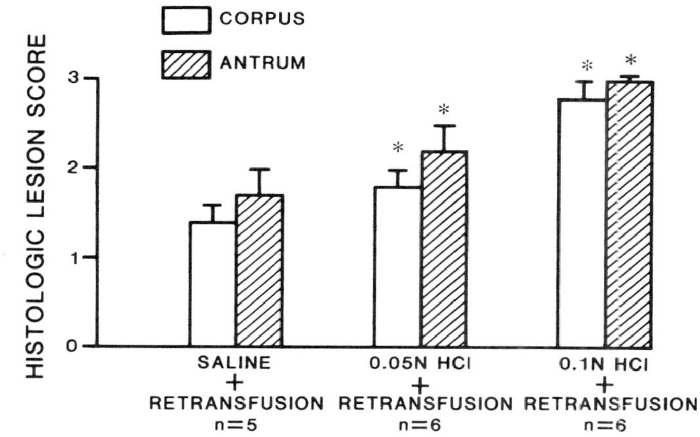

FIGURE 6. Effect of exogenous acid on the histological lesion scores in rats subjected to hemorrhagic hypotension and retransfusion. *Significantly different from saline group, $p < 0.02$ (ANOVA with contrasts).

may alter the gastric mucosal defense mechanism because of both decreased removal of back-diffusing hydrogen ions and/or decreased delivery of oxygen and energy substrates.

In their *in vivo* microscopic study, Morishita and Guth[41] observed gastric mucosal bleeding in hemorrhagic hypotension followed by reinfusion of shed blood only when HCl was present. Smith et al.,[45] however, found that scavenging of oxyradicals prevented leak of red blood cells from the gastric mucosal in a similar mode. Taken together, these findings suggest that there is a potential interaction between HCl and oxyradicals on the vessel damage which leads to mucosal bleeding as well as gastric mucosal cell damage. Thus, the effect of oxyradical on the gastric injury is augmented by the presence of intragastric HCl.

X. INTERACTION BETWEEN OXYGEN-FREE RADICALS GENERATED BY THE XOD SYSTEM AND THE NEUTROPHIL NADPH OXIDASE SYSTEM IN ISCHEMIA-REPERFUSION INJURY

Both the XOD system and the leukocyte NADPH oxidase system are sources of oxygen radicals. Oxyradicals generated by leukocytes also may play a role in mediating tissue injury. Grisham et al.[51] demonstrated increased neutrophil infiltration into the tissue during ischemia-reperfusion injury in the cat small intestine. They used the activity of myeloperoxidase (MPO) in the tissue as an indicator of neutrophil infiltration. MPO activity increased to a small extent in the ischemic period; however, there was an 18-fold increase above the control level in the postischemic period, and this increase of MPO activity was significantly prevented by the administration of allopurinol or SOD. Their findings suggest that oxyradicals generated by the XOD system during the ischemia-reperfusion period are responsible for neutrophil infiltration into the tissue. They postulated the following possible mechanisms of this relationship:

1. Superoxide per se or other oxygen metabolites may damage the intestinal mucosa and cause the release of certain tissue proteases capable of interacting with the complement system to yield potent chemoattractants
2. Superoxide may interact with certain lipoproteins to yield a potent chemoattractant

Infiltrating neutrophils then may play a role in mucosal damage. Their hypothesis is summarized in Figure 7.

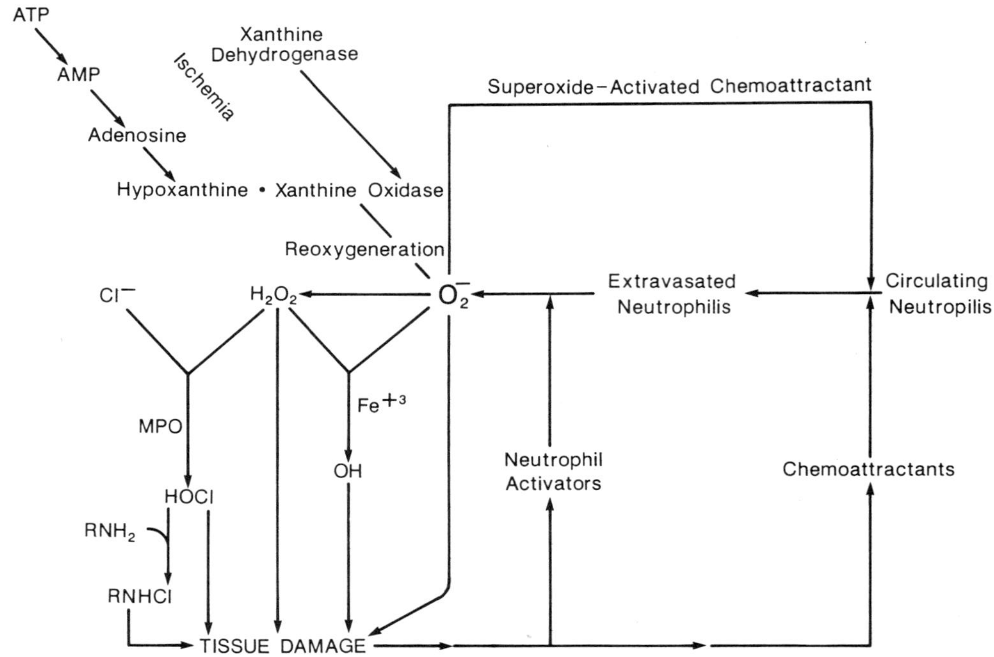

FIGURE 7. Proposed relationship between XOD-generated superoxide (O_2^-), neutrophil infiltration, and mucosal injury by Grisham et al.[51]

Possibly this hypothesis could also be applied to explain the role of oxyradicals in lesion formation in the upper gastrointestinal tract. During ischemia ATP is catabolized to hypoxanthine and xanthine dehydrogenase is converted to its oxidase form. During reperfusion, molecular oxygen is delivered to the tissue and reacts with hypoxanthine. This reaction is catalyzed by XOD and results in the generation of a burst of oxyradicals. Oxyradicals react with the polyunsaturated fatty acids of the cell membrane to set off a self-propagating chain reaction of lipid peroxidation. This reaction will occur in the vascular endothelial cells leading to the cell's inability to maintain its internal milieu, resultant cell disruption,[52] and release of endothelial cell products.[53] This phenomenon results in neutrophil adherence to the vascular endothelial cell.[40] Indeed, there are many reports that endothelial injury increases neutrophil adherence to endothelium,[54,55] and the endothelial cell products, such as platelet-activating factor (PAF), a potent neutrophil-activating agent, platelet-derived growth factor (PDGF), and other factors with chemotactic activity increase neutrophil adherence.[56-58] The adherent neutrophils are activated and release their own oxygen radicals, granule enzymes, and products of membrane phospholipases.[53] Oxyradicals generated by neutrophil and granule enzyme, such as elastase, cause further damage to the endothelial cell and the subendothelial hyaline matrix.[33] The lipoxygenase products and the phospholipase products have direct effects on microvascular permeability.[39,53,60] Vascular permeability increases, making neutrophil extravasation possible. Moreover, oxygen radicals yield a chemotactic factor in plasma, [61] This substance, activated complements as well as phospholipase reaction products, cause further neutrophil accumulation at the sites of vascular damage. This cycle results in the aggravation of vascular damage and the infiltration of neutrophils into the extravascular space. The observation that a specific leukocyte antibody largely prevented both neutrophil accumulation and neutrophil-dependent plasma leakage in inflammatory skin lesions supports this hypothesis.[62]

Simultaneously, gastrointestinal ischemia-reperfusion injury results in mucosal cell disruption and the formation of chemoattractants.[51,63] These chemoattractants cause further neutrophil infiltration. Infiltrated neutrophils have the arsenal for additional tissue injury, such as oxyradicals, various kinds of proteinases, and cationic proteins.[53,64] These substances act locally and cause further tissue damage. Thus, ischemia-reperfusion injury spreads from vascular injury to tissue injury. If other aggressive factors exist, such as HCl in the stomach, the damage will be aggravated. Further studies are needed to confirm the role of neutrophils in ischemia-reperfusion injury in the gastrointestinal tract.

XI. SUMMARY AND PROSPECTIVE

There is a growing body of experimental data indicating that reactive oxygen-derived free radicals play a role in mediating mucosal damage in the gastrointestinal tract in ischemia-reperfusion injury. Oxyradicals cause vascular endothelial cell damage as well as parenchymal cell damage. There are several possible links between microcirculatory disturbance and tissue damage. One candidate is infiltrating leukocytes. Gastric acid (and probably pepsin) is a potent aggressive factor in gastric mucosal injury. It markedly aggravates the injurious effect of oxyradicals. When the microcirculation is disturbed, there is failure to adequately carry away back-diffusing acid. Vigorous investigations are continuing in this field. There are still many problems to be clarified. For instance, what is the role of other blood elements, especially platelets, in lesion formation by oxyradicals? What is the role of other leukocytes in this process? Does prostaglandin I_2 or E_2, which are generated in the vascular endothelial cells as well as the mucosal cells, protect against this injury? Do oxyradicals per se alter the gastric secretion of HCl and pepsin? In addition, there are no reports as yet demonstrating the role of oxyradicals in duodenal lesion formation. These are fruitful fields for further investigation.

REFERENCES

1. **McCord, J. M. and Fridovich, I.,** Superoxide dismutase. An enzymic function for erythrocuprein (hemocuprein), *J. Biol. Chem.*, 244(22), 6049, 1969.
2. **Babior, B. M.,** Oxygen-dependent microbial killing by phagocyte, *N. Engl. J. Med.*, 298, 659, 1978.
3. **Hearse, D. J., Manning, A. S., Downey, J. M., and Yellon, D. M.,** Xanthine oxidase: a critical mediator of myocardial injury during ischemia and reperfusion, *Acta Physiol. Scand.* , 548(Suppl.), 1986.
4. **Johnson, K. J. , Fantone, J. C., III Kaplan, J., and Ward, P. A.,** *In vivo* damage of rat lungs by oxygen metabolites, *J. Clin. Invest.*, 67, 983, 1981.
5. **Vasko, K. A., Dewall, R. A., and Riley, A. M.,** Effect of allopurinol in renal ischemia, *Surgery*, 71, 787, 1972.
6. **Kogure, K., Morooka, H., Busto, R., and Scheinberg, P.,** Involvement of lipid peroxidation in postischemic brain damage, *Neurology*, 29, 546, 1979.
7. **Adkinson, D., Hollwarth, M. E., Benoit, J. N., Parks, D. A., McCord, J. M., and Granger, D. N.,** Role of free radicals in ischemia-reperfusion injury to the liver, *Acta Physiol. Scand.*. 548(Suppl.), 101, 1986.
8. **Manson, P. N., Anthenelli, R. N., Im, M. J., Bulkley, G. B., and Hoopes, J. E.,** The role of oxygen-free radicals in ischemic tissue injury in island skin flaps, *Ann. Surg.*, 198, 87, 1983.
9. **Weiss, S. J.,** Oxygen, ischemia and inflammation, *Acta Physiol. Scand.*, 548(Suppl.), 90, 1986.
10. **Weiss, S. J. and Lobuglio, A. F.,** Biology of disease. Phagocyte–generated oxygen metabolites and cellular injury, *Lab. Invest.*, 47(1), 5, 1982.
11. **Klebanoff, S. J. and Rosen, H.,** Ethylene formation by ploymorphonuclear leukocytes, *J. Exp. Med.*, 148, 490, 1978.
12. **Long, C. A. and Bielski, B. H. J.,** Rate of reaction of superoxide radical with chloride containing species, *J. Phys. Chem.*, 84, 555, 1982.
13. **Allen, R. C., Stjerholm, R. L., and Steele, R. H.,** Evidence for the participation of an electronic excitation state(s) in human polymorphonuclear leukocytes and its participation in bactericidal activity, *Biochem. Biophys. Res. Commun.*, 47, 679, 1972.
14. **Weiss, S. J., Lampert, M. B., and Test, S. T.,** Long–lived oxidants generated by human neutrophils; characterization and bioactivity, *Science*, 222, 625, 1983.

15. **Thomas, E. L., Grisham, M. B., and Jefferson, M. M.,** Myeloperoxidase-dependent effect of amines on functions of isolated neutrophils, *J. Clin. Invest.,* 72, 441, 1983.
16. **Granger, D., Rutili, G., and McCord, J.,** Superoxide radicals in feline intestinal ischemia, *Gastroenterology,* 81, 22, 1981.
17. **Granger, D. N. , Sennett, M., McElearney, P., and Taylor, A. E.,** Effect of local arterial hypotension on cat intestinal capillary permeability, *Gastroenterology,* 79, 474, 1980.
18. **Granger, D. N., McCord, J. M., Parks, D. A., and Hallmarth, M. E.,** Xanthine oxidase inhibitors attenuate ischemia-induced vascular permeability changes in the cat intestine, *Gastroenterology,* 90, 80, 1986.
19. **Parks, D. A. and Granger, D. N.,** Ischemia-induced microvascular changes: role of xanthine oxidase and hydroxyl radicals, *Am. J. Physiol.,* 245, G285, 1983.
20. **Parks, D. A., Grogaard, B., and Granger, D. N.,** Comparison of partial and complete arterial occlusion models for studying intestinal ischemia, *Surgery,* 92, 896, 1982.
21. **Parks, D. A. and Granger, D. N.,** Role of hydrogen peroxide in ischemic injury to the small intestine, *Gastroenterology,* 84 1207, 1984.
22. **Parks, D. A., Shah, A. K., and Granger, D. N.,** Oxygen radicals: effects on intestinal vascular permeability, *Am. J. Physiol.,* 247, G167, 1984.
23. **Parks, D. A., Bulkley, G. B., Granger, D. N., Hamilton, S. R., and McCord, J. M.,** Ischemic injury in the cat small intestine; role of superoxide radicals, *Gastroenterology,* 82, 9, 1982.
24. **Grogaard, B , Parks, D. A., Granger, D. N., McCord, J. M., and Forsberg, J. O.,** Effects of ischemia and oxygen radicals on mucosal albumin clearance in intestine, *Am. J. Physiol.,* 242, G448, 1982.
25. **Granger, D. M., Hollwarth, M. E., and Parks, D. A.,** Ischemia–reperfusion injury: role of oxygen-derived free radicals, *Acta Physiol. Scand.,* 548(Suppl.), 47, 1986.
26. **McCord, J. M. and Fridovich, I.,** The reduction of cytochrome C by milk xanthine oxidase, *J. Biol. Chem.,* 243, 5753, 1968.
27. **Olson, J. S., Ballou, D. P., Palmer, G., and Massey, V.,** The reaction of xanthine oxidase with molecular oxygen, *J. Biol. Chem.,* 249, 4350, 1974.
28. **Porras, A. G., Olson, J. S., and Palmer, G.,** The reaction of reduced xanthine oxidase with oxygen, *J. Biol. Chem.,* 256, 9096, 1981.
29. **Czapski, G. and Ilan, Y. A.,** On the generation of the hydroxylation agent from superoxide radical. Can the Haber–Weiss reaction be the source of OH· radicals? *Photochem. Photobiol.,* 28, 651, 1978.
30. **Halliwell, B. and Gutteridge, J. M. C.,** Oxygen free radicals and iron in relation to biology and medicine: some problems and concepts, *Arch. Biochem. Biophys.,* 246, 501, 1986.
31. **Winterbourn, C. C.,** Production of hydroxyl radicals from paraquat radicals and H_2O_2, *FEBS Lett.,* 128, 339, 1981.
32. **Kellogg, E. W., III and Fridovich, I.,** Superoxide, hydrogen peroxide, and singlet oxygen in lipid peroxidation by a xanthine oxidase system, *J. Biol. Chem.,* 250, 8812, 1975.
33. **Del Maestro, R. F., Thaw, H. H., Bjork, J., Planker, M., and Arfors, K. E.,** Free radicals as mediators of tissue injury, *Acta Physiol. Scan.,* 492, 43, 1980.
34. **McCord, J. M.,** Free radicals and inflammation: protection of synovial fluid by superoxide dismutase, *Science,* 185, 529, 1974.
35. **Fridovich, I.,** The biology of oxygen radicals. The superoxide radical is an agent of oxygen toxicity; superoxide dismutases provide an important defense, *Science,* 201, 875, 1978.
36. **Chance, B., Sies, H., and Boveris, A.,** Hydroperoxide metabolism in mammalian organs, *Physiol. Rev.,* 59, 527, 1979.
37. **Christopherson, B. O.,** Reduction of linolenic acid hydroperoxide by a glutathine peroxidase, *Biochem. Biophys. Acta,* 176, 463, 1979.
38. **Parks, D. A. and Granger, D. N.,** Xanthine oxidase: biochemistry distribution and physiology, *Acta Physiol. Scand.,* 548(Suppl.), 87, 1986.
39. **Del Maestro, R. F., Bjork, J., and Arford, K. E.,** Increase in microvascular permeability induced by enzymatically generated free radicals. I. In vivo study, *Microvasc. Res.,* 22, 239, 1981.
40. **Del Maestro, R. F., Bjork, J., and Arford, K. E.,** Increase in microvascular permeability induced by enzymatically generated free radicals. II. Roles of superoxide anion radical, hydrogen peroxide, and hydroxyl radical, *Microvasc. Res.,* 22, 255, 1981.
41. **Morishita, T. and Guth, P. H.,** Effect of exogenous acid on the rat gastric mucosal microcirculation in hemorrhagic shock, *Gastroenterology,* 92, 1958, 1987.
42. **Itoh, M. and Guth, P. H.,** Role of oxygen-derived free radicals in hemorrhagic shock-induced gastric lesions in the rat, *Gastroenterology,* 88, 1162, 1985.
43. **Itoh, M., Paulsen, G., and Guth, P. H.,** Hemorrhagic shock and acid gastric injury in the rat, *Gastroenterology,* 90, 1103, 1986.
44. **Perry, M. A., Wadhwa, S., Parks, D. A., Pickard, W., and Granger, D. N.,** Role of oxygen radicals in ischemia-induced lesions in the cat stomach, *Gastroenterology,* 90, 362, 1986.

45. **Smith, S. M., Gisham, M. B., Manci, E. A., Granger, D. N., Kvietys, P. R., and Russell, J. M.,** Gastric mucosal injury in the rat. Role of iron and xanthine oxidase, *Gastroenterology,* 92, 950, 1987.
46. **Von Ritter, C., Oosthuizen, M. M. J., Lambrechects, H., Hunter, S., Svensson, L. G., and Hinder, R. A.,** Free radical scavengers decrease reperfusion damage of the gastric mucosa in baboons, *Gastroenterology,* 90, 1682, 1986.
47. **Hiraishi, H., Terano, A., Ota, S., Ivey, K. J., and Sugimoto, T.,** Free radical damage to cultures gastric mucosal cells, *Gastroenterology,* 90, 1460, 1986.
48. **Cochran, T., Stefanko, J., Moore, C., and Saik, R.,** Dimethylsulfoxide protection against gastric stress ulceration, *Curr. Surg.,* 40, 435, 1983.
49. **Terano, A., Hiraishi, H., Ota, S., Shiga, J., and Sugimoto, T.,** Role of oxygen-derived free radicals in ethanol-induced damage in rat stomach, *Gastroenterology,* 90, 1661, 1986.
50. **Yasue, N. and Guth, P. H.,** Role of exogenous acid and retransfusion in hemorrhagic shock-induced gastric lesion in the rat, *Gastroenterology,* 92, 1703, 1987.
51. **Grisham, M. B., Hernandez, L. A., and Granger, D. N.,** Xanthine oxidase and neutrophil infiltration in intestinal ischemia, *Am. J. Physiol.,* 251, G567, 1986.
52. **Sacks, T., Moldow, C. F., Craddock, P. R., Bowers, T. K., and Jacob, H. S.,** Oxygen radicals mediate endothelial cell damage by complement-stimulated granulocyte. An *in vitro* model of immune vascular damage, *J. Clin. Invest.,* 61, 1161, 1978.
53. **Harlan, J. M.,** Leukocyte-endothelial interaction, *Blood,* 65, 513, 1985.
54. **Bowman, C., Butler, E., and Repine, J.,** Hyperoxia damage cultured endothelial cells causing increased neutrophil adherence, *Am. Rev. Resp. Dis.,* 65, 469, 1983.
55. **MacGregor, R., Friedman, H., Macarak, E., and Kefalides, N.,** Virus infection of endothelial cells increases granulocyte adherence, *J. Clin. Invest.,* 65, 1469, 1980.
56. **Camussi, G., Aglietta, M., Malavasi, G., Tetta, C., Piacibello, W., Sanavio, F., and Bussolino, F.,** The release of platelet-activating factor from human endothelial cells in culture, *J. Immunol.,* 131, 2397, 1983.
57. **Duel, T. F., Senior, R. M., Huang, J. S., and Griffin, G. L.,** Chemotaxis of monocyte and neutrophil to platelet-derived growth factor, *J. Clin. Invest.,* 69, 1046, 1982.
58. **Mercandetta, A. J., Lane, T. A., and Colmerauer, M. E. M.,** Cultured human endothelial cells elaborate neutrophil chemo-attractants, *J. Lab. Clin. Med.,* 104, 370, 1984.
59. **Dahlen, S., Bjork, J., Hedqvist, P., Arfors, K., Hammarstrom, S., Lindgren, J., and Samuelsson, B.,** Leukotrienes promote plasma leakage and leukocyte adhesion in postcapillary venules. *In vivo* effects with relevance to the acute inflammatory response, *Proc. Natl. Acad. Sci. U.S.A.,* 78, 3887, 1981.
60. **Humphrey, D. M., MacManus, L. M., Hanahan, D. J., and Pinckard, R. N.,** Morphologic basis of increase vascular permeability induced by acetyl glyceryl ether phosphorycholine, *Lab. Invest.,* 50, 16, 1984.
61. **Petrone, W. F., English, D. K., Wong, K., and McCord, J. M.,** Free radicals and inflammation: superoxide-dependent activation of a neutrophil chemotactic factor in plasma, *Proc. Natl. Acad. Sci. U.S.A.,* 77, 1159, 1980.
62. **Arford, K. E., Lundberg, C. L., and Lindbom, L.,** A monoclonal antibody to the membrane glycoprotein complex CD18 inhibits polymorphonuclear leukocyte accumulation and plasma leakage *in vivo, Blood,* 69, 338, 1987.
63. **Hill, J. K. and Ward, P. A.,** C3 leukotactic factors produced by a tissue protease, *J. Exp. Med.,* 130, 505, 1969.
64. **Henson, P. M. and Johnston, R. B., Jr.,** Tissue injury in inflammation: oxidants, proteinases, and cationic proteins, *J. Clin. Invest.,* 79, 669, 1987.

Chapter 10

ROLE OF SULFHYDRYLS IN GASTRODUODENAL DAMAGE AND PROTECTION

Sandor Szabo and K. D. Palitzsch

TABLE OF CONTENTS

I. INTRODUCTION

The pathogenesis of gastric mucosal injury (i.e., superficial mucosal erosions and deep ulcers) has been investigated from many perspectives.1 One of the major targets in ulcer research over the last 2 decades has been the demonstration of functional alterations (e.g., secretory changes) in ulcer patients and in animal models of the disease. In addition to gastric lesions, the pathogenesis of duodenal ulceration is also poorly understood.

The first compounds studied from biochemical and pharmacological points of view in ulcer disease were prostaglandins (PG). For many years, anti-inflammatory drugs (e.g., glucocorticoids, aspirin, indomethacin) were known for their potential to cause gastrointestinal ulcers in humans and in laboratory animals. PG, the mediators of inflammation,[2] on the other hand, inhibit gastric acid secretion, experimental ulceration, and exert acid-independent cytoprotection.[3] Measurement of PG levels in gastric mucosa may be used to correlate endogenous concentrations of PG with the effect of either exogenous PG synthesis inhibitors (e.g., cyclooxygenase inhibitors) or PG derivatives and their influence on gastric lesions. Irrespective of the development of gastric ulcers induced by PG synthesis inhibitors and their prevention by exogenously administered PG, changes in endogenous PG did not correlate closely with the formation of gastric mucosal lesions. Surprisingly, gastric mucosal injury did not develop until the endogenous PG levels decreased to 10% of normal levels.[4,5] This fact raised serious questions as to whether PG were indeed the common mediators of acute gastric mucosal injury.

The discovery of gastric mucosal protection by sulfhydryls (SH) provided an attractive and testable hypothesis where biochemical parameters and their correlations with functional and morphological changes in the pathogenesis of ulcer disease could be obtained. Relatively high levels of glutathione (GSH) have been found in the stomach and duodenum,[6,7] implying a certain role for SH in gastric and duodenal mucosal injury. Since gastroprotection is not a property unique to PG, but other agents also share this action,[8] we developed a hypothesis that endogenous SH mediate the gastric mucosal protection afforded by drugs with different structures and physicochemical properties. Further evidence for the effects of SH in gastric mucosal damage and protection originates from the fact that the SH-alkylator *N*-ethylmaleimide (NEM) abolishes gastroprotection induced by PG and other agents.[9] Recent work in our laboratory concerning the endogenous SH pool in gastric mucosal injury and protection[10] strongly suggests that protein SH may be involved in the mechanism of action of gastroprotective compounds. On the other hand, certain compounds containing SH groups may also cause or aggravate gastric or duodenal ulcers (Table 1). For example, cysteamine may prevent gastric mucosal injury, but it induces duodenal ulcer if administered in doses three- to fivefold higher.[11]

In this regard, the SH groups resemble other critical endogenous chemicals such as the PG which may offer gastroprotection or aggravate experimental esophagitis or gastric lesions under certain conditions.[12] The concentration of oxygen, hydrogen ion (pH), calcium, and other electrolytes are only a few of the many examples where only a narrow optimal level is compatible with life; disturbed concentration in either direction is detrimental and may cause cell and tissue injury.

In this chapter, the protective and damaging mechanisms of SH in the gastric and duodenal mucosa are reviewed on the basis of our own results and related studies from the literature.

II. SH AND GASTRODUODENAL DAMAGE

SH are very reactive functional groups but the molecular mechanisms of their action are still poorly understood. Most of the results obtained concern the gastroprotective effects of SH while little is known about the damaging action of SH in the gastric mucosa. In contrast, numerous studies were devoted to the damaging and ulcerogenic effects of SH compounds, especially

TABLE 1
SH-Containing Duodenal Ulcerogens and Gastroprotection by Compounds with Reduced SH or SH in Various States of Oxidation

Duodenal ulcerogens which also exert gastroprotection[a]	Gastroprotectors with: Reduced SH	Gastroprotectors with: Oxidized SH
Cysteamine	*N*-Acetylcysteine	Acetazolamide and derivatives
Cystamine	BAL	*S*-Adenosylmethionine
	Cysteine	Cystine
	Dimercaptosuccinic acid	Methionine
	Glutathione	Sucralfate
	Mercaptoethanol	Sucrose octasulfate
	Penicillamine	Sulfate (Na, K, or Mg)
		Thioctic (lipoic) acid
		Thimerosal
		Thiodipropionic acid
		Thiosulfate sodium

[a]The duodenal ulcerogenic dose is 3 to 5 times higher than the gastroprotective dose.

cysteamine in duodenal mucosa, whereas the protective action, if any, of SH on duodenal mucosa still needs to be further investigated.

A. DUODENAL ULCERATION

Initially our interest in SH had been focused on cysteamine, which is a SH-containing chemical. Cysteamine induces acute duodenal ulcer in the rat after administration of a single dose. In addition, cysteamine is useful for generating chronic duodenal ulcers.[11] The duodenal ulcerogenic properties of cysteamine are due to a 2-carbon backbone with adjacent nucleophilic groups such as SH and NH_2.[12] Chemicals which bear SH groups on one or both ends of their carbon chain are known to have similar duodenal ulcerogenic properties (e.g., allythiol, 1,2-ethanedithiol, 1,2-propanethiol).[13] Cystamine, the oxidized dimer of cysteamine, also causes rapidly developing duodenal ulcers in the rat.[13] Unlike for gastroprotection, the SH component is not the most important group for duodenal ulcer induction since other electronegative groups (e.g., -CN, $-NH_2$, -Cl) on 2-3 carbon alkyl chemicals also cause duodenal ulcer in rats.[13] Other compounds which do not contain SH groups but have the 2-carbon backbone may also initiate duodenal ulceration (e.g., propionitrile, *n*-butyronitrile, ethylamine).

Among the SH-containing duodenal ulcerogens, only the effects of cysteamine and cystamine have been investigated in detail. These chemicals exert many peripheral and central (e.g., brain) effects.[14,15] The adminstration of cysteamine leads to a transient increase followed by a decrease (for about 15 to 30 min) in blood flow in the adrenal glands, brain, and the duodenal mucosa.[14] The biochemical changes which follow the adminstration of cysteamine include depletion of norepinephrine in virtually all the tissues examined.[15] The effect was maximal 4 or 7 h after cysteamine or propionitrile, and norepinephrine levels had returned to normal by 24 h. Dopamine changes were selective and often biphasic, e.g., elevation in adrenals, biphasic in brain cortex, hippocampus, and midbrain, but uniformly decreased in the glandular stomach and duodenum.[15] In the median eminence, dopamine levels decreased by 131 and 324% at 15 and 30 min respectively, after cysteamine, but neither dopamine nor 3,4-dihydroxyphenylacetic acid was modified in the periventricular nucleus. Serotonin levels were relatively stable revealing slight elevations or no changes in most of the tissues. The turnover of norepinephrine was accelerated by both chemicals in virtually all brain regions, but dopamine turnover was

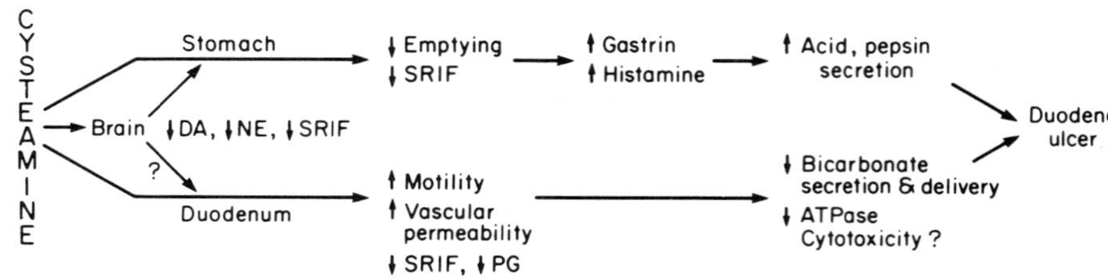

FIGURE 1. Pathogenesis of duodenal ulceration induced by the SH-containing cysteamine.

affected only in a few areas, e.g., in the corpus striatum and medulla oblongata cysteamine decreased dopamine turnover, whereas propionitrile first (at 1 h) accelerated then (at 8 h) significantly suppressed it. Correlation of duodenal ulcer intensity after a single dose of cysteamine with concentrations of monoamine revealed a significant negative association between dopamine levels in the brain and duodenal ulcer severity ($r = -0.633$, $p < 0.05$). Thus, the development of experimental duodenal ulcers is preceded and accompanied by changes in central and peripheral tissue levels of catecholamines. Somatostatin immunoreactivity is also depleted by cysteamine and other SH-containing duodenal ulcerogens in the glandular stomach, duodenal mucosa, pancreas, and hypothalamus.[16] The somatostatin depletion is followed by elevated serum gastrin levels[17-19] which was followed in most of the studies by increased gastric acid and pepsin output.[20-24] In one series of experiments, the effect of cysteamine on gastric secretion was not substantial,[23] and in another experiment the duodenal ulcerogen decreased gastric acid output.[25]

In the duodenum, the activities of ATPase and phosphoprotein phosphatase as well as alkaline phosphatase were decreased by cysteamine.[26,27] These enzymes seem to be involved in the secretion of duodenal bicarbonate, which is important for the neutralization of acid in the proximal duodenum. Indeed, cysteamine impairs acid disposal in the duodenal bulb because of decreased bicarbonate secretion[33-35] and/or diminished delivery of pancreatic bicarbonate from the proximal duodenum.[28-32] The impaired transport caused by the rapidly developing duodenal dysmotility and myoelectric changes caused by cysteamine affects not only gastric emptying,[36,37] but also the site of acid-base mix in the duodenal bulb, e.g., shift of "proper mix" to "misplaced mix".[24,33-35]

In addition to the duodenal dysmotility caused by cysteamine,[33,35,38,39] the SH-containing duodenal ulcerogens seem to exert direct cytotoxic effects on the duodenal mucosa, as indicated in our recent ultrastructural studies[40,41] and experiments with isolated duodenal mucosal cells.[119]

The pathogenesis of duodenal ulceration induced by SH-containing chemicals such as cysteamine seems to involve not only central and peripheral pathways, but damaging actions mediated through acid-base disbalance in the duodenal bulb (caused by secretory and motility changes) as well as direct damage to duodenal epithelium (Figure 1).[42] The mechanism of direct cytotoxicity is very poorly understood and it may involve free radical (e.g., thyil) generation, an ischemic component or other factors. The possibility of direct or indirect (e.g., by free radicals or other metabolites) chemical damage is also suggested by the early alterations in the tissue concentrations of the protective glutathione. The duodenal glutathione level was decreased 1 h after the administration of either cysteamine or the non-SH-containing propionitrile, while these changes were biphasic (i.e., increase at 1 h followed by decrease at 4 and 7 h) in the glandular stomach.[6] Glutathione concentration was also affected by the ulcerogens in the brain, i.e., it was first diminished then elevated in the cortex, medulla oblongata, and hypothalamus.[13]

These results thus indicate a complex pathogenesis of duodenal damage leading to ulceration caused by sulfhydryls such as cysteamine and its derivatives. In addition to local secretory and motility changes in the stomach and duodenum (which are also influenced centrally), direct or indirect cytotoxicity of duodenal ulcerogens in the duodenum and certain brain regions may also contribute to the pathogenesis of these experimental ulcers.

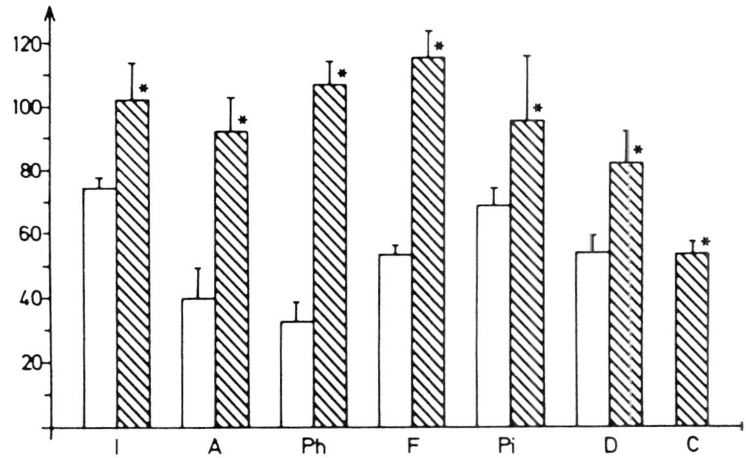

FIGURE 2. Influence of a pretreatment with DEM on the ulcerogenic activity of NSAID in rats. (□) Without pretreatment, (▨) with DEM pretreatment. Ph = phenylbutazone, A = acetylsalicylic acid, I = indomethacin, F = flufenamic acid, D = diclofenac, Pi = piroxicam, C = controls (DEM only), $^{*}p = 0.05$. (From Strubelt, O. and Hoppenkamps, R., *Arch. Int. Pharmacodyn. Ther.*, 262, 268, 1983. With permission.)

B. GASTRIC MUCOSAL INJURY

As is discussed on the following pages, numerous studies demonstrate the protective effect of sulfhydryls in the gastric mucosa. A few studies are related to the damaging action of these endogenous compounds.

Boyd et al.,[7] while working on gastric carcinogenesis found that diethylmaleate (DEM), which depletes gastric GSH levels, aggravates stress-induced gastric erosions. Strubelt and Hoppenkamps[43] reported that pretreatment with DEM enhanced the ulcerogenic effect of several nonsteroidal antiinflammatory drugs (NSAID) (Figure 2). The gastrotoxic effect of NSAID, on the other hand, was decreased by the adminstration of GSH precursor cysteine. These authors also documented the inverse correlation between the GSH concentration in the gastric mucosa after fasting and phenylbutazone administration and gastric ulceration (Figure 3).[43] Ghanayem et al.[44] recently reported that the development of acrylonitrile-induced gastric erosions was accompanied by a dose- and time-dependent depletion of nonprotein SH, presumably GSH (Figure 4).

We found[9,14] that the SH blockers iodoacetamide or NEM administered subcutaneously 10 min after protective agents such as $PGF_{2\beta}$, cysteamine, or dimercaprol (BAL), counteracted the gastroprotection in the ethanol model. Furthermore, ingestion of low concentrations of NEM or iodoacetamide in drinking water produced diffuse or severe acute and chronic gastritis in the rat.[45] The inflammatory lesions involved the glandular stomach, rarely extended into the antrum, and usually spared the forestomach.

These data indicate that depletion of gastric GSH aggravates the mucosal injury caused by stress, numerous NSAID derivatives, or acrylonitrile. Thus, GSH seems to confer certain protection in the gastric mucosa. On the other hand, chronic ingestion of GSH alkylating agents produces diffuse gastritis in the rat.

III. SH AND GASTRODUODENAL PROTECTION

Following the surge of interest in gastric "cytoprotection" by PG,[46] most of the studies performed with SH compounds were related to protection of gastric mucosa against erosions induced by stress or exogenous chemicals.[47,48] We are aware of only preliminary or unpublished

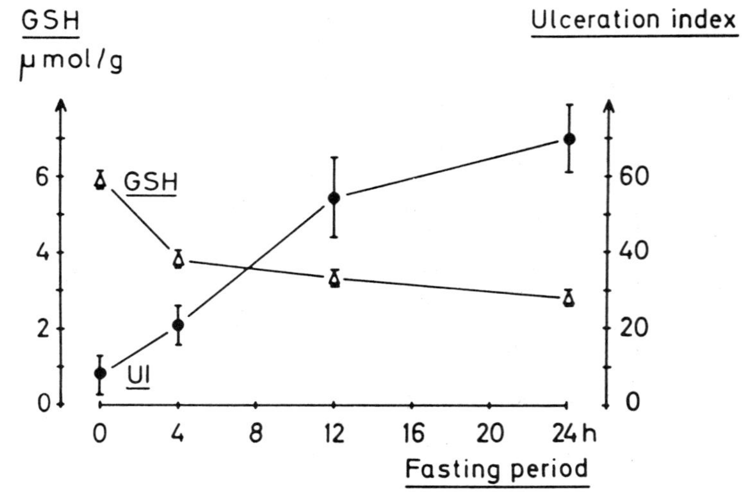

FIGURE 3. Gastric mucosal GSH concentration and ulceration in rats 4 h after oral treatment with 200 mg/kg phenylbutazone preceded by different fasting periods. (From Strubelt, O. and Hoppenkamps, R., *Arch. Int. Pharmacodyn. Ther.*, 262, 268, 1983. With permission.)

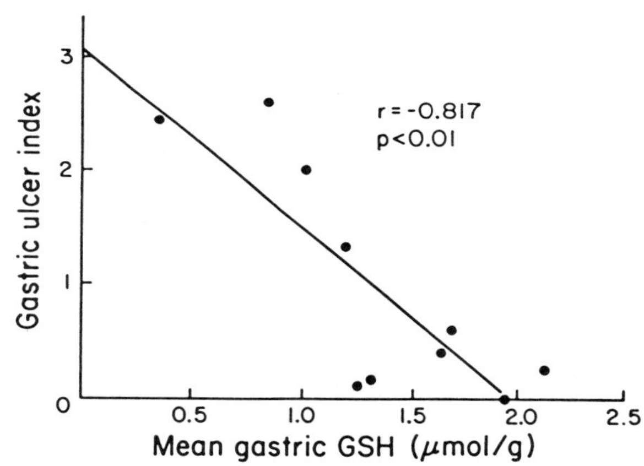

FIGURE 4. Inverse correlation between gastric concentration of GSH and ulcer index in rats given acrylonitrile. (From Ghanayem, B. I., et al., *J. Pharmacol. Exp. Ther.*, 232, 570, 1985. With permission.)

results indicating modest or no protection by SH against ethanol-induced acute duodenal lesions. Hence, in the subsequent section only pharmacological and biochemical results relevant to gastroprotection by SH are presented.

A. PHARMACOLOGICAL DATA

The gastroprotective effect of chemicals containing SH, as reduced form or in various states of oxidation (Table 1), has been confirmed and expanded after the initial observation.[9,43,47-58] Most of these studies used the ethanol-induced model of acute hemorrhagic gastric erosions.

The gastric ulcerogenic actions of other drugs, however, can also be modified by SH compounds. The gastric mucosal injury caused by indomethacin,[49,50] phenylbutazone, piroxicam, diclofenac,[43] aspirin,[58] or acidified ethanol[59,60] was also reduced by SH-containing agents

TABLE 2
The Biphasic Effects of the Glutathione Depletor DEM and SH Alkylators NEM or Iodoacetamide (IA) on Gastric Lesions

DEM		NEM or IA	
Aggravation by	Protection against	Antagonism (if injected s.c.) of protection by	Protection (if given i.g.) against
Stress	Ethanol	SH	Ethanol
NSAID		PG	
Phenylbutazone		Antacids	
Piroxicam		Metals	
Diclofenac		Polyamines	
		Sodium salicylate	
		Somatostatin	

(Table 1). The hemorrhagic mucosal lesions caused by 1 h exposure to restraint and cold were decreased in a dose-dependent manner by several SH drugs (e.g., cysteamine, *N*-acetylcysteine),[51] while the erosions and ulcers produced by immobilization for 24 h were either unaffected or aggravated by cysteamine, cysteine, or GSH given intragastrically.[49]

Chemicals which modulate the endogenous SH pool have also been shown to protect against ethanol-induced erosions. Divalent metals which bind to or oxidize SH groups *in vivo*[61] can prevent damage in the ethanol model.[10] The protection afforded against ethanol by the metals, copper, or lead could last up to 6 h after their administration. This effect was not reversed by the prior administration of indomethacin, indicating a PG-independent process, however, NEM blocked the protection caused by lead or copper when administered before the metals. On the contrary, when NEM was given after the metals, it had no effect.[10] This can be explained by the fact that lead has a strong affinity for SH groups[62] and copper strongly oxidizes SH.[63] Hence, NEM could not react with the already affected groups. Diamide, another strong SH oxidant, has also been shown to cause a significant dose-dependent reduction in ethanol-induced gastric erosions.[63] DEM, despite decreasing gastric GSH, was also shown to reduce ethanol-induced gastric erosions.[64] At first, this result was unusual since adminstration of SH compounds also prevents the ethanol-induced gastric erosions.[9,43,44,47-58] However, the gastroprotective effect of DEM against alcohol is still an SH-sensitive process interrupted by NEM,[65,66] implying that protein SH groups and not GSH may be involved in this gastroprotection. The protective effect of DEM seems to be also limited only against ethanol since DEM aggravates the gastric erosions caused by stress,[7] numerous NSAID[43,67] or acrylonitrile[44] (Table 2). Furthermore, gastric GSH levels have been shown not to be important in gastric mucosal protection against ethanol injury.[63,65] In fact, prior adminstration of the GSH synthesis inhibitor buthionine sulfoximine (BSO) resulting in gastric mucosal GSH levels of 6% of controls did not affect the DEM-induced protection, and BSO alone offered no gastroprotection.[65] Nevertheless, as discussed above, the DEM-induced gastric mucosal protection could be abolished by NEM.[65,66] Unpublished results from our laboratory indicate the small electrophilic compounds dibromoethane and dibromopropane, which may react with protein SH groups, also decrease ethanol-induced gastric erosions.[120]

These pharmacological data thus strongly support the hypothesis that protein SH and not nonprotein SH groups are involved in mediating gastric mucosal protection. The DEM studies, although they may have created some confusion, have actually helped to clarify the pharmacological role of SH in gastric mucosal protection, and have shifted the focus of attention from GSH and other nonprotein SH to mucsoal protein SH.[10,63,65,66] These seemingly unusual results also reinforced the specific pharmacological profile of ethanol-induced gastric lesions,[68] which are diminished by DEM but not affected by antisecretory agents, while the stress or NSAID-caused gastric erosions are worsened by DEM but decreased by drugs which inhibit gastric acid secretion[69] (Table 2).

The usual study design for investigating gastroprotective properties of various compounds was originally devised by Robert[46] with his cytoprotection studies. This protocol involved administering compounds intragastrically 30 min before the damaging agents. Most of the pharmacological studies with SH compounds were performed with this paradigm. More recently, in an attempt to evaluate ten SH compounds for efficacy in preventing aspirin-induced hemorrhagic gastric erosions when administered in parallel with aspirin, four compounds (i.e., *N*-acetylcysteine, methionine, sodium thiosulfate, and thiodipropionic acid) demonstrated a dose-dependent effect even in the coadministration regimen in rats.[58] These studies open new therapeutic possibilities where the protective SH compounds may be given together with aspirin-like drugs.

Studies with the SH alkylators NEM and iodoacetamine also contributed to the pharmacological characterization of gastroprotection by SH compounds. Iodoacetamide or NEM counteracted the gastroprotection not only by $PGF_{2\beta}$, but these SH alkylators were equally effective in reversing the protective action of SH drugs such as BAL and cysteamine in the ethanol model.

Adrenalectomy also interfered with the gastroprotection induced by PG or SH compounds in the ethanol model. In addition, the virtual loss of $PGF_{2\beta}$ or cimetidine-induced gastroprotection against ethanol in adrenalectomized rats was restored if the adrenalectomized rats were treated with glucocorticoids, but not with mineralocorticoids.[70,71]

We conclude that administration of SH drugs or SH-modulating drugs decreases the acute erosive effect of several damaging agents and the pharmacological studies implicate not only GSH, but most importantly protein SH in the stomach.

B. BIOCHEMICAL RESULTS

The biochemical studies involving the endogenous SH pool have been focused mainly on analyzing nonprotein SH and sometimes protein SH. The majority (about 90%) of nonprotein SH is composed of reduced GSH and a small fraction is made up from other naturally occurring SH compounds (e.g., cysteine, cysteamine, homocysteine). The protein fraction is mainly cysteine and its oxidized form, cystine, which compromise the SH content of the protein primary structure. Mixed disulfides also occur (e.g., interaction between protein cysteine and GSH or cysteine from the nonprotein SH fraction) (Figure 5).

Only a few correlative biochemical and pharmacological studies have been published with SH compounds in the stomach. For methodological reasons, in previous investigations, most of the biochemical analysis of SH compounds has been limited to the nonprotein SH fraction. The method to measure nonprotein SH employed the colorimetric determination of reduced SH groups[72,73] by reacting the supernatant of tissue homogenates after the precipitation of proteins (e.g., by trichloroacetic acid) with Ellman's reagent.[72] Boyd et al.[7] initially used this method to demonstrate the relatively high level of nonprotein SH in the gastric mucosa. In our past experience with ethanol, we also used this method and found that intragastric administration of 100% ethanol caused a time-dependent decrease in nonprotein SH concentration in the mucosa of the glandular stomach and proximal duodenum, without much change in liver nonprotein SH of these rats.[6,9,47,71] These studies, however, also revealed a decrease in gastric mucosal protein SH after adrenalectomy which is known to interfere with gastroprotection by PG or SH.[70,71] For us, these were the first indications that mucosal protein SH groups might also be involved in gastroprotection.

Other studies, however, remained focused on the nonprotein SH fraction. Ghanayem et al.[44] implicated GSH in the pathogenesis of acrylonitrile-induced gastric erosions. The acute gastric erosions caused by acrylonitrile were also accompanied by a dose- and time-dependent depletion of gastric nonprotein SH and the lesions were prevented by SH compounds (Figure

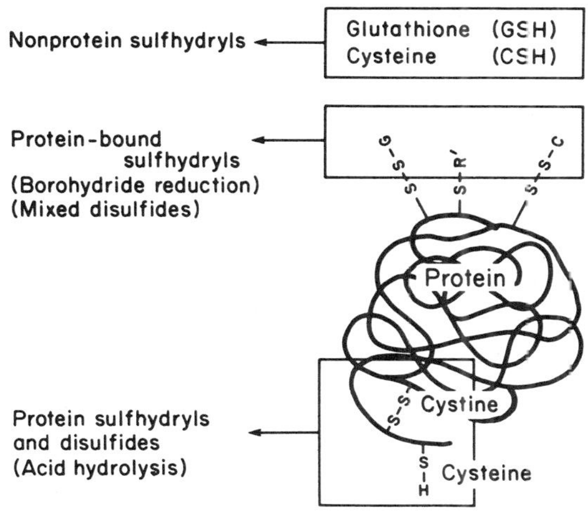

FIGURE 5. Tissue sulfhydryls and disulfides. (From Dupuy, D. and Szabo, S., *J. Liquid Chromatogr.*, 10, 107, 1987. With permission.)

4). Strubelt and Hoppenkamps[43,67] described diminished gastric GSH levels after fasting or NSAID adminstration in rats, and decreasing concentrations of GSH correlated with ulcer development. In other studies, Miller et al.[55] and Fumagalli et al.[52] demonstrated a rise in nonprotein SH of gastric mucosa when PG (e.g., PGE_2 or rosaprostol) were given with ethanol as compared to ethanol alone.

Contrary to studies which correlated decreased nonprotein SH levels with gastric mucosal injury, Robert et al.[64] reported a relationship between low gastric mucsoal nonprotein SH levels and prevention by DEM of ethanol-induced gastric erosions. These results were unexpected because the GSH depletor aggravated gastric ulcers induced by stress,[7] phenylbutazone, piroxicam, diclofenac,[18] or acrylonitrile.[44] The unexpected effect of DEM in the ethanol model has been in good part explained by very recent pharmacological and biochemical studies.

We developed a new technique which allowed the measurement of the separate components of the protein SH fractions.[74] This technique is a specific, sensitive, and quantitative method which allows the measurement of tissue SH and disulfide levels in nonprotein, protein, and protein-bound fractions by using high performance liquid chromatography (HPLC) with electrochemical detection. Recently, we demonstrated with this technique that DEM protects independently of GSH.[10,63] Protection afforded by DEM in ethanol-induced gastric erosions persists after GSH levels return to normal.[63,64] Furthermore, measurement of SH fractions in the rat stomach indicates that the protein SH and not the nonprotein SH levels are crucial for gastric mucosal protection, and in this respect the decrease in protein SH produced by DEM is virtually identical to those caused by other protective agents (e.g., cysteamine, metals, diamide).[10,63,69]

The new technique for obtaining isolated gastric mucosal cells[75] allowed us to implicate the localization of the protein SH affected. These methods, along with previous procedures used to measure cell surface SH groups[76,77] have implicated membrane SH groups as the target for protective agents. We found the cell surface protein SH to be approximately 35% of the total SH in isolated gastric cells.[120] The protective agents DEM, 16,16-dimethyl PGE_2, and a gastroprotective dose of iodoacetamide decreased cell surface protein SH concentrations. These new results indicate that the effect of agents that contain SH (e.g., cysteamine), deplete GSH (e.g., DEM), bind SH (e.g., divalent metals such as lead or zinc), or oxidize SH (e.g., diamide or copper) on endogenous nonprotein SH fractions is variable, but they all decrease the concentration of protein cysteine in the gastric mucosa.[10,63,65] Specifically, the new studies implicate cell surface SH. NEM, which antagonizes any form of mucosal protection, increased free cysteine in the protein SH fraction.[10]

The new biochemical and pharmacological studies indicate that a common effect of diverse protective agents including SH compounds seems to be the blocking of cell surface or other protein SH groups by disulfide or mixed disulfide formation as with cysteamine, oxidation with diamide, conjugation with DEM, or binding by metals. These endogenous SH groups that may be blocked seem to mediate cellular response to injury. The characterization of these sulfoproteins that modulate cell injury and their localization to cell types in the stomach remains to be elucidated.

IV. SH AND THE MECHANISMS OF ACTION OF GASTROPROTECTIVE AGENTS

Since PG were the first compounds studied extensively in gastric mucosal injury and protection, the question of whether PG mediated the effects of SH drugs or endogenous SH mediated the effects of PG needed to be answered. The fact that the SH alkylator NEM blocked the effect of $PGF_{2\beta}$ strongly suggested a SH-sensitive process in the mechanism of PG action.[9] The effectiveness of parenteral adminstration of SH drugs (e.g., by intramuscular route for BAL or subcutaneously for *N*-acetylcysteine) suggested a systemic effect devoid of local generation of PG due to mild irritation associated with the intragastric adminstration (i.e., adaptive cytoprotection). More direct evidence in regards to the role of PG in gastroprotection by SH compounds was found by using indomethacin, an inhibitor of cyclooxygenase. Adaptive cytoprotection caused by 20% ethanol was abolished by indomethacin; however, mucosal protection afforded by BAL or cysteamine was only reduced to about 50% by prior administration of indomethacin.[64,78] In addition, the metals, copper, and lead,[10] as well as DEM,[64] showed complete protection even in the presence of indomethacin. In other words, drugs that affect endogenous SH were able to offer substantial gastroprotection irrespective of PG synthesis inhibition. The partial interaction between SH compounds and PG is also supported by the demonstration of additive or potentiating effects of PGE_2 and *N*-acetylcysteine in diminishing the indomethacin-induced gastric erosions.[50]

Neuroendocrine factors are important in the mechanisms of action of PG or SH compounds in gastric mucosal protection. Adrenalectomy markedly reduced the protective properties of PG and SH drugs and this can be restored by glucocorticoid, but not mineralocorticoid treatment.[70,71] Henceforth, glucocorticoids are implicated by their permissive effects on gastroprotection by either PG or SH compounds.[70] The fact that adrenalectomized animals display a vascular fragility[79] led us to study vascular factors in elucidating the mechanism of action of protective agents. Furthermore, glucocorticoids have been shown to be involved in the cellular maintenance of membrane receptors[80,81] and possibly protein SH concentrations in the gastric mucosa.[71]

Functional studies on gastric secretion have shown that PG and SH compounds protect indepedently of antisecretory mechanisms. Most of the SH drugs do not influence gastric secretion. The few that cause duodenal ulcers in doses three to five times higher than the gastroprotective dose (e.g., cysteamine) actually stimulate gastric acid secretion.[20-24,82] Although cysteamine dose-dependently increased the release of both soluble and insoluble mucus glycoproteins in the rat stomach,[83] there are two lines of evidence against a major role for mucus in acute gastric mucosal protection. NEM counteracts the protective effect of cysteamine without modifying its actions as mucus secretagogue (Figure 6)[83] and *N*-acetylcysteine, like mercaptoethanol, which solubilizes mucus gel, offers gastric mucosal protection after either intragastric or parenteral administration in rats.[9,47,55]

Free radical generation and lipid peroxidation have been implicated in the pathogenesis of acute gastric mucosal injury. SH compounds scavenge free radicals and consequently prevent

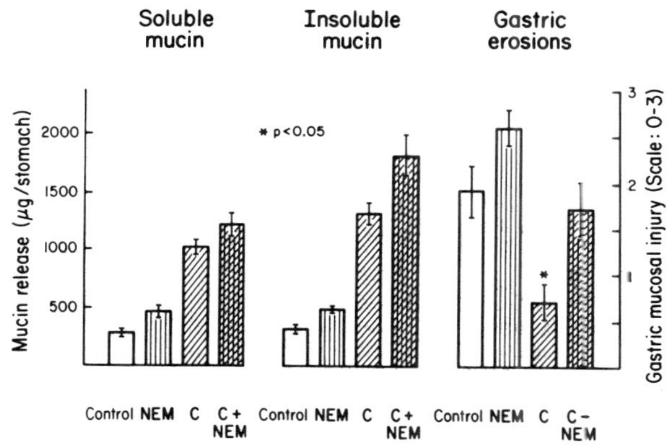

FIGURE 6. Effect of NEM on cysteamine (C)-induced mucus release and protection against ethanol-caused gastric erosions in the rat. (Adapted from LaMont, J. T., Ventola, A. S., Maull, E. A., and Szabo, S., *Gastroenterology,* 84, 306, 1983.)

membrane damage brought about by lipid peroxidation.[84] Surprisingly, there is little evidence, if any, for the involvement of lipid peroxidation in the pathogenesis of gastric mucosal damage caused by ethanol, aspirin,[85] HCl, NaOH, or postischemic reperfusion.[85] Even divalent cations which can promote lipid peroxidation protect against ethanol-induced gastric mucosal injury.[10] On the other hand, the enzymatic antioxidants superoxide dismutase (SOD) and catalase, as well as the nonenzymatic antioxidant propylgalate significantly protected against ethanol-induced gastric mucosal injury.[85,87] In addition, aspirin-induced damage to the gastric mucosa was reduced with sodium benzoate, butylated hydroxytoluene, and studies indicate that free radicals may play a role in gastric mucosal injury, but their mechanisms of actions probably do not involve lipid peroxidation. The fact low endogenous nonprotein SH levels do not necessarily lead to gastric mucosal damage suggests that free radical scavenging plays a limited role.

Activities of certain enzymes may also be involved in the mechanisms of gastroprotection by SH compounds. Polyamines offer gastroprotection through an SH-sensitive process,[60] which may be related to the recently demonstrated SH-dependence of ornithine decarboxylase activity,[88] the rate-limiting enzyme in the synthesis of polyamines. Proteases on the cell membrane of inflammatory cells have been shown to be SH sensitive.[89,90] Inhibition of these proteases or their specific endogenous inhibitors could lead to protection or damage, respectively, to the extracellular matrix.[91] One could envision the precise balance of protease activation and inhibition being offset in acute gastric mucosal injury and preserved or restored in gastroprotection. Thus, if the inhibitors were inactivated, the proteases could not be prevented from digesting the extracellular matrix leading to tissue injury. On the other hand, if proteases themselves are inactivated, digestion of the extracellular matrix will not occur. This system of proteases and their inhibitors has been shown to be involved in lung injury[91] and may well be a target for SH compounds in the mechanism of gastric mucosal protection. Indeed, we recently demonstrated a massive release of thiol proteases from the gastric mucosa after instillation of 50% ethanol.[92] Intragastric administration of iodoacetate prevented the alcohol-induced enzyme release and abolished the hemorrhagic erosions.[92] These results were confirmed by Robert et al.[93] The SH alkylator, NEM, and iodoacetamide thus counteract various forms of gastroprotection if they are injected subcutaneously,[9,47] but they prevent the ethanol-induced gastric mucosal injury after intragastric administration.[92,93] Other factors, however, may also contribute to their local gastroprotection.

What then are the pathways of mucosal protection at the functional and structural level of organization? First, one has to acknowledge that the gastric mucosal protection induced by either

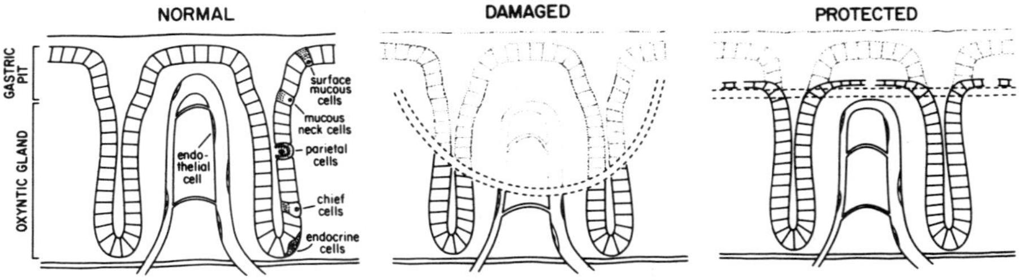

FIGURE 7. Normal, damaged, and "protected" (e.g., by SH compounds) gastric mucosa.

SH compounds or PG is initially not complete, but relative (Figure 7). The early superficial epithelial cell injury is not markedly altered even though the grossly evident hemorrhagic changes are prevented by PG or SH drugs and eventually rapid restitution will repair the surface epithelial damage as well.[47,71,94-97] Second, the main target of prevention seems to be the reduction of vascular injury and the massive increase in permeability induced by ethanol.[47,71,97] This indicates that the gastric vasculature could be the site of interaction of damaging and protective agents[71,97] and the structural preservation of microvasculature is accompanied by *maintenance* of blood flow which is crucial for the energy-dependent cell migration or restitution.[95-99] Protective agents such as sodium thiosulfate and 16,16-dimethyl PGE_2 prevented ethanol-induced vascular stasis while alone (without alcohol) they had opposite effects on mucosal blood flow per se.[98] Consequently, the reduction of severe vascular injury and the prevention microcirculatory stasis seem to be crucial steps in the mechanism of protection concerning SH compounds. If the blood flow is maintained by preventing or decreasing endothelial injury,[97-99] or preventing venoconstriction,[100,101] then mucosal necrosis will be prevented and the mucosal proliferative zone will be preserved for restitution and cell proliferation (Figure 7). Some of the steps of the pathway were proven with SH[71,97,98] and virtually all the points were tested with the examples of PG that maintained constant blood flow[98,99] and stimulated cell restitution and proliferation in ethanol-treated animals.[95,102]

Vascular injury in the stomach can be caused or prevented by direct or indirect factors. Direct effects are produced by the gastrotoxic chemicals and their metabolites. Indirect effects are induced when compounds or their metabolites liberate or modify the action of vasoactive products. SH compounds may then directly influence membrane permeability or enzymes in endothelial, smooth muscle, or epithelial cells; indirectly prevent the release of vasoactive substances (e.g., from mucosal and submucosal mast cells or macrophages); or hinder the access of exogenous damaging agents to epithelial and endothelial basement membranes. Mast cell degranulation accompanies ethanol-induced hemorrhagic erosions in the stomach,[103] thus supporting the idea of vasoactive product liberation leading to gastric mucosal injury. Preventing the release (by cromolyn or doxantrazole) or action (by diphenylhydramine) of vasoactive substances from mast cells decreased the ethanol-induced mucosal lesions.[103,104] In addition, these erosions were significnatly decreased in a mouse strain which are genetically deficient in mast cells.[105] Many receptors related to mast cell products and catecholamines are SH sensitive (e.g., cholinergic, adrenergic, dopaminergic) and the state of these membrane SH groups influences secretion, membrane permeability, and enzyme activities.[106-111]

Leukotrienes (e.g., LTC_4 or LTD_4) are much more potent in increasing vascular permeability[112] than biogenic amines (e.g., histamine, serotonin), and both are released when mast cells degranulate. GSH is a precursor for leukotriene synthesis. The reaction involves the combination of LTA_4 and GSH by the enzyme glutathione-*S*-transferase.[112] GSH levels have been shown to affect the synthesis of slow reacting substance (SRS).[113] It is tempting to postulate that the gastroprotective effect of GSH depletor such as DEM may be due, at least in part, to decreased production of certain leukotrienes because of the unavailability of GSH.

Although chemically induced extensive vascular injury and massive leakage lead to hemorrhagic or ischemic necrosis in the gastric mucosa of rats, the slightly increased vascular permeability caused by gastroprotective SH compounds, copper, or PG seems to contribute to mucosal protection. Namely, similar to the creation and role of a "mucoid cap" detected in the stomach after intragastric administration of ethanol,[114] a mildly enhanced vascular permeability also seems to produce a "histodilutional barrier" which dilutes the concentration of gastrotoxic agents in the lamina propria, especially perivascularly.[115-117] Since the LD_{50} of ethanol in cultured endothelial cells is about 6%, a small dilution (e.g., from 8 to 3%) means life or death for most of the endothelial cells.[118] Decreased endothelial damage in subepithelial capillaries means preservation of microcirculation, which allows the energy-dependent rapid resititution to repair the superficial epithelial injury. The functional status of gastric microcirculation thus seems to be crucial in the development of both gastric mucosal lesions and protection.

V. SUMMARY

In addition to PG, SH are the other endogenous group of chemicals whose role has been studied pharmacologically and biochemically, not only in causing cell and tissue injury but in cyto-, histo-, or organoprotection. PG, as mediators in inflammation, aggravate experimental esophagitis and certain gastric lesions, but in very low doses prevent, through a SH-sensitive process, the chemically induced acute hemorrhagic gastric erosions. A small group of structurally defined SH compounds (e.g., 2-3 carbon alkanes or alkenes bearing electronegative radicals, such as -SH, -CN, $-NH_2$, Cl, as in cysteamine or cystamine) induce acute and chronic duodenal ulcers in the rat. The pathogenesis of tissue injury in the duodenum involves a direct and an indirect centrally mediated influence on gastric acid and pepsin secretion, duodenal and pancreatic bicarbonate secretion, and delivery of bicarbonate from distal to the proximal duodenum. The other contributory factors include gastroduodenal dysmotility and probably some form of direct duodenal cytotoxicity which alone is not sufficient to cause ulceration, but this epithelial damage in the duodenal bulb can be aggravated by acid and pepsin.

Gastroprotection studies in the last few years demonstrated that not only SH-containing chemicals, but also agents that modify SH groups (e.g., DEM), oxidize SH groups (e.g., copper, cysteamine, diamide, *N*-acetylcysteine) or bind to SH groups (e.g., lead, zinc), afford protection against gastric mucosal injury induced by ethanol, NSAID, or stress in animal models. Contrary to earlier beliefs, the SH pool which seems to be the site of action of protective drugs is not GSH, but rather protein SH. These structural or enzymic sulfoproteins could influence vascular tone, vascular permeability, cell membrane permeability via ion transport, free-radical scavenging, or the release or action of enzymes in the gastric mucosa. The ultimate structural and functional target of acute gastroprotection by SH compounds seems to be prevention or reduction of vascular injury in subepithelial capillaries, maintenance of blood flow which allows the energy-dependent rapid restitution to cover initial epithelial surface damage. Studies with SH chemicals thus provide valuable new information concerning both tissue injury and histo- or organoprotection in the stomach and duodenum.

REFERENCES

1. **Guth, P. H.,** Pathogenesis of gastric mucosal injury, *Ann. Rev. Med.*, 33, 183, 1982.
2. **Vane, J. R.,** Inhibition of prostaglandin synthesis as a mechanism of action for aspirin-like drugs, *Nature (London) New Biol.*, 231, 232, 1971.
3. **Robert, A.,** Regulatory systems: prostaglandins, in *Bockus Gastroenterology*, Vol. 7, 4th ed., Haubrich, W. S., Kalser, M. H., Roth, J. L. A. and Schaffner, F., Eds., W. B. Saunders, Philadelphia, 1985, 4480.

4. **Garay, G., Carter, H., and Annesley, P.,** The incidence and the severity of experimentally induced gastroduodenal mucosal lesions by NSAIDs or by analgesic compounds do not correlate with the degree of the inhibition of prostaglandin (PG) biosynthesis in the monkey, *Dig. Dis. Sci.*, 30, 376, 1985.
5. **Ligumsky, M., Golanska, E. M., Hansen, D. G., and Kauffman, G. L., Jr.,** Aspirin can inhibit gastric mucosal cyclo-oxygenase without causing lesions in rat, *Gastroenterology*, 84, 756, 1983.
6. **Bailey, K. A. and Szabo, S.,** Effects of duodenal ulcerogens, cysteamine and propionitrile on tissue glutathione in rats, *Fed. Proc.*, 37, 302, 1978.
7. **Boyd, S. D., Sasame, H. A., and Boyd, M. R.,** High concentrations of glutathione in glandular stomach: possible implications for carcinogenesis, *Science*, 205, 1010, 1979.
8. **Guth, P. H., Aures, D., and Paulsen, G.,** Topical aspirin plus HCl gastric lesions in the rat. Cytoprotective effect of prostaglandin, cimetidine, probanthine, *Gastroenterology*, 76, 88, 1979.
9. **Szabo, S., Trier, J. S., and Frankel, P. W.,** Sulfhydryl compounds may mediate gastric cytoprotection, *Science*, 214, 200, 1981.
10. **Dupuy, D. and Szabo, S.,** Protection by metals against ethanol-induced gastric mucosal injury in the rat: comparative biochemical and pharmacologic studies implicate protein sulfhydryls, *Gastroenterology*, 91, 966, 1986.
11. **Szabo, S.,** Animal model of human diseases. Duodenal ulcer disease. Animal model: cysteamine-induced acute and chronic duodenal ulcer in the rat, *Am. J. Pathol.*, 93, 273, 1978.
12. **Takeuchi, K., Furukawa, O., Nishiwaki, H., and Okabe, S.,** 16,16-Dimethyl prostaglandin E_2 aggravates gastric mucosal injury induced by histamine in rats: possible role of the increased mucosal vascular permeability, *Gastroenterology*, 93, 1276, 1987.
13. **Szabo, S., Reynolds, E. S., and Unger, S. H.,** Structure-activity relations between alkyl nucleophilic chemicals causing duodenal ulcer and adrenocortical necrosis, *J. Pharmacol. Exp. Ther.*, 223, 68, 1982.
14. **Szabo, S., Horner, H. C., Gallagherg, G. T., Silver, E., Hollenberg, N. K., and Reichlin, S.,** Pathogenesis of duodenal ulcer induced by cysteamine and propionitrile in the rat, *Fed. Proc.*, 38, 326, 1980.
15. **Szabo, S., Horner, H. C., Maull, H., Schnoor, J., Chiueh, C. C., and Palkovits, M.,** Biochemical changes in tissue catecholamines and serotonin in duodenal ulceration caused by cysteamine opropionitrile in the rat, *J. Pharmacol. Exp. Ther.*, 240, 871, 1987.
16. **Szabo, S. and Reichlin, S.,** Somatostatin depletion by cysteamine: mechanism and implication for duodenal ulceration, *Fed. Proc.*, 44, 2540, 1985.
17. **Lichtenberger, L. M., Szabo, S., and Trier, J. S.,** Duodenal ulcerogens, cysteamine and propionitrile, stimulate serum gastrin levels in the rat, *Gastroenterology*, 73, 1305, 1977.
18. **Kirkegaard, P., Petersen, B., Skov Olsen, P., Poulsen, S. S., and Christiansen, J.,** The mechanism of gastrin release in cysteamine-induced duodenal ulcer, *Scand. J. Gastroenterol.*, 17, 609, 1982.
19. **McIntosh, C., Bakich, V., Trotter, T., Kwok, Y. N., Nishimura, E., Pederson, R., and Brown, J.,** Effect of cysteamine on secretion of gastrin and somatostatin from the rat stomach, *Gastroenterology*, 86, 834, 1984.
20. **Groves, W. G., Schlosser, J. N., and Mead, F. D.,** Acid hypersecretion and duodenal ulcer produced by cysteamine in rats, *Res. Commun. Chem. Pathol. Pharmacol.*, 9, 523, 1974.
21. **Ishii, Y, Fujii, Y., and Homma, M.,** Gastric acid-stimulating action of cysteamine in the rat, *Eur. J. Pharmacol.*, 36, 331, 1976.
22. **Kirkegaard, P., Poulsen, S. S., Loud, F. B., Halse, C., and Christiansen, J.,** Cysteamine-induced duodenal ulcer and acid secretion in the rat, *Scand. J. Gastroenterol.*, 15, 621, 1980.
23. **Gallagher, G. T. and Szabo, S.,** Secretory changes associated with chemically-induced duodenal ulceration: simultaneous measurements of acid, pepsin, base and pancreatic enzymes in rats with chronic gastric fistula, *Digestion*, 29, 73, 1984.
24. **Szabo, S.,** Biology of disease. Pathogenesis of duodenal ulcer disease, *Lab. Invest.*, 51, 121, 1984.
25. **Robert, A., Nezamis, J. E., Lancaster, C., and Badalamenti, J. N.,** Cysteamine-induced duodenal ulcers: a new model to test antiulcer agents, *Digestion*, 11, 199, 1974.
26. **Japundzic, I. and Japundzic, M.,** Cysteamine is a potent inhibitor of duodenal phosphoprotein phosphatase in rats: probable role of gastric acid hypersecretion, *Dig. Dis. Sci.*, 30, 382, 1985.
27. **Japundzic, I. and Levi, E.,** Mechanism of action of cysteamine on duodenal alkaline phosphatase, *Biochem. Pharmacol.*, 36, 2489, 1987.
28. **Ohe, K., Okada, Y., Fujiwara, T., Inoue, M., and Miyoshi, A.,** Cysteamine-induced inhibition of acid neutralization and the increase in hydrogenion back-diffusion in duodenal mucosa, *Dig. Dis. Sci.*, 27, 250, 1982.
29. **Adler, R. S., Gallagher, G. T., and Szabo, S.,** Duodenal ulcerogens cysteamine and propionitrile decrease duodenal neutralization of acid in the rat, *Dig. Dis. Sci.*, 16, 716, 1983.
30. **Bridén, S., Flemström, G., and Kivilaakso, E.,** Cysteamine and propionitrile inhibit the rise of duodenal mucosal alkaline secretion in response to luminal acid in rats, *Gastroenterology*, 88, 295, 1985.
31. **Poulsen, S. S., Kirkegaard, P., Skov Olsen, P., and Christiansen, J.,** Brunner's glands of the rat during cysteamine ulceration, *Scand. J. Gastroenterol.*, 16, 459, 1981.

32. **Kirkegaard, P., Poulsen, S. S., Olsen, P. S., Halse, C., Loud, F. B., and Christiansen, J.,** The effect of cysteamine on Brunner gland secretion in the rat, *Scand. J. Gastroenterol.*, 16, 93, 1981.
33. **Szabo, S., Pihan, G., Gallagher, G. T., and Brown, A.,** Role of local secretory and motility changes in the pathogenesis of experimental duodenal ulcer, *Scand. J. Gastroenterol.*, 19(Suppl. 92), 106, 1984.
34. **Pihan, G., Kline, T. J., Hollenberg, N. K., and Szabo, S.,** Duodenal ulcerogens cysteamine and propionitrile induce gastroduodenal motility alterations in the rat, *Gastroenterology*, 88, 989, 1985.
35. **Pihan, G., Gallagher, G. T., and Szabo, S.,** Biliary and pancreatic secretions influence experimental duodenal ulcer without affecting gastric secretion in the rat, *Dig. Dis. Sci.*, 30, 240, 1985.
36. **Lichtenberger, L. M., Szabo, S., and Reynolds, E. S.,** Gastric emptying in the rat is inhibited by the duodenal ulcerogens, cysteamine and propionitrile, *Gastroenterology*, 73, 1072, 1977.
37. **Poulsen, S. S., Kirkegaard, P., Skov Olsen, P., Kürstein Jensen, K., and Christiansen, J.,** Role of delayed gastric emptying in the pathogenesis cysteamine-induced duodenal ulcer in the rat, *Scand. J. Gastroenterol.*, 17, 325, 1982.
38. **Bakich, V., Brown, J., Kwok, Y. N., McIntosh, C., and Nishimura, E.,** Contractile effects of cysteamine on the guinea-pig ileum, *Br. J. Pharmacol.*, 82, 791, 1984.
39. **Okabe, S., Takeuchi, K., and Nishiwaki, H.,** Role of local motility changes in the pathogenesis of duodenal ulcers induced by cysteamine in rats, *Dig. Dis. Sci.*, 32, 295, 1987.
40. **Pfeiffer, C. J., Pfeiffer, D. C., and Szabo, S.,** Early ultrastructural changes in rat duodenal mucosa associated with cysteamine-induced ulcer, *Exp. Mol. Pathol.*, in press.
41. **Pfeiffer, C. J., Pfeiffer, D. C., and Szabo, S.,** Development of cystamine-induced ultrastructural surface changes on duodenal mucosa, *Lab. Invest.*, 56, 444, 1987.
42. **Szabo, S. and Cho, C. H.,** From cysteamine to MPTP: structure-activity studies with duodenal ulcerogens, *Toxicol. Pathol.*, in press.
43. **Strubelt, O. and Hoppenkamps, R.,** Relations between gastric glutathione and the ulcerogenic action of non-steroidal anti-inflammatory drugs, *Arch. Int. Pharmacodyn. Ther.*, 262, 268, 1983.
44. **Ghanayem, B. I., Boor, P. J., and Ahmed, A. E.,** Acrylonitrile-induced gastric mucosal necrosis: role of gastric glutathione, *J. Pharmacol. Exp. Ther.*, 232, 370, 1985.
45. **Szabo, S., Trier, J. S., Brown, A., and Schnoor, J.,** Sulfhydryl blockers induce severe inflammatory gastritis in the rat, *Gastroenterology*, 86, 1271, 1984.
46. **Robert, A.,** Cytoprotection by prostaglandins, *Gastroenterology*, 77, 761, 1979.
47. **Szabo, S.,** Role of sulfhydryls and early vascular lesions in gastric mucosal injury, *Acta Physiol. Hung.*, 64, 203, 1984.
48. **Szabo, S., Pihan, G., and Dupuy, D.,** The biochemical pharmacology of sulfhydryl compounds in gastric mucosal injury and protection, in *New Pharmacology of Ulcer Disease*, Szabo, S. and Mózsik, G., Eds., Elsevier, New York, 1987, 424.
49. **Balint, G. A. and Varro, V.,** On the cytoprotective action of sulfhydryl-containing substances, *Acta Physiol. Acad. Sci. Hung.*, 60, 139, 1982.
50. **Johansson, C. and Bergstrom, S.,** Prostaglandins and protection of the gastroduodenal mucosa, *Scand. J. Gastroenterol.*, 17(Suppl. 77), 21, 1982.
51. **Kanazawa, H., Oishi, T., and Szabo, S.,** Effect of cysteamine on gastric erosions induced by cold and restraint, *Pharmacologist*, 24, 248, 1982.
52. **Famagalli, R., Caponi, R., Corsini, A., Brambilla, A., Palmira, M., Bernini, F., and Valcavi, V.,** Nonprotein sulfhydryls as possible components of the protective effect of rosaprostol on the rat gastric mucosa, *Prostaglandins*, 29, 467, 1985.
53. **Henagen, J. M., Smith, G. S, Miller, T. A., and Schmidt, K. L.,** *N*-Acetylcysteine and prostaglandins, *Anal. Surg.*, 204, 698, 1986.
54. **Szelényi, I. and Brune, K.,** Possible role of sulfhydryls in mucosal protection induced by aluminum hydroxide, *Dig. Dis. Sci.*, 31, 1207, 1986.
55. **Miller, T. A., Li, D., Yuh-Jyh, K., Schmidt, K. L., and Shanbour, L. L.,** Protein sulfhydryl compounds in canine gastric mucosa: effects of PGE_2 and ethanol, *Am. J. Physiol.*, 85, G137, 1985.
56. **Laudanno, O.,** Cytoprotective effect of *S*-adenosylmethionine compared with that of misoprostol against ethanol-, aspirin- and stress-induced gastric damage, *Am. J. Med.*, 43, 1987
57. **Tobey, N. A., Orlando, R. C., Schreiner, V. J., and Powell, D. W.,** Cytoprotective effect of sulfate ions in acid-exposed rabbit esophagus, *Am. J. Physiol.*, 86, G866, 1986.
58. **Szabo, S., Trier, J. S., Brown, A., and LaRoque, M.,** Protection against aspirin-induced hemorrhagic gastric erosions and mucosal vascular injury by co-administration of sulfhydryl drugs, *Gastroenterology*, 88, 1604, 1985.
59. **Ezer, E.,** Orally administered aspirin prevents the severe gastric damage induced by acidified ethanol and sulfhydryl blocker treatment counteracts this protective effect in the rat, *Gastroenterology*, 88, 1377, 1985.
60. **Mizui, T. and Doteuchi, M.,** Effects of polyamines on acidified ethanol-induced gastric lesions in rats, *Jpn. J. Pharmacol.*, 33, 939, 1983.

61. **Friedman, M.,** *The Chemistry and Biochemistry of the Sulfhydryl Group in Amino Acid, Peptides and Proteins,* Pergamon Press, Oxford, 1983, 25.
62. **Klotz, I. M., Uruguhart, J. M., and Feiss, H. A.,** Interactions of metal ions with the sulfhydryl group of serum albumin, *J. Am. Chem. Soc.,* 74, 5537, 1952.
63. **Raza, A. and Szabo, S.,** Gastroprotection by glutathione depletors is not due to low gastric glutathione: role for protein sulfhydryl modification, *Fed. Proc.,* 46, 1453, 1987.
64. **Robert, A., Eberle, D., and Kaplowitz, N.,** Role of glutathione in gastric cytoprotection, *Am. J. Physiol.,* 247, G296, 1984.
65. **Raza, A. and Szabo, S.,** Biochemical changes in endogenous sulfhydryls in gastric mucosal injury and protection: studies with diethylmaleate and *N*-ethylmaleimide, *Dig. Dis. Sci.,* 30, 397, 1985.
66. **Konturek, S. J., Brzozowski, T., Piastucki, I., Radecki, T., Dupuy, D., and Szabo, S.,** Gastric mucosal protection by agents altering gastric mucosal sulfhydryls: role of endogenous prostaglandins, *Digestion,* 37, 65, 1987.
67. **Strubelt, O.,** The role of sulfhydryls in the ulcerogenic action of nonsteroidal antirheumatics, in *New Pharmacology of Ulcer Disease, Experimental and New Therapeutic Approaches,* Szabo, S. and Mózsik, G., Eds., Elsevier, New York, 1987.
68. **Guslandi, M.,** Effects of ethanol on the gastric mucosa, *Dig. Dis.,* 5, 21, 1987.
69. **Szabo, S. and Mózsik, G., Eds.,** *New Pharmacology of Ulcer Disease, Experimental and New Therapeutic Approaches,* Elsevier, New York, 1987.
70. **Szabo, S., Gallagher, G. T., Horner, H. C., Frankel, P. W., Underwood, R. H., Konturek, S. J., Brzozowki, T., and Trier, J. S.,** Role of adrenal cortex in gastric mucosal protection by prostaglandins, sulfhydryls, and cimetidine in the rat, *Gastroenterology,* 85, 1384, 1983.
71. **Szabo, S. and Trier, J. S.,** Pathogenesis of acute gastric mucosal injury: sulfhydryls as a protector, adrenal cortex as a modulator, and vascular endothelium as a target, in *Mechanism of Mucosal Protection in the Upper Gastrointestinal Tract,* Allen, A., Flemström, G., Garner, A., Silen, W., and Turnberg, L. A., Eds., Raven Press, New York, 1984, 287.
72. **Ellman, G. L.,** Tissue sulfhydryl groups, *Arch. Biochem. Biophys.,* 82, 70, 1959.
73. **Sedlak, J. and Lindsay, R.,** Estimation of total, protein-bound, and non-protein sulfhydryl groups in tissue with Ellman's reagent, *Anal. Biochem.,* 25, 192, 1968.
74. **Dupuy, D. and Szabo, S.,** Measurement of tissue sulfhydryls and disulfides tissue protein and non-protein fractions by high performance liquid chromatography using electrochemical detection, *J. Liquid Chromatogr.,* 10, 107, 1987.
75. **Spill, W. F., Pihan, G., and Szabo, S.,** New method of using isolated gastric mucosal cells for toxicity studies reveals differential sensitivity to ethanol and HCl, *Gastroenterology,* 94, A439, 1988.
76. **Grasseti, D. R., Murray, J. F., Jr., and Ruan, H. T.,** The interaction of 6,6-dithiodinicotinic acid with thiols and with Ehrlich ascites tumor cells, *Biochem. Pharmacol.,* 18, 603, 1969.
77. **Mehrishi, J. N. and Grassetti, D. R.,** Sulfhydryl groups on the surface of intact Ehrlich ascited tumor cells, human blood platelets and lymphocytes, *Nature,* 224, 563, 1969.
78. **Szabo, S., Maull, E. A., and Movahedi, S.,** Sulfhydryl drugs: a new type of gastric cytoprotective agent, *Gastroenterology,* 80, 1298, 1981.
79. **Zweifach, B. W.,** *Functional Behavior of the Microcirculation,* Charles C Thomas, Springfield, IL, 1961.
80. **Salhanick, A., Krupp, M. N., and Amatruda, J. M.,** Dexamethasone stimulates insulin receptor synthesis in cultured rat hepatocytes, *J. Biol. Chem.,* 258, 14130, 1983.
81. **McDonald, A. R., Maddus, B. A., Okabayashi, Y., Wong, K. Y., Hawley, D. M., Logsdon, C. D., and Goldfine, I. D.,** Regulation of insulin-receptor mRNA levels by glucocorticoids, *Diabetes,* 36, 779, 1987.
82. **Gallagher, G. T. and Szabo, S.,** Direct measurement of duodenal acid-pepsin exposure at the site of ulceration in rats, *Am. J. Physiol.,* 246, G660, 1984.
83. **Lamont, J. T., Ventola, A. S., Maull, E. A., and Szabo, S.,** Cysteamine and prostaglandin $F_{2\beta}$ stimulates rat gastric mucin release, *Gastroenterology,* 84, 306, 1983.
84. **Kosower, N. S. and Kosower, E. M.,** The glutathione status of cells, *Int. Rev. Cytol.,* 54, 109, 1978.
85. **Pihan, G., Regillo, C., and Szabo, S.,** Free radicals and lipid peroxidation ethanol- or aspirin-induced mucosal injury, *Dig. Dis. Sci.,* in press.
86. **Kusterer, K., Pihan, G., and Szabo, S.,** Role of lipid peroxidation in gastric mucosal lesions induced by HCl, NaOH, or ischemia, *Am. J. Physiol.,* 252, G811, 1987.
87. **Mózsik, G., Pihan, G., Szabo, S., Javor, T., Czeglédi, B., Tigyi, A., and Zoldos, T.,** Free radicals, non-sulfhydryl antioxidants, drugs and vitamins in acute gastric mucosal injury and protection, *New Pharmacology of Ulcer Disease,* Szabo, S. and Mózsik, G., Eds., Elsevier, New York, 1987, 197.
88. **Guarnieri, C., Framigni, F., Rizzuto, S., Vaona, I., and Caldarera, C. M.,** Altered thiol group status in the heart ornithine decarboxylase inactivated following perfusion with t-butylhydroperoxide, *Int. J. Biochem.,* 19, 931, 1987.

89. **Khar, A.**, Activation of collagenase production in a rat macrophage-like cell line, *Biochem. Int.*, 13, 565, 1986.
90. **Melloni, E., Sparatore, B., Salamino, F., Michetti, M., and Pontremoli, S.**, Cytosolic calcium dependent neutral proteinase of human erythrocytes: the role of calcium ions on the molecular and catalytic properties of the enzyme, *Biochem. Biophys. Res. Commun.*, 107, 1053, 1982.
91. **Campbell, E. J., Senior, R. M., and Welgus, H. G.**, Extracellular matrix injury during lung inflammation, *Chest*, 92, 161, 1987.
92. **Szabo, S., Pihan, G., Raza, A., Mullen, E. A., and Hauschka, P. V.**, Multiple mechanisms of cell injury in the gastric mucosa, *Fed. Proc.*, 46, 1987.
93. **Robert, A., Lancaster, C., Olafsson, A. S., and Gilbertson, S. K.**, *N*-Ethylmaleimide (NEM) either protects or damages the gastric mucosa depending on route and duration of administration, *Gastroenterology*, 94, A377, 1988.
94. **Lacy, E. R. and Ito, S.**, Microscopic analysis of ethanol damage to rat gastric mucosa after treatment with prostaglandin, *Gastroenterology*, 83, 619, 1983.
95. **Lacy, E. R. and Ito, S.**, Rapid epithelial restitution of the rat gastric mucosa after ethanol injury, *Lab. Invest.*, 51, 573, 1984.
96. **Wallace, J. L., Morris, G. P., Krausse, E. J., and Greaves, S. E**, Reduction by cytoprotective agents of ethanol-induced damage to the rat gastric mucosa: a correlated morphological and physiological study, *Can. J. Physiol. Pharmacol.*, 60, 1686, 1982.
97. **Szabo, S., Trier, J. S., Brown, A., and Schnoor, J.**, Early vascular injury and increased vascular permeability in gastric mucosal injury caused by ethanol in the rat, *Gastroenterology*, 88, 228, 1985.
98. **Pihan, G., Majzoubi, D., Haudenschild, C., Trier, J. S., and Szabo, S.**, Early microcirculatory stasis in acute gastric mucosal injury in the rat and prevention by 16,16-dimethyl prostaglandin E_2 or sodium thiosulfate, *Gastroenterology*, 91, 1415, 1986.
99. **Leung, F. W., Robert, A., and Guth, P. H.**, Effect of a cytoprotective dose of 16,16-dimethyl prostaglandin on gastric mucosal blood flow, *Gastroenterology*, 88, 1472, 1985.
100. **Oates, P. J. and Hakkinen, J. P.**, Studies on the mechanism of ethanol-induced gastric damage in rats, *Gastroenterology*, 94, 10, 1988.
101. **Janicek, M., Hollenberg, N. K., Lin, Y. S., and Szabo, S.**, Area of congestion in angiography and rise of intravenous pressure determine the localization and extent of chemically-induced gastric mucosal injury, *Gastroenterology*, 94, A206, 1988.
102. **Tarnawski, A., Hollander, D., Stachura, J., Krause, W. J., and Gergely, H.**, Prostaglandin protection of the gastric mucosa against alcohol injury — a dynamic time-related process. Role of the mucosal proliferative zone, *Gastroenterology*, 88, 334, 1985.
103. **Bose, R., Brown, A., and Szabo, S.**, Histochemical and pharmacological studies related to mast cells with ethanol- or aspirin-induced gastric erosions, *Fed. Proc.*, 44, 733, 1985.
104. **Wershil, B. K., Szabo, S., Bose, R., and Galli, S. J.**, Ethanol-induced acute gastric injury in mice: mast cell-associated augmentation of hemorrhagic lesions is diminished by H_1 antihistamines, *Fed. Proc.*, 46, 933, 1987.
105. **Galli, S. J., Bose, R., and Szabo, S.**, Mast cell dependent augmentation of ethanol-induced acute gastric damage in mice, *Dig. Dis. Sci.*, 30, 375, 1985.
106. **Carrier, G. O., Marshall, D. C., and Aronstam, R. S.**, Calcium uptake by intestinal smooth muscle: influence of alkylation, *Eur. J. Biochem.*, 89, 173, 1983.
107. **Heikkila, R. A., Cabbat, F. S., and Manzino, L.**, Stereospecific binding of ^{3}H-dopamine in neostriatal membrane preparations: inhibitory effects of sodium ascorbate, *Life Sci.*, 32, 2183, 1983.
108. **Le-Quoc, K. and Le-Quoc, D.**, Control of the mitochondrial inner membrane permeability by sulfhydryl groups, *Arch. Biochem. Biophys.*, 216, 639, 1982.
109. **Leszczynska-Bisswanger, A. and Pfaff, E.**, Effect of depletion of cellular glutathione on methotrexate influx, efflux and retention in hepatocytes, *Biochem. Pharmacol.*, 34, 1627, 1985.
110. **Severne, Y., Wemers, C., and Vanequelin, G.**, Agonist *N*-ethymaleimide mediated inactivation of β-adrenergic receptors, *Biochem. Pharmacol.*, 34, 1611, 1985.
111. **Dueticke, B.**, The role of membrane sulfhydryls in passive, mediated transport processes and for the barrier function of the erythrocyte membrane, *Membr. Biochem.*, 6, 309, 1986.
112. **Samuelsson, B.**, The leukotrienes: an introduction, in *Leukotrienes and Other Lipoxygenase Products*, Samuelsson, B. and Paoletti, R., Eds., Raven Press, New York, 1982.
113. **Parker, C. W., Fischman, C. M., and Wedner, H. J.**, Relationship of biosynthesis of slow reacting substance to intracellular glutathione concentrations, *Proc. Natl. Acad. Sci. U.S.A.*, 77, 6879, 1985.
114. **Wallace, J. L.**, Increased resistance of the rat gastric mucosa to hemorrhagic damage after exposure to an irritant, role of the "mucoid cap" and prostaglandin synthesis, *Gastroenterology*, 94, 22, 1988.
115. **Dupuy, D., Kronauge, J. F., Jones, A. G., and Szabo, S.**, Gastric mucosal protection may be mediated through increases in vascular permeability which create a histodilutional barrier, *Gastroenterology*, 94, A615, 1988.

116. **Palitzsch, K. D., Kronauge, J. F., Dupuy, D., and Szabo, S.,** Slightly increased vascular permeability may be a protective mechanism in the stomach creating a histodilutional barrier, *Proc. 13th Int. Congr. Gastroenterol.,* in press.
117. **Pihan, G. and Szabo, S.,** 16,16-DMPGE$_2$ and thiosulfate decrease gastric mucosal penetration of hypertonic NaCl and increase net transmucosal water flux, *Gastroenterology,* 94, A354, 1988.
118. **Szabo, S.,** Cellular approach to cytoprotection: conditional or no protection by prostaglandins (PG) and sulfhydryls (SH) against ethanol- or HCl-induced injury to isolated mucous, parietal and chief cells and cultured endothelial cells, *Gastroenterology,* 94, A451, 1988.
119. **Palitzsch, K. and Szabo, S.,** manuscript in preparation.
120. **Raza, A., et al.,** manuscript in preparation.

INDEX

A

B

C

H

R

S

T

U

V

X

Z